*the All-In-One Guide to™*

# Natural Remedies and Supplements

the *All-In-One Guide* to™

# Natural Remedies and Supplements

Herbs • Vitamins • Minerals • Fats
Enzymes • Amino Acids
Aromatherapy • Homeopathy • Flower Remedies
Leading Edge Discoveries
Nutraceuticals • Phytochemicals

**Dr. Elvis Ali, N.D. • David Garshowitz, B.Sc., Pharm., F.A.C.A.**
**Dr. George Grant, Ed.D. • Dr. Gordon Ko, M.D.**
**Dr. Joseph Levy, Ph.D. • Ehab Mekhail, B.Sc., Pharm.**
**Dr. Selim Nakla, M.D. • Dr. Alvin Pettle, M.D.**

***AGES*** Publications™
Niagara Falls, New York

The authors of this book do not prescribe the use of any technique as a form of treatment, nor do they dispense medical advice as a form of treatment, for medical problems without the advice of a physician, either directly or indirectly. The only intent of the authors is to offer knowledge of a general nature to help you and your doctor cooperate in a joint quest for health. In the event you use any of the knowledge in this book for self-care, you are prescribing for yourself, in which case you are exercising your constitutional right, but the author(s) and publisher assume no responsibility for your actions. Dr. Gordon Ko, M.D. contributed Chapter 19. Dr. Pettle, M.D. contributed the section in Chapter 10, on menopausal symptoms and therapies.



The statements and information in this book, have not been evaluated by the American Food and Drug Administration.

**The All-In-One Guide to™ Series**
**The Love Living & Live Loving® Series**
**The Love Living & Live Loving Health Series™**

Library of Congress Cataloging-in-Publication Data

Natural remedies & supplements : the all-in-1 guide to herbs, vitamins, minerals, enzymes, amino acids, fats, herbs ... / Elvis Ali ... [et al.].
p. cm. — (The love living & live loving series)
Includes bibliographical references and index.
ISBN 1-886508-28-3
1. Naturopathy. 2. Dietary supplements. 3. Functional foods.
I. Ali, Elvis A. II. Series.
RC440.N364 2000
615.5'35—dc21 99-41819
CIP

Book Design by Inside Bestsellers Design Group™ 1 800 595-1955
http://www.800line.com/

Quantity discounted orders available for groups. Please make enquiries to
Bulk Sales Department – toll free within the U.S.A. & Canada call 1 888 545-0053, or
E-Mail: ages@800line.com

Printing history 05 04 03 02 01 ** * 8 7 6 – first printing
Printed in Canada. Simultaneously released in the U.S.A. and Canada.

We dedicate this book to you, the reader.

To those seeking self-health care and safe natural alternatives for healing, health and well-being.

To those enhancing their lives using the mind-body-soul transformational path outlined in *The Ultimate Power* for study groups.

You make a difference, each and every day.

Mission Statement

*We vow each and every day, to share with you the miracles we have found in this greatest of gifts called life. Our mission is not to change the world but fine tune it for our children, all children.*

*Helping restore the natural balance to our physical world and your well-being.*

Elvis Ali, David Garshowitz, George Grant, Gordon Ko, Joseph Levy, Ehab Mekhail, Selim Nakla, Alvin Pettle & Ken Vegotsky

We acknowledge with thanks:

The medical, health care and numerous other professionals who made this book possible.

Patricia McKenzie, Vice-President, Swiss Herbal Remedies Ltd. for her encouragement and support of natural remedies and supplements and the science of Naturopathic medicine and healing.

James Maranda, B.Sc., Chemist, President and CEO Swiss Herbal Remedies Ltd.

Aloe and the incredible design team at Inside Bestsellers Design Group. The editors: Sharon Crawford, Testaguzza and Martha Ayim.

Daniel Tamin, a student whose interest in the field of human physiology and all that it encompasses, who will one day become tops in whatever profession he finally settles on. His suggestions, ideas and research are greatly appreciated and incorporated into this book.

The alternative and traditional print, radio and TV media, who support our efforts to make this a better world. We are forever thankful to these fine folks who started the ball rolling. Tony, Chris and Charlette of KSON; Deborah Ray and Tom Connolly of the nationally syndicated show *Here's To Your Health;* Jana & Ted Bart and Karlin Evins of the show *Beyond Reason* on the Bart Evins Broadcasting Co. Network; Greg Lanning and Dr. Joseph Michelli of the *Wishing You Well Show* on the Business Radio Network; Kim Mason of *The Nightside Show* on 1010 AM; Willa and Bob McLean of *McLean & Company, Canada AM* and *Eye On Toronto*; *Concepts Magazine*; Tony Ricciuto of *The Niagara Falls Review*; Julia Woodford of *Vitality Magazine*; Susan Schwartz of *The Gazette*; Casey Korstanje of *The Spectator*; Tess Kalinowski of *The London Free Press*; Len Butcher and Dr. David Saul of *The Tribune*; Joanne Tedesco of *The Arizona Networking News*; Andre Escaravage of *The Journal of Alternative Therapies*; Tony Trupiano, host of *Your Health Alternatives* WPON 1460 AM; Joe Mazza and Sabastion the Wonderdog of *The Joe Mazza Show* on Talk America, and Danielle, Elvis, Elliot, Christine, John, Anthony and Greg T. at Z-100, the tri-state areas best morning show.

The support of Mark Victor Hansen, New York Times #1 co-author of the *Chicken Soup for the Soul series*; Brian Tracy, author of *Maximum Achievement*; Jerry Jenkins of *Small Press Magazine*; Barry Seltzer, Lawyer and author of *It Takes 2 Judges to Try a Cow and Other Strange Legal Twists*; Dr. J. Siegel, Psychologist; Cavett Robert, Chairman Emeritus of the *National Speakers Association;* Hennie Bekker, *Juno Award Nominee*; Dr. Michael Greenwood, M.B., B. Chir., Dip. Acup., C.C.F.P., F.R.S.A., co-author *Paradox and Healing;* Dottie Walters, President of Walters Speakers Bureaus International and author *Speak & Grow Rich.*

Dave, Nancy and Ian Christie, Karen, Mark Field, Marilyn and Tom Ross, Barbara Cooper, Sam Seigel...

...along with a host of others, too numerous to list.

# Preface

The All-In-One Guide to™ natural self-health care remedies and supplements takes your health as seriously as you do. We share your interest in identifying the best natural self-care products. We share your interest in safety and purity. We respect the power of an informed consumer, and this book does something about it. We are making a long-term commitment to natural health care in the twenty-first century. Use Dr. Joeseph Levy's self-care health list of Do's and Do not's:

***Do*** talk to your pharmacist or health care provider about any supplement that may help you. If they do not respect and honor your right to know, then find professionals who do.

***Do*** read all labels carefully. Pay attention to warnings, side effects and contra-indications.

***Do*** follow dosage instructions precisely, unless instructed to do so differently by your pharmacist or health care provider.

***Do*** listen to your body for signs of positive, negative and no effects due to the natural remedy or supplement.

***Do*** consult your pharmacist or health care provider if you have any concerns or questions.

***Do not*** take natural remedies or supplements in larger quantities than recommended, unless directed to do so by your pharmacist or health care provider.

***Do not*** take herbal products for longer than directed.

***Do not*** assume natural remedies or supplements are substitutes for medications your health care provider has prescribed.

Be patient when using natural remedies and supplements. The difference between alleviating symptoms and healing takes time. Alleviating symptoms may offer short-term relief, yet result in the need for long-term use of medications to deal with the symptom or underlying problem.

Natural remedies and supplements nourish the body, so the body can function at an optimal level. When necessary, these remedies can cause the appropriate healing response(s) in the body. The focus shifts toward prevention and helping the body with effective nutrition and supplementation.

The need for supplementation and detoxification surrounds us every day. Polluted water and air. Foods grown in soils depleted of the very substances, trace minerals and other ingredients, needed for sound bodies and minds. Excessive stress, due to chemical, environmental, social, emotional and other factors too numerous to mention, which slowly erodes and overwhelms our body's natural abilities to cope.

Ask an honest medical internist, and they will tell you the greatest health secret generally unknown to the public is that the body heals itself. Use the information provided in this book to tap into your body's wisdom to heal itself, using natural remedies and supplements today!

# Table of Contents

chapter 1

# Toward a New Model of Health and Healing

## The healing ladder to optimal health™

The foundation of optimal self-health care and healing is a sound mind-body-soul. From the traditional crisis intervention medicine practiced in America since the beginning of the twentieth century, to the ancient healing systems of China, India, Native Americans and other societies worldwide, the twenty-first century offers a gateway to a new and exciting self-care health and healing reality. It is one which offers the opportunity for a longer and better quality of life, at all stages of the lifecycle. *Natural Remedies and Supplements* will help you discover how to use nature's gifts to attain, maintain and achieve optimal self-health care and healing, using *the healing ladder to optimal health™*.

You will discover what you can use, when and how to take the supplements or natural remedies for maximum benefit. You will also find life enhancing resources that you and your health care practitioner can access in your mutually beneficial quest for a long life of self-care and healing.

When disease, illness or injury strikes, the modern allopathic medical approach uses diagnostic tools, prescription drugs and surgery. The system is based on a rigid scientific perception of medicine. If one is having a heart attack, has a hernia or experiences physical trauma requiring immediate attention, allopathic medicine is tops. In terms of prevention and long-term quality of life, this system pays little attention to the powerful roles of the mind, body and soul, preferring to focus on the symptoms, not the underlying cause that must be addressed.

Chinese, Indian and other healing models focus on the most powerful healing source, your body's own wisdom to heal itself by helping you attain and maintain a state of optimal well-being. They use a more integrated approach, one that values the balance of the mind, body and soul.

The new model of self-health care and healing integrates the best of all the models with a primary focus on prevention and healing by using less intrusive approaches. Symptoms are seen as signs of deeper problems that have to be resolved, otherwise the symptoms might return and negatively impact the quality of one's life or age the body more rapidly than normal.

The foundation of *the healing ladder to optimal health™* combines organically produced, nutrient-dense foods with exercise and gentle, mind-calming techniques.

The information in this book can help you compensate for the highly processed foods we eat, the increasingly unhealthy environment we live in and the crisis intervention medical approaches we typically use. You will discover gentle, natural self-health care aids to help you live longer and enhance your body's natural abilities to heal itself.

## An Example of the Different Approaches to Self-Care Health & Healing

Gray, balding and thinning hair provide an excellent example of how traditional American versus other medical models work. Modern medicine treats the symptoms as natural signs of aging. The treatments cover up the symptoms by coloring or transplanting hair. Both methods mask the potentially dangerous underlying deficiencies that may be causing the problems. In fact, they are warning signs that could mean many things. A very simple solution is available using a combination of vitamins, European herbal formulas and Indian or Chinese medicine herbs. Graying, thinning or balding hair may indicate:

> decreasing levels of the good testosterone and the formation of an unhealthy type of testosterone called dihydrotestosterone (DHT) which affects the libido (sex drive) in men and women.
>
> a lack of one or more vitamins: vitamin A or beta-carotene, vitamin B complex, the stress vitamins (vitamin $B_1$, vitamin $B_2$, vitamin $B_5$, vitamin $B_6$, biotin, folic acid), vitamin E, essential fatty acids (vitamin F), choline, Para Aminobenzoic Acid (PABA). For example, nervous breakdowns due to excessive stress can result in loss of some or all body hair.

a copper deficiency or imbalance. The trace mineral copper keeps your veins and arteries supple and flexible, possibly preventing strokes and brain aneurysms.

a silicon deficiency.

a sulfur deficiency.

too much of the potentially toxic trace element cadmium or too much mercury.

a need for iodine.

a need for the quasi-essential amino acid Cysteine (N-acetyl-L-cysteine) or one of the essential amino acids Lysine or Methionine.

Gray, thinning or balding hair signals internal changes that could affect your physical and emotional states of being. You should and can do something about it now, before the problem worsens. The long-term answer is Indian Ginseng or Chinese Ho Shou Wu, commonly known as Fo-Ti, see page 206, to restore and nourish your hair. Take it with saw palmetto to help rebalance your testosterone levels. Add a B complex vitamin and you have a well rounded hair restoration package. Other things you can do include:

supplementing with copper, but before you do, consider its possible benefits and dangers on page 128.

supplementing with one, some or all of the vitamins and minerals your body may lack.

supplementing with chamomile or rosemary in a tea or hair rinse, see page 196.

supplementing with horsetail, or silica as it is commonly known, page 213.

promoting hair health with jojoba oil, see page 251.

using apple cider vinegar, see page 283.

using methylsulfonylmethane (MSM) organic sulfur, see page 312.

using lecithin, see page 307.

## The Focus of This Book

This book informs you about natural self-care and leading edge choices, so you can choose what is best for your health and healing. As in all matters of health, we suggest you share this information with your pharmacist or health care professional in your mutual quest for optimal health.

*Natural Remedies and Supplements* focuses on the substances that naturally orientated doctors and healers use to create a powerful internal healing environment. They do this with the understanding that symptoms often reflect a deeper problem that needs attention.

A cold is no longer seen only as being sick, but also as the body's signal to strengthen its immune system. Symptoms of disease and illness signal that the body is internally unbalanced. The key is to alleviate the symptoms and promote the necessary response in the hopes of effecting both short- and long-term enhanced states of wellness and health. This is a critical shift in thought for the public, patients and doctors using the medical systems we have created.

The foundations of optimal self-health care were laid long before doctors existed. Science and medicine acknowledge the role of nutrition and natural remedies for optimal health.

To minimize your efforts and maximize the self-health care benefits, we initially share important ideas about key systems and bodily functions that affect you daily. Then we show you keys to unlocking the powers of herbs, vitamins, minerals, amino acids, fats and oils, homeopathy, flower remedies, aromatherapy and leading edge supplements. In addition, we include many old tried, tested and true natural remedies used for hundreds, even thousands, of years.

***Tip:*** When seeking answers or choices to specific problems or conditions, use the index at the back of the book.

chapter 2

# Why Use Natural Remedies and Supplements?

## The truth about drugs versus natural remedies

The case for self-health care using natural remedies and supplements is being made daily. The benefits and drawbacks of pharmacological and surgically orientated modern medicine are being exposed. In the early 1990s, Ralph Nader's consumer advocacy group revealed that across America, up to 300,000 medically induced deaths occur in hospitals each year. This is more than five times the number of soldiers killed during the entire Viet Nam war.

In 1998, according to the American Association of Poison Control Centers, Centers for Disease Control, FDA Reports, Journal for the American Medical Association, March of Dimes Consumer Product Safety Commission and the National Center for Health Statistics, the following summarizes other causes of death.

**Annual Average Causes of Death in the U.S.**

| | |
|---|---|
| Adverse Drug Reactions | 60,000 to 140,000 |
| Automobile Accidents | 39,325 |
| Contaminated Food | 9,100 |
| Boating Accidents | 2,064 |
| Cleaners (Household) | 20 to 24 |
| Pesticide Poisoning | 9 to 12 |
| All Vitamins | 0 |
| Homeopathic remedies | 0 |
| Amino acid products | 0 |
| Aromatherapy products | 0 |
| Commercial Herbal Products | 0 |

## *Why pharmacological drugs replaced natural healing methods?*

The Second World War began the era of synthetic germicides. It wasn't until the 1960s that awareness of the hazardous side-effects of many synthetic drugs, as well as their questionable costs and environmental implications, came under scrutiny by members of the medical research community. Their negative effects upon the kidneys, liver and other body parts were becoming known. Researchers or doctors who dared to speak out faced lawsuits, persecution and loss of their livelihoods.

The economic reality of the marketplace also contributed to the lack of interest in natural alternatives by pharmacologically based medical businesses. Pharmaceutical monopolies charge high prices, over long periods of time, to recoup their costs and make substantial profits on patents and patented medicines. Because naturally occurring substances in an unprocessed state cannot be patented, pharmaceutical monopolies could not benefit enough from them to meet their high monetary expectations.

Today, it is estimated to cost between $100 million and 500 million to develop and test for a new synthetic drug, before bringing it to the marketplace. That does not guarantee the company will ever recover its costs, let alone make a profit on its labors.

In the United States and Canada, this resulted in a lack of funding for medical and drug research into natural remedies. Even though research into alternative therapies continued around the world, particularly in the Far East, Europe and Australia, the findings were not reported in North America. The result is that the United States and Canada account for roughly 70 percent of the money from the world's pharmacological drug sales, yet represent only 5 percent of the world's population! Even in Europe, the comparative sales of pharmacological synthetic drugs are significantly smaller.

The awakening of the 1960s resulted in new North American research into, and reports about the numerous benefits of natural remedies. Unfortunately, the media paid little attention to these findings due to limited money to publicize and advertise them. Both the public and media embraced sensationalism and the quick-fix mentality. In America, financial resources and groups large enough to support and promote this research did not exist. The public was not informed of findings through the mass media.

In addition, American and Canadian government agencies and regulations were created to sustain and maintain the pharmacologically based medical businesses, which are highly profitable and excellent sources of tax revenues, jobs, and are heavy financial supporters of traditional medical schools and associations.

### *Are Vitamins and Minerals Drugs?*

The difference between vitamins and minerals versus drugs is that vitamins and minerals are tolerated over a wide range of dosages, while even slightly high levels of drugs can be toxic. Vitamins and minerals play biochemical roles in the body, whereas drugs do not become part of the tissue or biochemical processes.

Vitamins and minerals are nutrients. Drugs are foreign matter in the body, broken down and usually discharged from the body's systems when their work is done.

Vitamins and minerals are involved in a wide range of processes in the body, such as converting food into energy and building bones and tissues. Consequently, according to G. Ambau, author of *The Importance of Good Nutrition, Herbs and Phytochemicals,* they are constantly depleted and must be replenished.

### *A question of toxicity?*

Vitamins and minerals must be taken for a long time, before the possibility of adverse reactions or symptoms arises. G. Blackburn's article, in the August 26, 1997 National Research Council's *HealthNews,* on the *Safe Amounts of Vitamins* indicates the following: a onetime megadose of vitamins is unlikely to harm the body; Children may have adverse effects from ingesting large amounts of iron supplements; Even too much water can kill.

As in all things, moderation is the best course for self-care. The bottom line is that the overwhelming majority of herbs, vitamins and minerals, in appropriate amounts and even in very large dosages, have generally shown no troubling side effects.

### *Can more vitamins and minerals help your supplementation program?*

Higher dosages of the antioxidant vitamins C, E and beta-carotene result in more protection for the body, in particular from damaging free radical molecules. While the RDAs (Recommended Daily Allowances) serve as a point of reference, exceeding those levels may offer better health protection.

### *But by how much should you exceed these RDAs?*

In 1997, *The Annals of Internal Medicine* reported that one man and three women had lost bone mineral density by taking too much vitamin D. They were all ingesting many supplements daily, some having 3600 IU (International Units) of vitamin D. Calcium needs adequate levels of vitamin D to be absorbed by bones, yet excessive amounts of vitamin D have the opposite effect.

Cases like these have resulted in the National Academy of Sciences' work towards creating new guidelines for levels of vitamin and mineral supplementation – yet even these guidelines will have their weaknesses, as they will be based solely on the sex and age of a man or woman or on whether a woman is pregnant. They still do not account for many variables such as weight, exposure to UV (ultraviolet) rays from sunshine – necessary for your body to naturally produce vitamin D – or the effects of accidents, illness, disease, diet and lifestyle choices.

You know your body and the effects of these and numerous other variables better than anyone else. Educating yourself or working with a nutritionally orientated health care provider, before you develop problems, can help you attain and maintain a state of optimal health.

### *How Natural Remedies and Supplements Fell out of Favor;*

*a brief history using one natural remedy example, Tea Tree Oil.*

Archeological investigations indicate Australian Aboriginal people have lived on the continent over 40,000 years. Their existence depended on their peaceful coexistence with their environment and the plant and animal life that flourished there. Learning to live in harmony with their environment, they took what they needed from the land, waters and forests, and no more. When injured or sick, they found healing remedies in the strong medicinal properties of the continent's plant life.

In 1770, Captain Cook arrived in Australia on a journey of exploration for the British. The Western world's first known collector of tea tree leaf samples was Sir Joseph Banks who accompanied Captain Cook on his journey. He apparently was not aware of the healing properties of the plant. For many years, only the Aborigines and a few settlers living in New South Wales knew of the therapeutic value of the tea tree. It was not until the twentieth century that the scientific community began to take notice of *Melaleuca alternifolia*.

In 1922, a government chemist, Dr. Arthur Penfold, working as the curator and economic chemist for the Museum of Technology and Applied Sciences in Sydney, started a series of laboratory studies examining the antiseptic power of tea tree oil. He announced his results in 1925. According to the generally accepted standards of the time, tea tree oil exhibited bactericidal and antiseptic qualities 13 times stronger than carbolic acid. In addition, his research showed it was non-toxic and non-irritating.

In 1925, Penfold announced his findings to the Royal Society of New South Wales. In 1929, Penfold and Morrison published their work in the *Technological Museum Bulletin*. This generated a burst of research in general medical practices and by the scientific community.

During the years following Penfold's initial research, his colleagues in the medical community put tea tree oil to the test. At first, it was tested as an antiseptic/bactericidal agent for numerous problems.

In 1930, the *Medical Journal of Australia* featured an article by E. M. Humphrey about tea tree oil, titled 'A New Australian Germicide.' He wrote:

> *The results obtained in a variety of conditions when it was first tried was most encouraging, a striking feature being that it dissolved pus and left the surfaces of infected wounds clean, so that its germicidal action became very effective without any apparent damage to the tissues. This was something new, as most effective germicides destroy tissue as well as bacteria.*

Other conditions that Humphrey indicated tea tree oil was good for included:

use as an antiseptic mouthwash in dentistry,

treating infections of the naso-pharynx,

its powerful antibacterial deodorant properties,

its strong disinfecting properties on the typhoid bacilli illustrating it was more than 60 times stronger than ordinary hand soap.

**_Naturally occurring substances in an unprocessed state cannot be patented._**

In the following years, many applications were tested and studied, examining the therapeutic and numerous other claims about tea tree oil. Initially, papers were published in *The Australian Journal of Dentistry, The Medical Journal of Australia, The Manufacturing Chemist, Soap and Sanitary Chemicals, Perfumes, Cosmetics and Soap* and *The Australian Journal of Pharmacy.* As tea tree oil's reputation grew, additional studies were reported in *The Journal of the National Medical Association of America* and *The British Medical Journal*. In 1936, a severe life threatening case of diabetic gangrene was successfully treated and documented in *The Medical Journal of Australia*.

Worldwide interest increased and numerous reports from other countries noted tea tree oil's power in treating mouth and throat infections, gynecological problems, parasitic and fungal skin conditions as well as its incredible antiseptic properties. Toward the end of the 1930s, tea tree oil became known as a 'miracle healer.'

## *How highly did that era's medical establishment and government regard tea tree oil?*

At the outbreak of the Second World War, tea tree oil was standard issue in the Australian armed forces first-aid kits. Growers and processors were exempted from military service to ensure adequate supplies. Even ammunition plants used it in a 1 percent dilution in machine cutting oils to reduce skin infections to the hands, due to injuries caused by metal filings.

Unfortunately, tea tree oil's popularity waned with the pharmacological industry's rise to power. The general public and medical establishment looked to manufactured chemicals as the answer to their health care needs. The shift from inexpensive natural remedies to highly profitable and patentable synthetic drugs began. Only in Australia did tea tree oil remain popular as a natural remedy.

The 1960s saw a resurgence of research into the numerous benefits of tea tree oil. *The Tea Tree Oil Bible* cites many studies that support the extensive research on tea tree essential oil from the *Melaleuca alternifolia* tree.

In the 1990s, industry and consumer awareness of this essential oil's powerful properties fuels a growing world wide market. The Australian Tea Tree Industry Association raised $60 million for a research and product development facility for tea tree oil. The research facility is run by Southern Cross University in Lismore, Australia.

In 1998, an American consumer direct marketing company, with over 60 products using tea tree oil, generated over $400 million of business and is expanding its market share into Canada, Taiwan, Japan, Argentina and elsewhere. Colgate-Palmolive tested a tea tree oil toothpaste, but could not secure sufficient supplies of tea tree oil to launch the product in other countries. They discontinued its production. Hospitals in Australia, use tea tree oil to control mold and other pathogens in their environments.

Tea tree oil provides one example of the numerous safe and effective natural remedies and supplements in this book.

Parts of the above are excerpted from *The Tea Tree Oil Bible,* with permission of the authors and copyright holder. To order your copy, please refer to the back of this book.

## *More Evidence for Natural Remedies and Supplements*

Food affects mood according to registered dietitian, Elizabeth Somer in her book *Food & Mood: The Complete Guide to Eating Well and Feeling Your Best, How the nutrients in food improve memory, energy levels, sleep patterns, weight management and attitude.*

In addition, researchers discovered that diet can reduce violence in jails. Professor S. Shoenthaler of California State University found that when prisoners were given balanced meals, the level of violence was cut in half. His research covered the effects of diet in over 1000 prisons. The guidelines for a balanced diet were those set out by the World Health Organization, British Health Authorities and the National Academy of Science. Inmates usually lacked 14 to 15 nutrients in those prison situations where violence was more rampant.

The Great Ormand Street Hospital Study in Great Britain found a link between hyperactivity, processed foods and the chemically laden water children consumed. Many parents and school boards resisted further examination of this problem, even after it was brought to their attention. Researchers supplied families of hyperactive children organically grown foods, without any additives, and distilled re-mineralized water. The results were astounding. Within two weeks, all the children in the study showed dramatic improvements in behavior.

Our bodies have not kept pace with our ability to change our environment. This results in stress. Food and its nutrients provide a primary means of dealing with stress. Studies indicate that stress stimulates the breakdown of serotonin, a mood-affecting hormone in the body.

> ***"Inmates usually lacked 14 to 15 nutrients in those prison situations where violence was more rampant."***

To replenish serotonin levels and aid in reducing your response to stress, eat complex carbohydrates produced without additives. A few examples are whole-grain bagels, whole wheat breads, cereals and pastas. In addition, these snacks can help soothe stressful moments: apricots, baked apples with cinnamon, broccoli, black beans with cilantro, blueberries, carrots with raisins and poppy seed dressing, cantaloupe, dried figs, lentil soup, mixed dried fruits, mangoes, oranges, papaya, canned peaches in their own juice with nonfat yogurt, raspberries, strawberries and wheat germ sprinkled on anything.

Comfort foods really work! These foods are nutrient rich. They positively affect the neural transmitters that are adversely affected by stress. Natural remedies and supplements, when used appropriately, help restore inner balance by boosting deficient nutrient levels in the body. You may try supplementing with the master hormone melatonin or 5-HTP. They can promote inner harmony of the body's operating systems, so the body functions at a higher level.

## A Quick Summary of Key Nutrients for Optimal Health

### What are the key nutrients your body uses?

The body needs carbohydrates for fuel, which basically means simple and complex sugars in many forms – fruits, vegetables, legumes (beans), pasta, bread and others. Carbohydrates contain fiber for good digestion and bulk, glucose for brain function and energy, water for detoxification, enzymes for digestion and vitamins and minerals for good health.

### Why have fiber in your diet?

Think of fiber as a toothbrush for your digestive system. Fiber helps remove toxins, which are a major source of stress to the body. Fresh, unprocessed plant life contains fiber, which helps stabilize your weight or aid in weight loss. Fiber's bulk lets you know when your stomach is full. The result is that you eat less. A body at its optimal weight places less stress on the heart, back, knees, feet and all those body parts where excess weight can cause unnecessary wear and tear.

### Feel bloated after that heavy meal?

Introduce this friendly bacteria to your digestive system – Lactobacillus acidophilus. Later, you will meet a bunch of friendly bacteria.

***Tip:*** Antibiotics do not discriminate, they kill the bad and good bacteria, particularly in your stomach. Counteract this negative side-effect by returning the friendly bacteria you need when taking antibiotics. This helps restore the body's internal balance. Ask your pharmacist to recommend a bacteria supplement, when you should have it and what it will do.

***Food Tip:*** Eating plain yogurt with active bacterial cultures is another way to get those user friendly bacteria. Check the label to make sure the yogurt has those active friendly bacteria!

### Your state of being can effect your physical well-being.

Today, some hospitals use the healing and de-stressing power of laughter in their cancer departments. This idea is based on the work of Norman Cousins, author of *Anatomy of An Illness*, who was diagnosed as terminally ill from cancer. His doctor expected he would not live more than a few months. He challenged their negative prognosis, using the power of his mind combined with his body's natural wisdom to heal itself.

He isolated himself from the outside world. He rented classic comedy films and laughed his way to wellness. Laughter plus nutritional supplements, primarily vitamin C, and changes to his diet cured his cancer. He lived decades beyond the doctor's prognosis. In the last eight years of his life, he taught at the world renowned Harvard Mind/Body Clinic in Boston, Massachusetts.

Many physical disorders are caused by stress. In extreme or potentially extreme cases, it is necessary to alleviate these problems with proper diet. Someone suffering anxiety may find it very difficult, if not impossible, to relax. Nutritional deficiencies are a result of the body's inability to handle nutrients well during those times. University of Texas researchers believe excess amounts of the ACTH (adrenocorticotrophic hormone) are produced when the brain is under stress. In turn, the white blood cells vital to fighting disease are reduced by the presence of this hormone.

### *How do you restore the nervous system's ability to function properly at times like these?*

The quick answer is B-complex vitamins to help restore the proper functioning of the nervous system and reduce the damage to your immune system. Self-supplementation is possible, using B-complex in pill form with an extra helping of $B_5$ (pantothenic acid), the anti-stress vitamin. In some cases, intramuscular injections are used for quick results, and sometimes under the supervision of a doctor, injections of liver and $B_6$ (pyridoxine) are used.

Supplementation with other nutrients is also an option. The key is to reduce the negative effects upon your body and enhance its capacity for peak performance. By pro-actively addressing extreme cases of stress related symptoms before they turn into major illnesses, you will greatly improve your life.

For example, smokers need more vitamin C. It is said that one cigarette depletes the body of 25 to 100 milligrams of vitamin C, draining the body of this vitamin. Your current state of health, your body type, your age and a whole slew of other possibilities are important to consider and account for when supplementing. A qualified health-care practitioner can help you consider the variables to insure you set up the best self-care nutrient supplementation program for your body.

## *Here is a partial list of other supplements that are beneficial in dealing with stress*

Calcium and magnesium – builds bones, muscle relaxants.

The amino acid L-Tyrosine – a sleep aid.

Vitamin C with bioflavonoids – essential for adrenal gland functioning.

Brewer's yeast or Bio-Strath. (Bio-Strath is a tonic with concentrated yeast, enzymes, amino acids, minerals and vitamins.)

Extra fiber, such as oat bran or Aerobic Bulk Cleanse (ABC), to cleanse and improve bowel functioning, helping remove toxins from your system.

The amino acid GABA (gamma-aminobutyric acid) with Inositol, as a tranquilizer.

Kelp, a seaweed containing minerals, vitamins and trace elements. Kelp's iodine content aids and promotes thyroid function, as well as promoting other interactions with various drugs.

Lecithin, a naturally occurring group of compounds found in every living cell, coats the nerves, very important for brain functions such as memory; it protects against cardiovascular disease and provides cellular protection.

L-Lysine plus vitamin C and zinc gluconate treat cold sores, one of the first indicators of stress in many people.

Multivitamins with vitamin A, mineral complex and potassium. Potassium is for the adrenal gland and heart functions.

Proteolytic enzymes which destroy free radicals released by stress.

Vitamin E and zinc for immune system functioning.

Raw thymus and raw adrenal to stimulate functioning of those glands which are important in helping the body deal with stress.

## *Cost is important*

Your money may be wasted if the supplement you take does not do the job. The biological availability of different forms and delivery systems for supplements is shown in the chart on page 70. It clearly indicates that the form and type of delivery system you select greatly affects the amount of nutrients available for your body to use. This chart will help you better choose your supplements, maximize the benefits to your body and minimize your costs. Two critical points to remember are that labels can be misleading, unable to deliver sufficient information within their limited space, and that the information is generalized, based on an average person of average weight and height, not individualized or case specific.

In the following chapters you will find condensed information sections revealing key elements that affect your body's ability to get what it needs, when it needs it, in a way it can use it best.

chapter 3

# The Digestive System

## A key to unlocking the power of Natural Remedies and Supplements

### *Digestion – Where it all begins*

Improper digestion can cause gas, allergic reactions, heartburn and numerous other problems. When you eat, your body may get unnecessarily stressed. Signs of this type of stress include bloating or flatulence. The most important signs of improper digestion, that may take days, months or years to present themselves, are diseases due to insufficient nutrient assimilation by the body. One example is scurvy, caused by a lack of vitamin C.

Lethargy can result from a large meal. Your stomach uses energy to convert food and drink into usable states so that the vitamins, minerals and a multitude of nutrients can be utilized by your body.

Enzymes are nature's magical transformational chemicals and a vital part of the process. The main sources of enzymes are fresh fruits and vegetables. Because cooking and processing foods destroys enzymes, supplemental digestive enzymes may be required, depending on your diet.

Digestive enzymes allow the complete digestion and assimilation of nutrients. They are the bridge between food and your body's nutritional needs, helping the nutrients become available for use by the body. Lack of the appropriate enzymes leads to putrefaction and fermentation, which produces an overgrowth of pathogenic bacteria and toxins.

Lactose intolerance, the inability to digest the sugar in milk (lactose), is due to a lack of the appropriate digestive enzyme. Around age 12, many people start having a problem digesting milk products containing lactose. Digestion can be facilitated by using lactase or a full spectrum enzyme with enough lactase in it. Properly used, enzymes reduce stress in the digestive tract, better enabling your body to get the critical nutrients it needs from the food you eat.

## *When does digestion begin?*

Digestion begins the moment you anticipate or smell food. Your brain signals your stomach to start secreting digestive juices. The juices start your pancreas and gallbladder working.

Your mouth prepares to breakdown food with enzymes in saliva. Amylase breaks down starches and is one of the most important enzymes.

The mouth's soft inner tissue, the mucous membranes, absorbs fat-soluble nutrients and signals the digestive system to produce certain digestive juices and enzymes. The more you chew your food, the clearer the signals will be, which means less strain on the system and easier absorption of the nutrients you are consuming.

Twenty is the usual number of times you want to chew a bite of food. When you swallow, the special muscles of the esophagus tighten and loosen to move the food into your stomach.

The stomach is a large flexible bag that does not absorb anything, except for alcohol, through its walls. A regular meal usually remains in the stomach for three to five hours before heading to the small intestines. Fats take much longer to leave the stomach. Enzymes, mucus, hydrochloric acid (HCl) and a specific chemical that helps dissolve vitamin $B_{12}$ are produced by glands and the stomach wall lining.

Normally the stomach is very acidic. On top of producing hydrochloric acid, it secretes pepsin, an enzyme that breaks down proteins into amino acids for use by the body. The hormone gastrin promotes the release of these secretions.

Hydrochloric acid does many things: it breaks down foods, kills parasites and kills bacteria, prepares the small intestines for absorption of vitamins $B_{12}$ and folic acid, and helps the body absorb minerals. Heartburn usually results from lack of hydrochloric acid, so food is not fully digested and may come back up into the esophagus.

To stimulate HCl production, drink 2 to 3 teaspoons of cold-pressed organically grown apple cider vinegar with 'mother', the nutrient rich cloudy sediment in apple cider vinegar, with a glass of lukewarm water before meals. Cold water inhibits the production of digestive juices.

Next, the partially digested food enters the small intestines where most of the nutrients are absorbed. Now your digestive system starts extracting thousands of nutrients, using digestive enzymes to break them down, sending them through the blood to the liver. The liver is like a traffic cop. It distributes the nutrients throughout the body, targeted to the correct areas so they can do their job. Doctors who focus on natural approaches to health and healing, believe the liver is one of the keys.

The small intestines have a slightly alkaline environment, are about 21 to 23 feet long and comprises over 2000 square feet of surface area. This area is composed of tiny finger-like protrusions, called villi, which are the gate keepers controlling the flow of nutrients between your intestines and your liver. The alkalinity stimulates the pancreas to produce digestive enzymes and the gallbladder to release the bile needed to break down fats. Poor nutrient absorption is usually a result of damaged intestines.

The liver plays an important role in the process. It breaks down and gets rid of the toxins in the body. The liver stores the fat-soluble vitamins A, D, E and K as well as glycogen, the digested carbohydrate. Glycogen sustains blood sugar levels. The liver changes the chemical structure of nutrients, so they can be used or discarded as needed by the body. It makes cholesterol, enzymes and blood coagulation factors, produces bile and turns beta-carotene into vitamin A. The salts in bile act like a detergent, to help fats become efficiently digested in the gallbladder. The water-soluble materials that are not passed on to other body parts, or are not needed, are then excreted in the urine.

The gallbladder is about 3 inches long. It is a small storage organ that holds and processes bile, increasing the bile's strength by a factor of 10. The taste, sight or smell of food can cause the gallbladder to empty itself.

The pancreas is a gland approximately 6 inches long, resting inside the duodenum, the first section of the small intestines below the stomach. It produces vital enzymes for the body. It secretes insulin into the bloodstream, which helps transport sugars in the blood into cells. The vital enzymes and bicarbonate found in pancreatic juices neutralize stomach acids.

By the time the remaining food materials get to the large intestines, almost no nutrients remain. The large intestine is a 5 foot long by 1.5 inch wide diameter tube. It expels food wastes, which are mainly made up of food matter that was not broken down or absorbed. The enzymes produced by the bacteria found in the colon, act on the undigested cells, fiber and mucous that the upper gastrointestinal tract could not effectively process and use. The remaining unusable materials are combined with water, and excreted through the anus.

chapter 4

# Enzymes and Carbohydrates

## Key Energy Factors

### *Enzymes*

Every cell in the body uses enzymes. They facilitate the millions of biochemical reactions occurring every minute. Each enzyme has a particular job to do. Vitamins, minerals, and oxygen all need enzymes to make them useful. Without enzymes plants and animals would not be able to live.

Digestive enzymes catalyze the breakdown and absorption of the nutrients we consume. While they cause change, the enzymes themselves do not change. They convert food into its components: sugars, amino acids, fats, starches, vitamins, minerals and numerous nutrients. These enzymes direct the right nutrient into the correct cell. Enzymes of one type cannot be substituted for enzymes of another type.

Dr. Anthony Cichoke, author of *The Complete Book of Enzyme Therapy*, states that enzymes are critical to sustaining life. The absence or lack of enzymes can cause everything from allergies, to heart disease, to a weakened immune system, to stress, to indigestion.

Enzymes are categorized according to their purpose in the body. We focus on the digestive enzymes known as the hydrolases group. A particular enzyme acts on a specific food component, and is known by what it acts on. The suffix 'ase' is added to the end of the substance's name. For example one of the enzymes that acts on sugar is referred to as sucrase, one that acts on proteins is called protease (also known as 'proteolytic enzymes' just to drive us all a little crazy), one that acts on cellulose is called cellulase, for the enzyme acting on the milk sugar 'lactose' is lactase, and so on. In some cases the Latin term for the substance is used as the root word, and things become a little more confusing, that is unless you know Latin.

Four basic digestive enzyme types are:

Amylolytic or amylase, in the intestines, pancreas and saliva, which breaks down carbohydrates.

Cellulase, which breaks down cellulose.

Lipolytic or lipase, which breaks down fats.

Proteolytic or protease in the stomach, intestines and pancreas, which breaks down proteins.

Starch digesting amylase enzymes include the following:

Alpha-amylase and beta-amylase process starches into sugars. Alpha-amylase is in the saliva and pancreastes.

Beta-amylase is in unprocessed raw vegetables and grains.

Glucomylase and mylase process starches in the small intestines. They digest thousands of times their own weight in starches.

Protein digesting protease enzymes include:

Bromelain, from pineapple.

Pancreatin, from animal pancreas,
which works best in the small intestines.

Pepsin, from animal enzymes,
breaks down proteins into amino acids.

Prolase, from the papain in papaya.

Protease, from papaya.

Renin, which converts casein, the milk protein, into a usable form for the body and helps release the calcium, potassium, phosphorous, iron and other minerals found in milk.

Chymotrypsin and trypsin, produced by the pancreas, aid in breaking down proteins.

A full spectrum enzyme supplement should contain enzymes that breakdown proteins, fats, carbohydrates, fiber and milk sugars. Here is a sample of what a full spectrum digestive system enzyme capsule needs to have:

Pancreatic protease, with acid stable protease,
to break down protein.

Lipase to break down fats.

Alpha amylase to break down carbohydrates.

Amyloglucosidase to break down carbohydrates.

Cellulase to break down cellulose.

Hemicellulase to break down fiber.

Lactase to break down milk sugar (a type of carbohydrate).

Excellent food sources for enzymes are the aspergillus plant, avocados, bananas, papaya (papain), pineapple (bromelain), mangoes and sprouts. All uncooked fresh fruits and vegetables are sources of enzymes.

***Note:*** Digestive enzymes are critical for optimal health, and found in foods such as vegetables, fruits and raw milk. When foods are processed, cooked at high temperatures (generally over 118 F), irradiated, exposed to electromagnetic or radiation fields, microwaved, contain or exposed to fluoridated water, genetically engineered, use bovine growth hormone for milk production, exposed to heavy metals, hybridized, pasteurized, treated with synthetic herbicides or pesticides it is almost certain the enzymes are destroyed. The result is your body is unable to draw nutrients from food. Over the long term this creates deficiencies resulting in illness and disease.

***Tip:*** If you are using a digestive enzyme, check if fillers are used. It is preferable to have no artificial preservatives, color, milk, soya, wheat or yeast in the supplement. These are full spectrum digestive enzyme blends: *Swiss Natural Sources Full Spectrum Digestive Blend, Gastroprotective Enzymes, Chirozyme Enzymes, Flora's Ultimate Digestive Enzyme Blend.* Also try any of the following whole green super food supplements with digestive enzymes: *Green Power by Swiss Herbal, ProGreens, Nu-Greens Profile, Green Magic, Green Vibrance, Pure Synergy.*

## *Carbohydrates*

Carbohydrates are the body's main source of energy. Digestion breaks the main carbohydrates, starches and sugars, into blood sugars, also known as glucose. This is critical for your brain and central nervous system to function.

You find carbohydrates mainly in plant foods such as vegetables, fruits, legumes (beans) and peas. The only animal foods that have a lot of carbohydrates are milk and milk products.

With too little carbohydrate, your body uses protein for energy, rather than allowing the proteins to do their tissue repair jobs. That is when ketosis, an acidic environment in the blood occurs, rendering your own body fat the main energy source.

With too many carbohydrates, the excess gets processed into glucose and glycogen, then eventually is stored as fat. The liver stores the glucose and glycogen, converting them into fat for future use as energy. The liver changes the chemical structure of nutrients, so they can be used or discarded as need be.

There are two types of carbohydrates – simple and complex. Simple carbohydrates, also known as simple sugars, include the following: table sugar (sucrose), fruit sugar (fructose), milk sugar (lactose) plus other sugars. Complex carbohydrates are sugar molecules linked together to form longer more complex chains of sugar. Foods containing complex carbohydrates include vegetables, beans, peas and whole grains.

Only the fiber, which is not digestible, cannot be changed into glucose or glycogen. This fiber is critical to your long-term health. It prevents constipation, hemorrhoids and colon cancer, keeps blood sugar levels balanced and aids in removing toxins from the body.

The rate at which carbohydrates are processed into fuel for the body is called the glycemic index. High glycemic foods are high in sugars and starches. The glucose derived from them rapidly enters the bloodstream. Your pancreas works hard to produce the insulin your body needs to use the glucose for energy. In turn the insulin converts the excess into fat for future energy use.

Low glycemic foods are high-fiber, slowly digested carbohydrates. They are gentler on the pancreas and your body, providing energy in a more constant and even flow.

Your daily food intake, in terms of calories, should be about 60 percent carbohydrates, the majority of them complex carbohydrates. If that is the case, then you will be getting the 30 grams of fiber your body needs to function optimally.

***Health Tip:*** A short list of high glycemic foods to avoid or cut back on: refined white sugar, corn flakes, white flour pastas, candies, cakes, cookies, potato chips, bagels, carrots, parsnips, instant mashed potatoes, honey, pretzels, soft drinks, white rice, potatoes, brown rice, white bread, biscuits, bananas, raisins, sweet corn, yams, sucrose.

***Health Tip:*** A short list of low glycemic foods to eat more of for optimal health: whole wheat bread, oatmeal, bran, whole grain pasta, high fiber fruits (fresh oranges, apricots, mangoes, etc.), high fiber vegetables (brussels sprouts, broccoli, onions, etc.), hard beans such as mung, pinto and soy as well as other soy products.

***Important Fact:*** Not all enzymes are for digestive purposes. Many facilitate other biochemical processes in the body. For example, Coenzyme Q10 is found in every cell of the human body with the greatest concentration in the heart muscles. In Japan and other countries it is used to strengthen the heart muscles. It acts to help energy from outside sources become available at a cellular level in the body. It is one of the supplements we recommend.

# chapter 5

# Fats and Oils

## The Good, the Bad & the Ugly

### *A Quick Course on Good versus Bad Fats*

Are your body's natural biorhythms stressing you out? Physical problems taxing you? Biological concerns are a major source of stress. Premenstrual syndrome, menopausal flashes, arthritis, psoriasis and eczema, angina, strokes, coronary heart disease, multiple sclerosis and cancer can destroy the quality of your life. In many cases, they are a cause or symptom of stress. In these cases, de-stressing your body may require the use of dietary or supplemental changes. Lignans, a fiber that friendly bacteria in the gut change to a cancer-fighting substance, may be the answer. They have been scientifically proven to reduce the incidence of breast cancer. Lignans also regulate hormonal levels and reduce menopausal symptoms, such as yeast infections, vaginal dryness and hot flashes. The problem is how do you get this miraculous substance into your system? It's easy and cheap.

Consume essential fatty acids (EFAs), also known as vitamin F, the nutritional component found in dietary fats and oils. They are essential fats we must get from food. Essential means every human being, regardless of age, needs sufficient amounts of these fats for optimal functioning. They support the following vital functions:

Help transport and metabolize triglycerides and cholesterol and have been shown to greatly reduce the levels of both of these substances.

Improve the body's functioning by increasing metabolic rate, energy production and oxygen uptake.

Contribute to cell membrane flexibility, fluidity and selective permeability by keeping crucial products in, and harmful products out of cells.

Maintain and enhance normal brain development and functioning.

Manufacture eicosanoids, including hormone-like substances called prostaglandins that regulate critical functions such as arterial muscle tone, the transport of oxygen in the blood, sodium excretion through the kidneys, inflammatory response and immune system functions.

These fats are vital for human nutrition, they improve your body's ability to deal with external stress. Here's a quick primer and short list of types of healthy fats and foods they are found in.

Omega-3 Fatty Acids (essential)– Alpha Linolenic Acid (ALA) is found in flax and hemp oils.

Eicosapentaenoic Acid (EPA) is found in fish oil.

Docosahexaenois Acid (DHA) is found in fish oil.

Omega-6 Fatty Acids (essential) – Linoleic Acid (LA) is found in flax, hemp, borage and evening primrose oils.

Gamma Linolenic Acid (GLA) is found in borage, hemp and evening primrose oil.

Omega 9 monosaturated fatty acids are not essential. They are processed by your body and break down into the Omega 3 and Omega 6 essential fatty acids in the body.

Monosaturated fatty acids promote optimal health and are found in avocado, borage, flax, olive, peanut and evening primrose oils. They stay liquid at room temperature and get harder at colder temperatures. They raise the levels of the good HDL cholesterol.

Polyunsaturated fatty acids are being linked to higher incidence of cancer and are found in corn, sesame, soy, safflower and sunflower oils. They stay liquid at room temperature and at colder temperatures.

Saturated fatty acids are associated with high cholesterol readings, many diseases and illnesses. They stay solid at room temperatures. Food sources include butter, beef, chicken, coconut, palm kernels, veal and dairy products. They raise the levels of the bad LDL cholesterol.

Trans-fatty acids are being connected to heart disease, cancers, obesity and an increasing list of negative affects upon the body.

***Tip:*** One of the least expensive sources for these essential fatty acids is gently processed flax seeds.

Physicians and researchers are discovering that by changing the blend of dietary oils they can positively change the body's supply of beneficial prostaglandins, altering body function and, in some cases, treat disease. It is estimated that North Americans and other countries eating a Western-style diet get only 20 percent of the essential oils that are required, while eating excessive amounts of harmful saturated fats. Furthermore, activities such as alcohol and caffeine consumption, chemical exposure, air pollution, increased use of drugs and a stressful lifestyle easily deplete Omega-3 fatty acids, only compounding the problems.

***Health Tip:*** Here's a fat that helps you lose weight. According to Sam Graci, author of *The Power of Superfoods,* high quality soybean lecithin granules can aid in weight loss. They are also known as phosphatidyl choline, one of the most important foods that support your health. It is an unsaturated fat that improves the quality of human life and longevity. In addition, soybean lecithin granules reduce high blood pressure, lower bad LDL cholesterol levels, increase absorption of vital fat-soluble vitamins A, E and D by up to 100 percent, add sheen to hair, maintains skin elasticity, reduce health threatening levels of homocysteine by transforming them into non-toxic compounds, and support brain function and the nervous system. Graci recommends 2 tablespoons (30 grams) daily in your food.

## *Now for the nitty gritty*

When you eat, your body stores the unused energy from foods as fat. One gram of fat contains nine calories of banked energy, just waiting to be released. It takes very little energy to maintain fat, whereas muscle requires and uses much more energy to maintain itself, even when you are at rest. This is only a small part of the story, because not eating the right fats can destroy your health and help make you obese!

## *The hidden killers*

The last hundred years have seen a massive increase in cardiovascular disease and cancer deaths in Western cultures. Our diet has changed dramatically. The types of oils and fats we eat now did not exist back then. Changing diets, food processing methods and technological manipulations without sufficient long-term studies are leading to a health care crisis, in young and old alike.

Canola oil was derived from irradiated rapeseed, a seed oil that was toxic to animal and human life before it was treated with radiation. Canola oil did not exist in our diets, until the latter half of the twentieth century, which means we have not evolved over thousands of generations using this oil. Is it healthy, in terms of monosaturated content: Yes, without question. In terms of genetically altered foods, no one appears to be publicly examining this issue at this time.

Trans-fatty acids are another synthetic fat, generally suspected of causing many illnesses and diseases. They are common in most processed foods and in fast food restaurants using prepackaged foods. The main benefit of trans-fatty acids is to extend the shelf-life of a product. Unfortunately, it may decrease the length and possibly the quality of your life at the same time.

Trans-fatty acids also did not exist a hundred years ago. Evolutionary biology is uncovering the partnership that slowly evolved between humankind and the earth over thousands of generations, millions of years. We can change our environment, but can our minds and bodies adapt and adjust to these changes at the same speed? The answer is, "No!" This is evidenced by the increasing amounts of cardiovascular diseases, cancers and attention deficit disorder (ADD) problems in Western societies.

### *Why you need good fats*

Your body needs fat for energy, to transport and store the fat soluble vitamins (A, D, E, F and K), which are critical to your health and wellness. Your brain is approximately two-thirds fat. Your nerves are protected by an outer layer of fat. Your body is wrapped in a layer of fat, critical to helping you maintain the right body temperature. Recent studies prove ADD and ADHD (Attention Deficit Hyperactivity Disorder) can be positively influenced with nutritional supplementation using essential fatty acids. The right fats help you lose weight. The wrong fats help you gain weight. Fake fats, such as Olestra™, rob your body of nutrients critical to sustaining and maintaining your health. To lessen some of the potential negative health effects of Olestra™, vitamins and other nutrients are added to it. Yet over time, a body slowly robbed of nutrients will exhibit illnesses, diseases and eventually death.

Prevention is the key. Using the right types of fat in your diet can improve the quality of your life. There are four types of fats: three are good, one should be discarded, and the fake fats, like Olestra™, should be avoided at all costs!

### *How do fats help your body?*

Every cell in the human body needs fat to continue the process of cell regeneration. Cell membranes are greatly affected by the types of fats they are supplied with, to grow and be in a state of optimal health.

As time passes, small negative changes at a cellular level, result in poor health over the entire body as it attempts to compensate for this assault upon it.

Saturated and trans-fatty acids are bad fats which make very poor quality cell membranes. They can also interfere with your internal organ functions, which may lead to a host of illness and diseases. A list of health problems resulting from essential fatty acid deficiencies is at the end of this chapter.

When consumed in the correct proportion, good fats promote proper cell regeneration and internal organ functions. The best ratio is one part Omega 3, with three parts Omega 6, and one part Omega 9 fatty acids.

Most problems are created by the overconsumption of saturated fat and usually too much Omega 6 and 9 fatty acids. This interferes with the proper metabolism of Omega 3.

### *What is cholesterol?*

Cholesterol is a common steroid found primarily in most animal cells, blood, nerve tissue, and bile. It is essential to your health. Your liver or intestines produce from 66 percent to 85 percent of the cholesterol the body needs.

The bad news about cholesterol is that it can cause blockages leading to arteriosclerosis and heart attacks, in addition to a host of illnesses. But that is only part of the story. You need cholesterol and all the good things it can do for you. Cholesterol:

aids in carbohydrate metabolism. The more carbohydrates you eat, the more cholesterol you produce.

helps the skin convert the sun's ultraviolet rays into the essential vitamin D.

is the main supplier of adrenal steroid hormones, for example cortisone.

is the critical part of every membrane and required for producing female and male sex hormones.

Cholesterol is transported through the blood stream, by hitching a ride and bonding with proteins. Three main varieties of protein are used by cholesterol for its transportation in the blood system. They are low-density lipoproteins (LDL), very-low density lipoproteins (VLDL) and high-density lipoproteins (HDL).

Currently the ratio between LDL and HDL is used to determine whether or not you have a healthy balance. The overall percentages of these proteins in the system is as follows: 65 percent LDL, 15 percent

VLDL and 20 percent HDL. Studies indicate that HDL, which is made up mainly of a very important fat, lecithin, is the blood system's internal scrubber, which breaks up and prevents the plaque byproducts of LDL from causing arterial blockages.

Blood test's for cholesterol usually include measuring your triglyceride fat levels. High triglyceride levels do not mean you will have high cholesterol readings. Low triglyceride levels do not mean you will have low cholesterol readings. However, it does appear that if you manage to lower your triglyceride levels, your cholesterol levels fall.

Modern science has found a better test predictor for your cardiovascular system's health status – testing for elevated levels of the amino acid homocysteine. There are many natural remedies and supplements you can use, including vitamins, minerals and herbs covered in this book. Health care practitioners have successfully used high doses of vitamins $B_6$, $B_{12}$ and folic acid, and sometimes $B_3$ (niacin), to reduce homocysteine levels.

Recent research proves bioflavonoids reduce LDL levels while increasing HDL levels. Bioflavonoids also reduce the LDL oxidation that leads to artherosclerosis.

J. D. Holt of the University of Wisconsin-Madison Medical School, in the *Journal of Investigative Medicine* wrote: 'Commercial mixture of flavonoids, Provex CV™, inhibits in vivo thrombosis and ex vivo platelet aggregation in dogs and humans.' This was the first time in America that a natural remedy's effectiveness for cardiovascular health was proven, and the findings were presented at the 47th and 48th annual conventions of the American College of Cardiology.

## *What are the main differences between the fat types?*

The three naturally occurring fats are saturated, polyunsaturated and monosaturated. Saturated fats are more stable and less chemically active than the unsaturated oils. In your body the unsaturated oils increase fluidity by being anti-sticky and easily moving apart. The saturated oils tend to stick together in our bodies. The body can manufacture most of the fats it needs, except for the Omega 3 and Omega 6 fats, which are called essential fatty acids since they must come from our diets. Our need for the right fats, in the right ratio, helps determine how well the body functions.

Of the essential fatty acids, North Americans get too much of their fat requirements from the Omega 6 group and too little from the Omega 3 essential fatty acids. Our body requires more Omega 3 essential fatty acids. One part Omega 3 to three parts Omega 6 essential fatty acids is the ideal daily consumption ratio.

In addition, chemically altered and processed foods unnecessarily add to the stress on your body. Trans-fatty acids are toxic, and come hidden in oils and foods we use, such as french fries, margarine, ice creams, donuts, corn chips, potato chips, the vast majority of chemically altered and processed foods. Supplementation can lessen the impact of these bad fats.

### *How can I get more of the Omega 3 fats I need?*

A good idea is to take 1 tablespoon of cold-pressed flax seed oil each day, since it is such a rich source of Omega 3 essential fatty acids. Sprinkle it on salads, use it in cereals (if they are hot let them cool down), use it on breads, instead of butter. Flax seed oil has a delicious flavor and loads of nutritional benefits for your health.

### *How are good oils made and recognized?*

Expeller processed quality oils are produced at temperatures below 118 degrees Fahrenheit in light- and oxygen-free environments. Next they are stored and refrigerated in amber or dark colored, light-resistant containers. Heat, light and oxygen destroy the beneficial properties of oils, which in turn can negatively impact your health.

### *Is there another oil that is good for you?*

Monosaturated and polyunsaturated oils, fats that are liquid at room temperature, are better for you than saturated oils, which are usually solid at room temperature. If a food contains significantly more of one type of fat than another, the food will adopt the behavior of the predominant fat in terms of your health. The most beneficial oil is the monosaturate one, abundant in certain nuts, seeds and salmon.

Cold-pressed organically grown monosaturated fats are an excellent choice for a fat in your diet. This is what researchers discovered in the 1980s when they studied the Mediterranean diet and learned of the power of olive oil. Other monosaturated fats are found in the oil from macadamia nuts, hazelnuts, almonds, avocados, and pistachios. Research on monosaturated fats indicates it does not increase your risk of heart disease – but too much of a good thing can lead to weight gain, and that can add unnecessary stress to your body.

Monosaturated fats can reduce total cholesterol while improving the ratio of the HDL (good cholesterol) to LDL (bad cholesterol) and lowering the levels of the other fat in the blood, triglycerides. Studies have shown monosaturated fatty acids can help diabetics improve control over their blood sugar levels, possibly resulting in significant reductions of the amount of insulin they require daily.

Medium Chain Triglycerides (MCTs) are getting a lot of coverage, as the fat you can take without the worry of weight gain. While this may be true, MCTs are not good for cooking and using them unthinkingly ignores your body's need for the good fats that you require to achieve an optimal state of health and well-being. Balance is the key. Occasional use may be helpful, but if you deprive your body of the needed fats, you deprive it of the vehicle that transports the powerful and life enhancing fat soluble vitamins A, D, E, F and K. In essence, you leave your body open to the ravages resulting from deficiencies in these vitamins.

Medium Chain Triglycerides are purported to be a good energy source which can increase athletic endurance, reduce cholesterol levels, and help lose weight. If supplementing with MCTs, follow label directions, supplement with the fat soluble vitamins A, D, E and F. For vitamin K, use natural sources such as green leafy vegetables and alfalfa. It is prudent to consult your doctor or natural health care provider if you plan to use MCTs for prolonged periods. People with diabetes or high blood cholesterol levels should NOT use medium chain triglycerides, MCTs.

### *How do fats and oils become bad?*

Processing using high temperatures destroys the beneficial components of many oils and can create poisonous substances. For instance, adding preservatives, chemical solvents, using high temperatures and excessive sunlight all combine to destroy the beneficial properties of the unsaturated Omega 3 and Omega 6 essential fatty acids during processing. The result is the creation of rancid and poisonous trans-fatty acids, which are thought to be responsible for many diseases and illnesses.

Although heat destroys the beneficial properties of Omega 3 and Omega 6 essential fatty acids, you can use fats and oils in baking at temperatures up to 325 degrees Fahrenheit. Boiling, deep-frying and frying alter the chemistry of oils, negatively impacting their composition in terms of beneficial health properties. If you must fry, it is preferable to use the oils with the highest saturated and monosaturated fatty acids content.

### *What happens during the manufacture of vegetable oils?*

Shortening, margarine and the vast majority of processed foods using vegetable oils create partially hydrogenated or hydrogenated fats, called trans-fatty acids. Studies indicate these trans-fatty fats are the main cause of many types of cancer and heart disease. They lower the levels of the good cholesterol (HDL) and increase the levels of the bad cholesterol (LDL), disrupting the ideal ratio between the two, needed for optimal health. In addition, they interfere with your body's ability to utilize and metabolize essential fatty acids.

Saturated fats, on the other hand, found in margarine won't lower HDL but will increase LDL levels. This makes nut butters a better choice, even cow's butter is better than margarine. Oils that remain liquid at room temperature are the best choice. Try using extra virgin olive, flax or hemp oil by putting them on a plate and dipping your bread into them or sprinkling them over your food once it has cooled down to 118 degrees Fahrenheit or less.

In the 1940s, grocery stores generally had 300 to 400 food items, relatively few were processed. Today, a supermarket has between 30,000 to 100,000 items, most of which are processed. It is these processed foods which contain the potentially life- and health-threatening fats.

These are the bad fats in the processed foods such as hot dogs, hamburgers, sausages, wieners, cold meats, cakes, donuts, candies, ice creams, french fries and much of what the modern life offers. The cheap fats used are refined, deodorized and toxic. They usually are partially hydrogenated to prolong shelf life and have become oxidized or rancid.

### *What are some examples of toxic fats and oils?*

All vegetable oils that are hydrogenated or partially hydrogenated should be avoided. Read the labels and if dining out, ask to see the type of fats and oils they use. Here are the top three oils used in commercially made products:

*Cottonseed oil* – cotton is one of the most heavily sprayed crops. It contains manufactured and natural toxins. The fast food industry extensively uses this inexpensive toxic oil.

*Corn oil* – toxic solvents and high temperatures are usually used when processing it. Usually the commercial grades used become rancid. If using corn oil, look for unrefined corn oil from corn germ that is organically grown and mechanically cold processed.

*Soybean oil* – due to the difficulty in extracting oil from soybeans, the oil is usually damaged in the process. High temperatures and toxic solvents are used to produce the oil.

### *Here are some recommended oils and fats for cooking:*

*Extra Virgin Olive Oil* – after processing it lasts the longest of the cold-pressed oils, about two years. If stored in the refrigerator it may turn cloudy. If frozen, it makes an excellent solid spread that quickly liquefies at room temperature. For cooking or salads, you can substitute 2 tablespoons for each 3 tablespoons of the other oils you would use, since olive oil is a fat with flavor.

*Macadamia oil, hazelnut oil, almond oil, avocado oil, pistachio oil* along with extra virgin olive oil are mainly monosaturated fats which according to research do not increase your risk of heart disease – but too much can lead to weight gain.

*Sesame oil, Ghee or Butter.*

***Caution:*** If butter browns when frying or cooking with it, don't use it. The change in its chemical composition is not beneficial to your health.

***Healthy Cooking Tips:*** Sulfur rich foods such as garlic and onions help minimize the damage caused by free radicals, when frying. Combine them with the oils and fats which are recommended for cooking.

Wok cooking is a quick frying technique, which damages vegetables and food less than other methods of frying. First add water to the wok, then vegetables, then the oil. The trick is to stir frequently to prevent scorching. Use the sides of the wok for cooking. Add spices and oil mixtures after main dishes and vegetables are cooked.

For salads and cut vegetables the best choice is fresh oils or seeds with the oil still in them.

## *How much fat and oil should I have in my daily allowance of calories?*

For an average healthy human being, it is estimated that between 15 percent and 20 percent of your total daily calories should come from fats and oils. This is usually between 2 and 5 tablespoons of fat or oils from all sources. Each tablespoon is 120 calories. If you eat 1500 calories a day, that means you need between 225 to 300 calories of the good fats and oils each day.

Dr. Dean Ornish, author of *Reversing Heart Disease,* suggests 10 percent as the daily intake combined with other nutritional and lifestyle changes. This is part of the healing heart health program he promotes.

## *What is the best ratio of Omega 3 to Omega 6 essential fatty acids?*

The best ratio is one part Omega 3 essential fatty acids to three parts Omega 6 essential fatty acids.

## *What are the best sources?*

Hemp oil is the closest to the one-to-three ratio the body best utilizes. Next is flax seed oil, then canola oil, then walnut oil. In all cases, we refer to cold-pressed, mechanically extracted oil only, preferably from organically grown sources. Cold-pressed, mechanically extracted olive oils are generally labeled 'extra virgin'.

Good sources of Omega 3 essential fatty acids include: flax oil, hemp oil, soya, herring, mackerel, salmon, sardines, seafood, shellfish and dark green leafy vegetables.

Good sources of Omega 6 essential fatty acids include: borage oil, corn oil, evening primrose oil, hemp oil, safflower oil, sesame oil, sunflower oil, beef, chicken, eggs, lamb, legumes, nuts, pork, seeds.

## *Bad fats to decrease in your diet*

- hydrogenated margarine
- dairy products**
- prepared luncheon and deli meats
- commercial peanut butters
- fried and deep fried foods
- red meat
- nonorganic butter
- potato and corn chips
- pastries and candies

** Especially if they might have been produced using bovine growth hormones, antibiotics, or unnaturally genetically altered cows

## *Goods fats to increase in your diet*

- nuts and seeds
- whole grains
- sea vegetables
- cold water fish
- fresh organic vegetables
- soy products
- lentils
- flax, hemp and borage oils
- legumes**
- seafood
- lean meats

** beans, seeds – plants having seeds that grow in pods

If you can afford organically grown and cold processed plant foods or organically fed free-range animal meats, that is the best choice for your health and healing. A major concern is the use of genetically engineered food crops. Adulterated modified foods may not have the short- and long-term benefits, if any at all, that are the healing properties of organically grown foods.

Genetically altered, irradiated and hormone enhanced foods are considered potentially hazardous to the health. No long-term multi-generational studies have been done on humans with these foods. It has not been determined how they affect other plant, animal, insect, and microscopic life forms. Independently funded groups to monitor these changes do not exist. There is insufficient protection, in the form of international and local laws to hold individuals and corporations accountable. Unbiased bureaucracies for monitoring and enforcement, do not exist. These are some of the issues arising from genetically altered and synthetic chemically enhanced foods. In Great Britain and throughout Europe, consumers and government agencies are demanding that these foods be clearly labeled to enable clear choices.

Laboratory studies compared a control group of rats that ate naturally grown potatoes with rats fed genetically altered potatoes. The control group suffered no side effects, while the entire group that ate genetically altered potatoes died.

John Losey, a Cornell University entomologist, dusted milkweed, the main plant food source for Monarch butterflies, with genetically altered BT corn pollen. His report, in the journal *Nature,* indicated half the Monarch butterfly caterpillars died within four days of eating the milkweed and those that did not die had eaten significantly less of the food. It is feared hundreds of species of butterflies and moths worldwide will be wiped out by this genetically engineered corn that is being widely distributed since 1996.

Independent laboratory tests, done for consumer advocacy groups (e.g. Consumer's Report), prove unmarked genetically altered ingredients are in baby foods, restaurant meals and on your grocery store shelves.

If you are concerned, write or speak to your local, state and federally elected representatives. Ask them what specific actions they will undertake on behalf of your community. Protect yourself, your family and your community, take action today to protect your supply of food.

### *Essential fatty acid deficiencies are evident in the following health conditions*

Acne, AIDS, allergies, Alzheimer's, angina, atherosclerosis, autoimmunity, behavioral disorders – such as ADD (attention deficit disorder), ADHD (attention deficit hyperactivity disorder), dyslexia, cancer, cartilage destruction, cystic fibrosis, depression, dermatitis, eczema, *e. coli* infection, heart disease, high blood pressure, hyperactivity, hypertension, immune disorders, inflammation, intestinal problems, kidney dysfunction, learning problems – see behavioral disorders, leprosy, leukemia, Lupus, menopause, mental illness, multiple sclerosis, myocardial infarction, neurological disease, obesity, osteoarthritis, painful menstruation, premenstrual syndrome (PMS), post viral fatigue, psoriasis, Reye's syndrome, rheumatoid arthritis, schizophrenia, stroke, vascular disease, vision problems.

# chapter 6

# Water

## Water everywhere, and not a single drop to spare

Water makes up about 70 percent of your body's composition. It lubricates and transports nutrients throughout the body. Water helps cleanse by taking waste products out of the body. It helps maintain your biochemical balances. It is a critical component of the heating and air conditioning system that maintains your body temperature. Water performs a host of other beneficial activities. The type and quality of water you get, can significantly affect your health. Here is a quick guide to water.

### *Tap water and safety issues.*

The advantages of tap water are ease of access, low cost and hopefully constant monitoring and accurate testing by public authorities. The disadvantages vary, depending on whether you live in the city, or the country. Drinking, bathing, swimming and showering in water are the key ways you absorb some of these potentially hazardous chemicals. Here are some of the negatives.

*Chlorination* – Chlorine has numerous negative health side effects, from skin irritation to possible cancer causing properties, that are as yet unexplored. Whether absorbed through the skin, inhaled through the nose or drunk through the mouth, chlorine invades and affects the body. Europeans, whose water resources are significantly less than ours, use ozonation as their primary method of cleaning water. It is a significantly safer and healthier method than adding this potentially toxic chemical which stresses your body.

*Fluoridation* – The unnatural fluorides used in our water supplies are very dangerous to handle. They are linked to and may be the cause of a mottling of the teeth (discoloration and bumpy surfaces called dental fluorosis), as well as cancer, and Down's Syndrome. Recent studies indicate fluoridation does not reduce the incidence of cavities and may even cause a loss of bone density over time, resulting in osteoporosis and osteomalacia.

The two types of fluoride generally used to treat water are fluorosalic acid and sodium fluoride, both are man made industrial byproducts not found in nature. They are so toxic, they must be stored in special containers and are used in rat poison. Unfortunately, the naturally occurring non-toxic calcium fluoride is not the one used in our water supplies.

Fluoride is now found in most of the processed foods we consume, since it is in our water systems. This may result in increased symptoms of fluoride overload in the coming years. *Methods exist to remove most of the fluoride from your water, they are:* distillation, reverse osmosis and activated alumina filtration systems.

Inappropriate dumping of industrial and household waste into the water system. Laundry detergents, cleaning products, paint, solvents, left over food, et cetera. The potential for dangerous chemical interactions increases as we keep spoiling this valuable and limited life giving resource.

A hidden source of toxic chemicals such as arsenic, are due to the byproducts of manufacturing.

Untreated farm sludge is a breeding ground for disease and illness, since it is composed primarily of the waste matter from overcrowded agri-business farms.

Excessive or unnecessary use of fertilizers, pesticides and other products seep into and become part of the water system.

Transportation methods provide breeding grounds for bacteria.

Air pollutants and chemicals that return, carried on the backs of rain drops, and become part of the municipal water system.

Parasites that use the water system to survive.

This is a small sample of what we are doing to our water and what we may be getting out of the tap. Water analysis may give you a sense of only some of the hazardous chemicals, parasites and other agents lurking in your water. It cannot test for everything.

The message is clear, you would not clean your food, utensils, floors, yourself or your car with dirty water, so do not expect your body to maximize its healing properties if all you use is polluted and/or dirty water. You do have choices.

### *Soft Versus Hard Water*
### *It's all about mineral content!*

Hard water refers to water with higher amounts of the minerals magnesium and calcium. It does not easily form suds or lather when using soaps. The result leaves a filmy deposit on what the soap contacts. Some believe the magnesium and calcium in hard water are beneficial for the arteries, bones and heart. In addition, the taste of the water is affected.

Soft water may be hard water that has been treated to remove the magnesium and calcium, or it may be naturally soft. Water treated to make it soft water has the following problems:

greater chance of dissolving pipe linings than hard water. In the case of older buildings with lead pipes, this can be a serious threat to your health.

a similar threat exists in galvanized or plastic piping that contains the toxic heavy metal cadmium.

artificially softened water can also leach out the arsenic, copper, iron and zinc found in copper piping.

The issue here is that your water can be the underlying cause of illness or disease. Your body may have to constantly work to counteract the affects of toxic overload. This may prevent your body from doing what it needs to do to achieve and maintain optimal health.

### *Ways to improve your tap water*

Hardware and general merchandise stores carry many types of water filtration systems. They can be easily added onto your existing water system at home. However, some just remove chlorine and other chemicals that cause water to taste bad. Here are the options we suggest:

Bring your tap water to a rolling boil for at least five minutes to kill parasites and bacteria. Unfortunately, this requires time to cool the water in your refrigerator and may increase concentrations of other byproducts. Exposing water for hours or aerating it in a blender can reduce the taste caused by chlorine and other chemicals. These methods do not really clean the water.

Nature cleans water by filtration. The bacteria are deposited into rocks and the water is re-mineralized with trace minerals such as magnesium and calcium, from the rocks. Many man-made systems use this idea to produce cleaner water. Here are three:

1. absorbent filters, using carbon to remove impurities from the water. They may be attached to the water system or used in containers that you store in the refrigerator.
2. micro filtration systems run the water through tiny pores of the filtering system, which picks up and eliminates contaminants.
3. ion-exchange and other specialized methods using various media to clean the water.

Reverse osmosis and ceramic filtration systems are widely used and considered among the best of the household water purification methods. A carbon filter is recommended, to trap and prevent the toxic gases that escape purification from reentering the clean water. It should be noted that none of these systems can get rid of all the impurities in your water.

## *What other choices and treatment methods do you have?*

### *Bottled water*

Classified by its source, mineral content and/or by the method of treatment. It could come from a variety of places, such as a spring, well, spa, even your municipal water supply! The mineral content indicates a minimum of 500 parts per million of dissolved parts. If the water has been steam-distilled, demineralized, deionized or undergone any type of treatment, the bottle's label should indicate this.

The major problem with bottled waters are that they are not regulated and tested like the public system water is. California has some of the strictest requirements for bottled waters, yet most other government bodies take a lax attitude towards pollutants in the water, such as arsenic and bacterial levels. This can result in misleading labeling and potentially false claims on the labels.

### *Demineralized and Deionized Water*

Demineralizing and deionizing mean neutralizing the electric charge of a water molecule. The process of deionization removes the nitrates, magnesium, calcium and other heavy metals such as barium, cadmium and lead compounds.

***Mineral, Natural Spring and Sparkling Waters – C'est la vie! Translation: This is the life! Or is it?***

Years ago Perrier, one of the world's top brands of mineral water, had to recall all of its bottled water because a breakdown in its filtration system prevented the removal of benzene, a carcinogen, from the water source it used for bottling. Yet this and other less notable incidents have not stopped the growing popularity of bottled waters. If you are using mineral waters as a dietary source of minerals, read the labels and make sure you are getting what your body needs. Drinking mineral waters with minerals your body does not lack, can harm you. Inorganic minerals can also be harmful for you. Moderation is the key.

Many mineral waters are carbonated, yet they are only called mineral waters because the producer added citrates, bicarbonates and sodium phosphates to distilled or filtered tap water. Club soda is an example of a sparkling carbonated mineral water – and usually a lot cheaper than other packaged brands.

Natural spring waters only mean the the mineral content of the water has not been manipulated or changed. It may or may not have been treated. It may or may not have come from a spring. All the above problems arise due to legal definitions and requirements or lack thereof. Read the label to discover the source of the water and its mineral content.

Sparkling water is water that has been carbonated. It is plain, without fillers such as sugars, artificial sweeteners and other additives. It is a healthy choice compared to a daily consumption of soda pop and alcoholic drinks.

Some carbonated waters are natural, some are synthetic. This does not reflect the quality of the water or its mineral content. Check the labels before buying.

***Warning***: If you suffer from ulcers or intestinal problems, do not drink sparkling or other carbonated waters as they can cause irritation to the gastrointestinal tract.

***Steam-distilled Water... really cleaning up your act!***

Distillation heats water and condenses the resulting steam to produce a nearly pure water. It removes nasty impurities like parasites, bacteria, chemicals, viruses, pollutants and, unfortunately some helpful minerals. A carbon filter is recommended for preventing organic gases such as benzene, carbon tetrachloride, trichloroethylene and trihalomethanes from re-entering the distilled water. When consumed, distilled water cleans out the system by leaching the inorganic minerals from the tissues and cells.

We recommend remineralizing the water with low sodium ConcenTrace® Trace Mineral drops. Use a quarter of a teaspoon (20 drops) for each gallon of water. Other healthy additives include lemon juice and the organic apple cider vinegar from Omega Nutrition of Bellingham, WA. They also add flavor and aid the digestive system.

The preferred storage medium for distilled water are glass bottles or containers. Water may leach compounds from plastic containers.

When buying commercially prepared drinking water we recommend distilled water.

chapter 7

# Fiber & Good Bacteria

## Keeping the body's systems in balance

Fiber is a thread-like structure that combines with other similar materials to create plant tissue. Fiber gives plants their shape. It is the part of food that is not digested, has no calories and the bulk it provides is very beneficial. In the body, fiber keeps things moving through the digestive tract providing bulk for stools. During this process it passes unscathed through many chemicals and enzymes in the gastrointestinal system.

There are two types of fiber. Soluble fiber becomes jelly-like and gluey in water while insoluble fiber does not change in water. Most vegetable and fruits have both types of fiber.

Fiber picks up and carries toxins harmlessly through the intestines and colon, where they are expelled. A lack of fiber can result in constipation. About 100 million Americans suffer from constipation, an uncomfortable and potentially health-threatening problem. Another main cause is age, as our bodies become less efficient in processing foods.

*Fiber can help with:* breast cancer, colectoral cancer, colitis, diabetes, diverticulitis, diverticulosis, excessive estrogen (fiber helps balance this good hormone), gallstones, hemorrhoids, irritable bowel syndrome (IBS), menopausal symptoms, obesity, premenstrual syndrome (PMS), varicose veins.

*Quick benefit facts about soluble and insoluble fiber:* improves digestion; helps cleanse and clear the digestive system; lowers blood pressure; lowers cholesterol; prevents colon and breast cancers; alleviates PMS and menopausal symptoms; keeps gallbladder healthy; prevents appendicitis; stabilizes blood sugars, promotes weight loss, and detoxifies your system.

### *Soluble fiber:*

Lowers cholesterol.

Lowers blood pressure.

Stabilizes blood sugar levels.

Gives the good bacteria in your digestive tract a good medium to grow in.

May lessen the amount of time food is in the digestive tract.

Detoxifies.

Reduces the intake of fat, since, by increasing the volume of food, it helps you feel full.

*Good sources of soluble fiber:* Fruits (especially oranges, apricots, mangoes), vegetables (especially any of the following cooked: brussels sprouts, parsnips, turnips, peas, broccoli, onions and carrots) fresh okra, cereals (especially cooked or cold oat bran and uncooked oatmeal), legumes i.e. plants having seeds that grow in a pod (especially cooked butter nut beans, black beans, canned baked beans, navy beans, canned white or kidney beans and chickpeas), gums from nuts, and oat bran.

### *Insoluble fiber:*

Prevents constipation.

Provides bulk for feces (stool).

Lessens the amount of time food is in the digestive tract.

Transports toxins from the bowels, detoxifies.

Helps scrub clean the intestines.

Reduces fat intake by helping you to feel full.

*Good sources of insoluble fiber are:* all vegetables, beans, whole grains such as wheat, barley, rye.

Insufficient fiber can cause the diverticula to malfunction. The diverticula are sacs opening out from the walls of the large intestines. Straining, or trying to force a movement, can cause fecal matter into these sacs, which in turn results in them becoming inflamed and enlarged, causing digestive matter to leak into the body.

The large intestine is full of waste matter and potentially harmful bacteria. This can cause abscesses and infections in the surrounding tissues. When the waste matter and bacterial byproducts get stuck in the diverticula, they ferment, rot, and become toxic to you and become an excellent breeding ground for parasites. All sorts of toxins and waste products can gather in these sacs. The result can be diverticulosis, uninflamed diverticula protruding from the intestines, or diverticulitis, which includes inflammation of these protruding sacs.

Reducing the amount of time food takes to go through your body is key to avoid problems such as these. The healthy average transit time is 12 to 24 hours in societies that eat fiber rich foods. In America, most people's digestive systems hold foods between 45 to 65 hours. If you want to check your own digestive systems transit time, eat corn and watch for it to appear in your feces.

Increase your daily fiber intake into the 30 to 35 gram range if you want to rid yourself of constipation and the resulting potential health problems.

### *Quick facts about constipation you should know*

Over-the-counter remedies do not deal with the underlying problem of constipation; they alleviate the symptoms. Overuse of any laxatives can cause "lazy-bowel" problems, acute, short-term bouts of constipation possibly becoming chronic, long-term conditions.

Constipation can be caused by any of the following: processed foods (especially those lacking fiber), pharmaceutical drugs (anti-histamines, anti-depressants, pain-killers, decongestants and tranquilizers), iron tablets, dairy products such as cheese, stress, change in hours awake, excessive alcohol, oral contraceptives, insufficient fiber, water, exercise or sleep.

Here are some ways you can deal with constipation: Drink more water; Increase your consumption of bran, prunes, prune juice, and psyllium powder; Try Metamucil or Correctol, both use psyllium as their main ingredient; drink lots of water whenever you use any bulk-forming laxatives; A cup or two of coffee may help; Try 300 mg of magnesium for constipation.

Once the problem is resolved, make the following routine part of your daily life: Drink 8 to 10 cups of clean water daily; Consume 30 to 35 grams of fiber daily; Do 30 minutes of gentle exercise, such as walking, to help keep your digestive system and mind tuned up. Since emotional stress can be an underlying cause of constipation, practice relaxation techniques or meditation.

Herbs and natural remedies that help alleviate constipation should only be used occasionally, or they can become habit forming like over-the-counter laxatives, and your bowels can become lazy. Try cascara sagrada, senna, organic prune juice, soaking flax seeds in water overnight then taking a tablespoonful in the morning, or aloe vera juice.

Excellent fiber rich foods include fruits, fresh or dried vegetables, barley, dried beans, brown rice, wheat bran, oats, rye, seeds, nuts and our all time favorite, popcorn – with a sprinkling of extra virgin olive or flax seed oil, please.

## *Good bacteria – fighting the good fight!*

Just as your body needs fiber to function optimally, it also needs good bacteria. These friendly bacteria defend your body against disease and infection. They keep bad bacteria in check, preventing them from overtaxing your body's immune system. They keep hormone levels within a normal range. They help prevent fungal and yeast infections from overwhelming the body. They are instrumental in producing B vitamins. They help the digestive system, plus a host of other activities beneficial to your health and well-being.

When you use pharmaceutical antibiotics, you disturb the natural balance of good and bad bacteria. Antibiotics are akin to using an atomic bomb to deal with a simple problem. Unfortunately, synthetic antibiotics destroy all the bacteria, good and bad, with which they come into contact. This may offer temporary relief from bacterial problems, but there is a price beyond immediate relief. Your immune system weakens, and you are more susceptible to diseases and infections until your body rebuilds it natural defense mechanism. Bad bacteria become resistant to antibiotics, which is part of the reason we are having outbreaks of 'super resistant bad bacteria' which are life threatening. The answer is to restore the good bacteria levels in your gut, as gently and as soon as possible.

Probiotics are an answer to this problem. At the very least, one should supplement with acidophilus when taking antibiotics. Generally you do not need a prescription for this. Ask your pharmacist what to use to restore your internal bacterial balance.

Probiotic supplementation should continue for at least 30 days after you finish taking the antibiotic.

Take your probiotics half an hour before each meal. Gas or bloating indicates your system is adjusting to the probiotics. Fermentation is occurring in your gut. The gas or bloating usually clear up within 10 days. If the problem persists, consult with your nutritionally orientated health care provider.

Dietary fiber is a feeding and breading ground for bacteria. They metabolize the fiber, turning it into acids which reduce the growth rates of bad bacteria.

Yogurt with live bacterial cultures support and restore your internal bacterial levels. Plain unsweetened yogurt, without any fruit is the easiest to digest and best type to use. Years ago scientists discovered a group of Russians who lived exceptionally long lives. The key was their high consumption of plain yogurt. In America, a major brand of yogurt used this information in their advertising.

*If you have problems digesting milk based products, do not be concerned, dairy free probiotics are available. Ask your pharmacist for your best choices. Supplementing with a full spectrum digestive enzyme or lactase, the digestive enzyme for lactose intolerance, may also help. Increasing your intake of fiber and fructo-oligosaccharide (FOS) improves the growth of good bacteria.*

# chapter 8

# Antioxidants

## Nature's Powerful Healers

Antioxidants are the scavengers which protect your body from free radical damage. Antioxidants are those amino acids, enzymes, minerals, vitamins and supplements that prevent or control the oxidative process. The oxidative process rusts the body from the inside out and outside in.

Free radicals are the negative byproduct created when the body produces energy or reacts to air pollution, sunshine, diseases, illnesses, food carcinogens like nitrates and smoke from charcoal barbecues, emotional or mental stress and almost all activities of daily life to one degree or another. They are responsible for the destructive process caused by uncontrolled oxidation and damaged cells, as well as weakening the immune system.

Free radicals are atoms that have at least one electron missing. Electrons are negatively charged components of atoms. The missing electrons create unstable atoms, which seeks a component to complete them. A chemical reaction occurs as free radical atoms bond with the molecules or atoms which are attracted to and easily able to bond with them. This process happens very quickly and can cause a lot of damage to the body. Over time, the body tires and can no longer compensate for this, resulting in diseases or illnesses.

Antioxidants freely give up an electron to a free radical. This stabilizes the free radical and keeps it from causing too much damage.

Not all free radicals are bad. Like weights are to a weight lifter, free radicals are to body systems. They help keep your immune system tuned up and running better by destroying bacteria and viruses. Free radicals help produce energy. They are critical for production of hormones and enzymes. Many substances the body needs requires the intervention of free radicals. The problem emerges when there are too many free radicals and the body's harmonious functioning, on a cellular level, is thrown completely out of whack. Many things and processes can cause a lack of antioxidants.

As we age, our body produces less antioxidants, thereby hastening the aging process. Aging can result in degenerative diseases and illnesses, as well as things like weakened eyesight and wrinkles. Even though food is the main source of antioxidants, individual needs exceed what food provides. Aging and the many stresses we endure increase our need for antioxidant supplementation which detoxifies our bodies.

Here is a partial list of known free radicals: hydrogen peroxide, hydroxy radicals, superoxide, hypochlorite radicals, nitric oxide, single atoms of oxygen and some lipid peroxides.

These are a few of the causes that create free radicals in the body:

Sunshine.

Radiation.

Exposure to toxic chemicals like cigarette and cigar smoke.

Exhaust from trucks and cars.

Environmental stressors, such as pesticides and fertilizers contaminating our food and water.

Chemicals in water whether they be industrial or used for water treatment, such as chlorine and fluoride.

According to Sam Graci, author of *The Power of Superfoods*, over 100,000 xenobiotics (foreign chemicals) are in use today. While the thousand or so new chemicals created each year may test negatively for causing birth defects or cancer, their affects upon reproductive systems and the human endocrine system are unknown. These chemicals are believed to be responsible for many wildlife and human health problems. The encouraging news is that antioxidants abound in nature.

## *Antioxidant Sources*

Antioxidants take the form of pigments in plants, as well as hormones, vitamins, minerals and enzymes. They even reside in the bark of the pine tree. The following is a sampling of antioxidants:

Antioxidant enzymes include: Superoxide dismutase (SOD), glutathione peroxidase, methionine reductase.

Antioxidant vitamins include: vitamin A, beta-carotene, vitamin C, vitamin E (alpha, beta and gamma tocopherols). Only natural vitamin E should be used for therapeutic purposes.

Selenium and zinc are antioxidant minerals. The hormone melatonin, produced by the pineal gland in the brain, is a powerful antioxidant.

### *Nutraceuticals can be antioxidants in foods, for example:*

quercetin (apple)

lycopene (best absorbed from cooked tomatoes with a little olive oil)

lutein (a carotenoid)

glutathione (produced in the body)

and zeaxanthin (a carotenoid in spinach, okra, and other vegetables). They are found in flavonoids (i.e. reserveratrol, catechins, proanthocyanidins, anthocyanidins) and isoflavones (such as those found in soy products like genistein and daidzein).

### *Other antioxidants you will want to check out:*

| | |
|---|---|
| Alpha-lipoic acid | bilberry |
| chlorella | coenzyme Q10 |
| ginkgo biloba | grape seed extract |
| green tea | DHEA |

cysteine and other amino acids

oligomeric proanthocyanidins (OPCs) like pycnogenol which can be extracted from pine tree bark.

### *Food sources high in antioxidants include*

red grapes – red wines and purple grape juices

yellow and red onions

raw or very lightly cooked broccoli, cabbage, cauliflower, spinach, okra, beet greens, Swiss chard, watercress

raw crushed garlic

fresh vegetables, especially dark green leafy ones

pink grapefruit

fresh whole fruits

extra virgin (means from the first cold pressing) olive oil**

herbs used in cooking such as thyme and rosemary

and carrots, pumpkins and sweet potatoes - the deeper the orange color the more antioxidants they have.

** Those using organically grown olives are tops.

Combinations of antioxidants are now easily available. They combine nutrients that work better together than they do when taken separately. In addition, they are usually less expensive and easier to take than if you combine the products together on your own. A formulation called 'ACES', is an example of a good synergistic blend. It usually has beta-carotene which converts to vitamin A, as well as vitamin C, vitamin E, and selenium. Some formulations include zinc and/or other beneficial nutrients.

The key is to get enough antioxidants to protect your body and neutralize free radicals. Your body produces antioxidants naturally, but polluted environments, nutrient deficient foods and stressful unhealthy lifestyle choices almost guarantee the body will not make enough of them.

The prescription integrates eating a wide variety of uncooked, organically grown and unprocessed foods with supplementation using a wide variety of antioxidants. Follow these self-care guidelines to enhance the quality of your life.

# chapter 9

# Price versus Value

## The question of bio-availability

## Are you getting what you pay for?

## Quick Reference Chart Bio-availability of Supplements

## How to get the most out of your supplements

There are important considerations to keep in mind when buying supplements. How much of the nutrient in the supplement is available for use by your body? Is the nutrient in the supplement one your body can effectively use? How much of the nutrient does your body actually get to use? These address the question of bio-availability. By the end of this chapter you will be equipped with the information you need to make better buying decisions.

Consider this example: A regular tablet (hard pill) with fillers may say it has 1000 units of vitamin C. Your body, however, only uses 5 to 10 percent (50 to 100 units) of the available vitamin C in the pill and eliminates the remainder through urination or defecation. So, even though you paid for a certain amount of a nutrient or active ingredient in a natural remedy or supplement, your body may not necessarily receive that amount. We want to simplify bio-availability for you.

### *What is bio-availability?*

Bio-availability concerns the body's ability to adapt (homeostatic regulation), using its moderating mechanism, to the available trace-element levels. The two key factors are physiological (intrinsic) variables and dietary (extrinsic) variables.

The adaptation process is a physiological regulatory variable which responds to metabolic, functional interactions either positively or negatively. Examples include copper and iron levels in catecholamine metabolism, selenium in iodine utilization and zinc levels in protein degradation or synthesis. These co-factors can increase or reduce the body's ability to maximize the benefits you get from a supplement.

These metabolic interrelationships can reduce the availability of stored elements to work effectively or they can enhance the release of the stored elements. The aim of this, is to bring vitamin and mineral balances into a harmony that can best benefit your health.

### *Do nutrients interact with each other?*

Yes. Some positively, others negatively. When taking vitamins, it is critical your body have enough trace minerals, otherwise the vitamins cannot be properly absorbed and used by the body.

Dietary variables include synergistic relationships, where two or more elements work more effectively inside the body. For example citrate- or histidine-enhanced zinc increases absorption, by maintaining and supporting the body's supplement transportation system and the mobility of the elements.

Antagonists limit the mobility of elements by decreasing gastrointestinal lumen volubility of elements and/or competing with element receptors involved in transport, absorption, storage and function. For example, excessive amounts of cadmium or copper can greatly undermine the capacities of zinc, a mineral critical for health and healing. Excessive iron affects copper and zinc balances.

Researchers are only beginning to fully understand and scientifically document these important issues. The bottom line is that with proper self-care supplementation you can fine-tune your body's natural abilities to attain a state of optimal health. Hopefully the medical professionals of the future will focus more on disease prevention and good health by correcting imbalances in the body.

### *Can labeling cover up the true nature of a problem?*

Yes. The use of the word 'genetics' is a good example. When you label something as a genetic defect, in many cases the tendency is to not look for the underlying cause of the problem, unless there is seen to be great monetary reward. This results in the health problem happening again and again. It means the underlying cause of a problem may not be examined, or even thought of.

Our overuse and desire to blame forces beyond our control as the basis of our problems, does not absolve us of the havoc we are causing to our food, water and air supplies. These used to be abundant with enough nutrients to help our bodies. Today, that is no longer the case.

In the 1800s, Harvard Medical School's teaching hospital had few cases of heart disease and cancer. Since then, the quality and preparation of our food has changed for the worse. Now, heart disease and cancers are leading causes of death and reduced quality of life.

In the 1950s, as Japanese immigrants embraced the American way of life including the typical American diet, heart disease and cancers became the leading causes of their deaths. Our diets and the amount, quality and type of nutrients we get from what we eat and drink, has radically changed over the last century.

Blaming genetics for problems such as attention deficit disorder, heart disease, cancer of the breast and a host of other health problems is not the best course of action, nor is it the correct answer in many cases. It would be wise to look at the changes to the world around us.

Our schools have become dispensers of fats that kill. The trans-fatty acids in potato chips, junk and processed foods were not so common 50 years ago. Combine this with the caffeine, fat and sugar in chocolate bars, as well as the phosphorous and caffeine in soda pop, which deplete our children's bodies of vital nutrients, and you awaken to the problems for which we are now laying foundations. Our children are being set up for heart disease and cancers from the moment these foods become part of their daily intake.

Junk food machines in schools only worsen the problem. Our children's long term health is being dealt a persistent and powerful blow. Short-term financial gains may cause significant long-term problems. Are all these children genetically predisposed to heart disease and cancer? Such perspectives divert us from the real problems and inappropriately shift blame. We can lessen the impact of these threats upon their health. Effective supplementation is part of the answer. The intimate relationship between our bodies and our environments is no longer questioned. We live in a world where self-care using appropriate supplementation is critical to our immediate and long-term health.

Some genetic conditions can be viewed as the body's inability to adapt to its environment. In the last century, humanity has radically changed the physical world, affecting its natural mechanisms to the point that even the air we breath or water we drink can kill us. The fast speed at which the world is changing is decreasing our quality of life. The mind and body have not had enough time to evolve so as to completely adapt to the rapidly changing environment. The outcomes are increasing occurrences of asthma, Alzheimer's, attention deficit disorder (ADD), attention deficit hyperactivity disorder (ADHD), heart disease, certain cancers and a list of illnesses and diseases that grows daily.

Recently, the critical role of folic acid supplementation for women before getting pregnant was discovered. Sufficient amounts of folic acid prevent the life threatening and crippling condition in newborns called spina bifida. Glucosamine and chondroitin heal and reduce the severity of many arthritic conditions. Vitamin E helps prevent heart disease and cancer. St. John's Wort is a safe and effective anti-depressant compared to many pharmacological alternatives. In essence, when the body's internal balance is disrupted, diseases and illnesses manifest themselves more readily. Self-care supplementation prevents harm to our bodies, heals us and enhances our quality of life.

### *Bio-availability: Are you getting what you want?*

*Medical and Clinical Research Summary*

Vitality, youthfulness, energy and clear thinking are greatly enhanced with proper nutrition and supplementation. The problem is the amount of misinformation and hidden agendas that veil the best forms of supplementation.

Unfortunately, the farming and food processing techniques of the last fifty years have created foods depleted of much of their nutritional value and containing toxic chemicals such as pesticides. These negative properties may greatly affect the healing and health promoting properties of foods, so they no longer offer sufficiently nutrient-dense levels needed for optimal functioning.

This subtlety affects your life and the lives of those around you. A critical point is not what you consume, but how much of it actually gets used by your body and how quickly it gets to where it has to go in your body.

The delivery system and how it's administered determines the rate of absorption and the percentage of nutrients that are actually available for use by your body. The label may say one thing, but reality says only what the body can and does use is effective. The *Physicians Desk Reference #49* gives information about the bio-availability of supplements. Use the chart on the following page the next time you go to buy your supplements.

### *What does the term 'standardized' mean, when used to describe herbal and other supplemental products?*

'Standardized' refers to the guaranteed minimum potency of the active ingredient in the product. For example, the standardized potency for 5-hydroxytryptophan (5-HTP), the active ingredient in Griffonia Simplicifolia, a calming neuro-nutrient and mood enhancer, is usually 5 percent (5-HTP). That means a 500 mg capsule, contains at least 25

Summary From

**The Physicians Desk Reference #49**

With Updated Information On

The Bio-availability of Supplements

| *Type* | *Method* | *Time to Absorb* | *% Nutrients Absorbed* |
|---|---|---|---|
| Tablets, regular | drink & swallow | 2–4 hrs. | 5%–10% |
| Gel caps | drink & swallow | 1–3 hrs. | 15%–20% |
| Pills citrate & chelated | drink & swallow | 4–6 hrs. | 25%–30% |
| Patches | apply to skin | 3–5 hrs. | 45%–50% |
| Liquids | sublingual through the mouth | 30 min. | 60%–70% |
| Patented fructose compounded tablets | through the mouth | | 80%** |
| Injections | intramuscular through the skin | 10 min. | 70%–80% |
| Liposome oral sprays | through the mouth | 30 sec. | 90%–95%** |

** Patented fructose compounded tablets and liposome oral sprays information provided by Dr. George Grant.

mg of 5-HTP. This is becoming the standard way of expressing the effectiveness of an herbal product.

When buying, ask yourself, *"Do my supplements do the job I bought them for?"* If your body does not get to use what a supplement offers, or the nutrients offered are not in the supplement, then you cannot use them to achieve optimal health or healing. Here is a consumer's quick tip list of what to look for in a natural remedy or supplement:

- Does the label clearly indicate the name and contact information for the supplier?
- Who stands by the product's quality? Is it independently verified?
- If it is a herbal product used for therapeutic purposes, does it show the percentage of standardized extract of the herb?
- If it is an herbal product, are directions for use clear?
- Is the form of the product you are buying, the most bio-available form, so your body will get what it needs?

- Is it worth it to spend more for a better quality and more user friendly form of the supplement?

If in doubt, call the manufacturer or ask the health food store staff or a naturally orientated pharmacist if they have any recommendations. Unfortunately, many consumers shop for supplements using price as the key to their decisions. Private label and major brands in their quest to give you the best price, may cut corners and not offer you the most absorbable and effective form of supplement. You get what you pay for, but you may not get what is best for your body.

### *What is the difference – synthetic versus natural vitamins?*

The majority of vitamins are synthetic. Vitamin C and E are usually available in natural forms. Natural vitamin E is the best choice versus synthetic vitamin E, since the body does not absorb synthetic vitamin E very well.

### *What are the best times to take vitamin and mineral supplements?*

Generally supplements are best taken during or at the end of a meal. It takes time for pills, tablets and other delivery systems to breakdown in your digestive tract. Since the food is first, it sets the pace at which everything following it travels through the digestive system. This gives them more time to be absorbed by the body.

If you experience digestive problems, or are in your late forties or older, make sure your multi-vitamin and multi-mineral supplement have natural digestive enzymes, or that you take digestive enzymes at the same time. As we age, our production of digestive enzymes decreases, resulting in nutritional deficiencies that cause diseases and illnesses. These enzymes help your body break down and absorb the nutrients in your supplement.

### *When is the best time to take other supplements?*

It depends on the reason for taking them. If you have a cold, you may want to supplement with zinc lozenges throughout the day, in combination with echinacea, astragalus, goldenseal or the many other options from aromatherapy to homeopathy that are explored in this book. The choice you make determines the best time to use that supplement. If a specific time is mentioned, it is for good reason.

The choice of remedy is a personal one. The information in this book will help you make better and more informed choices. The wisest choice is to refer to information about the specific supplement and follow the directions.

Amino acids should be taken on empty stomachs, at least an half-hour before eating or two hours after a meal. Herbs should be taken on empty stomachs, at least an hour before eating or two hours after a meal. Homeopathic remedies are best taken on a empty stomach, unless your health care practitioner or the products label directs otherwise.

Herbs, homeopathic remedies, aromatherapy, phytochemicals, nutraceuticals and other leading edge supplements have optimum times. Each depends on what the product is being used for and what the nature of the condition is. While it may appear confusing at first, the information guidelines in individual chapters will help you determine the best time and amounts to use for your health and well-being. The following sample of other options, which you will find more fully explained in their chapters, shows you why the question of timing depends on the option you choose:

Energizing supplements are best taken in the morning and during the day, not when you want to sleep.

Hormones such as DHEA are best in the morning, because your testosterone levels peak in the late morning, and this more naturally follows your body's rhythm. However the hormone melatonin is best taken at night, up to two hours before going to sleep.

Aromatherapy using the essential oil of lemon might be just what you want to perk you up in the morning and help you feel good during the day. The essential oil of ylang-ylang might set the mood for a romantic evening.

The all-natural remedy Tiger Balm® is best used when you have sore or sprained muscles.

Homeopathic flower remedies are best used when you recognize the emotional state or problem you want to deal with. Rescue Remedy® can be used whenever you have an emotional state that is beyond your ability to analyze at that moment, or is of such an extreme nature you need help rebalancing your emotional well-being immediately.

### *What about time-released pills?*

The problem with hard-coated time-released pills is they may not dissolve in time or in the right part of your digestive system to absorb what your body needs. Different spots in the intestinal tract absorb specific nutrients, your pill could miss its spot.

### *What vitamin and mineral supplemental delivery systems are best absorbed by the body?*

The inexpensive plain hard pills and tablets are not very well absorbed by the body. In many cases Di-Calcium-Phosphate (DCP) is used as a binding agent to hold the tablet together. DCP is unable to breakdown completely in the body. Thus only 5 to 10 percent of the nutrients get absorbed since the pill cannot completely dissolve. The undissolved remainder is voided from the body. Hard tablets and pills that have citrated or chelated ingredients are better absorbed by the body.

Chelated minerals, meaning bound to amino acids or other ingredients, are the best absorbed from your digestive system, into the body. The most effectively absorbed minerals have been bound to one of these: malate, phosphate, ascorbate, ethanolamine, citrate, fumarate, peptonate, sysinate, succinate, glycinate, picolinate, acetate. Minerals containing oxide or carbonate are the least absorbable. Labels list ingredients from most to least quantity, so it is best to choose those supplements that list the more absorbable forms at the beginning.

We prefer capsules, loose powder, and soft gel capsules since they dissolve more rapidly. Liposome oral spray is a fast effective nutrient delivery system. If you choose pills make sure the ingredients are chelated, citrated, or fructose compounded for greater absorbability.

# chapter 10

# Pharmaceutical Drug Therapies versus Natural Healing Choices

## Choices for 22 Health Conditions

## Naturopathic Doctor Elvis Ali's Prescription for You and Your Family's Daily Nutrient Supplementation

Over 11,000 scientific studies have been published documenting natural medicines' safe and effective uses for treating diseases and illnesses. Around the world, billions of people daily use these safer, successful and inexpensive natural medicines.

This chapter summarizes twenty-two health related problems in fifteen categories, their pharmaceutical therapies, and natural healing choices. Use the summary wisely with your physician or naturally orientated health care practitioner in your mutually beneficial quest for optimal health and healing.

Generally, pharmaceutical drug therapies stress your liver, kidneys, digestive system, and body in general, essentially suppressing symptoms. Often, they do not evoke a healing response yet cause many negative side effects.

Natural remedies work in partnership with the body, helping promote the body's own wisdom to heal itself. Natural remedies may offer relief of symptoms. The key is to give the natural remedy and your body enough time to foster the healing response.

For every year a condition has been developing, it takes roughly one month to generate a healing response. Most diseases and illnesses develop over long periods of time, progressing from a short-term acute condition to a long-term potentially chronic or permanent condition.

The following examples are in no way complete representations of all the drug or natural remedies and supplement choices available. In general we omit from this summary the aromatherapy essential oils, homeopathic and flower remedies plus natural remedies which are mentioned in the Leading Edge Supplements Chapter 18. For particular conditions refer to the index at the back of the book. These examples are a starting point for you to practice your constitutional right of self-health care and health care intervention with the professional of your choice.

## *Allergies*

*Pharmacological Drug Therapy:* Antihistamines such as Allerest, Dimetapp, Benadryl, Hismanol, Sinutab, Seldane. The new Claritin, may have no side effects.

*Potential side effects:* Drowsiness, allergic reactions, nausea, dry mouth, headache, reaction when consuming alcohol.

*Natural Choices:* Ephedra*, nettles, echinacea, ginkgo, goldenseal, bee pollen, bromelain, pycnogenol, quercetin, essential fatty acids (EFA's), B complex with additional $B_5$, $B_6$, $B_{12}$, vitamin C, vitamin E, selenium.

*Potential side effects:* *Do not use ephedra if you have thyroid problems, heart disease, high blood pressure or enlarged prostrate (BPH). Do not take ephedra if you are on antihypertensives or antidepressants. For all other natural choices, refer to specific chapters in this book.

## *Anxiety/Insomnia*

*Pharmacological Drug Therapy:* Benzodiazepines (i.e. Valium, Xanax)

*Potential side effects:* Allergic reaction, blurred vision, constipation, dizziness, drowsiness, headache, it might cause low or high blood pressure, impaired coordination, indigestion, lethargy.

*Natural Choices:* Chamomile, kava kava*, lemon balm, St. John's Wort*, passionflower*, valerian*, skullcap, wild oat, vitamin B complex, magnesium, melatonin.

*Potential side effects:* *Kava Kava, St. John's Wort, valerian and passionflower are not recommended during pregnancy, unless under professional health care supervision. St. John's Wort should not be taken at the same time as antidepressants unless under medical supervision; it can also cause photosensitivity to sunlight. For all other natural choices, refer to specific chapters in this book.

***Auto-immune diseases:*** – Asthma, Colitis, Lupus, Multiple Sclerosis (M.S.), Rheumatoid Arthritis.

*Pharmacological Drug Therapy:* Corticosteroids (i.e. Prednisone).

*Potential side effects:* Weight gain, increased appetite, water and salt retention, high blood pressure, blood clots, acne, facial hair growth on women, osteoporosis, depression, diabetes, peptic ulcers, insomnia, weakened immune system, muscle cramps, muscle weakness.

*Natural Choices for all the above:* Bromelain, curcumin (turmeric), vitamin E, pancreatin, essential fatty acids (EFAs), grape seed extract.

*For Asthma include:* Blessed thistle, blue cohosh, coltsfoot, elecampane, ginkgo biloba, goldenseal, horehound, licorice*, mullein, platycodon, wild cherry, magnesium, selenium, quercetin, B complex with extra $B_6$ and $B_{12}$, vitamin C, DHEA.

*For Colitis include:* vitamin A, bioflavonoids, magnesium, zinc. *For Lupus include:* Proteolic enzymes, calcium, magnesium, L-cysteine, L-lysine, L-methionine. *For M.S. include:* B complex with extra $B_{12}$, selenium, organic sulfur (MSM), essential fatty acids (EFAs), ginkgo biloba.

*For Rheumatoid arthritis include:* Alfalfa, black cohosh, devil's claw, ginger, glucosamine, sarsaparilla, tea tree oil, white willow, wild yam, licorice*, ginseng*, quercetin B complex with extra $B_3$ and $B_5$, vitamin C, manganese, copper, selenium, sulfur (MSM), zinc, glucosamine, chondroitin, betaine HCl, DHEA, L-methionine.

*For arthritic pain, exclude these trigger foods:* corn, wheat, pork, oranges, milk, oats, rye, eggs, beef, coffee, malt, cheese, grapefruit, tomato, peanuts, sugar, butter, lamb, lemon, soybeans.

*Potential side effects:* *Licorice and ginseng are not recommended during pregnancy, unless under professional health care supervision. For all other natural choices, refer to specific chapters in the book.

***Constipation***

*Pharmacological Drug Therapy:* Laxatives that stimulate movements (Ex-Lax, Correctol)

*Potential side effects:* Electrolyte deficiencies, fluid deficiencies, severe cramping, poor nutrient absorption, dependency, lazy bowel syndrome. Not recommended for use over 7 days.

*Natural Choices:* Aloe Vera juice, senna*, cascara sagrada*, goldenseal**, yellow dock, licorice root**, rhubarb, high fiber diet, psyllium husks, acidophilus, flax seeds soaked overnight, 8 to 10 glasses pure water daily. (Don't forget prunes and prune juice.)

*Potential side effects:* *Cascara sagrada and senna are a main component of some over-the-counter stimulating laxatives and may cause electrolyte deficiencies, fluid deficiencies, severe cramping, poor nutrient absorption, dependency, lazy bowel syndrome. Not recommended for use over 7 days. **Licorice root and goldenseal are not recommended during pregnancy, unless under the directions of a professional health care provider. For all other natural choices, refer to specific chapters in this book.

### *Diabetes*

*Pharmacological Drug Therapy:* Oral hypoglycemic prescription drugs: Glipizide (Glucotrol), Glyburide (DiaBeta, Micronase), Chlorpropamide (Diabinese), Tolbutamide (Orinase), Tolazamide (Tolinase).

*Potential side effects:* Low blood sugar (hypoglycemia), poor or decreased ability to function mentally (confusion, depression), headaches, blurred vision, heart palpitations, hunger, sweating, weakness.

*Natural Choices:* Chromium, vanadium, magnesium, manganese, potassium, selenium, zinc, gymnema sylvestre, banaba leaf, ginkgo, panax ginseng*, bilberry, spirulina, B complex (with extra $B_3$, $B_6$, $B_{12}$, inositol, biotin), vitamin C, vitamin E, alpha lipoic acid, carnitine, essential fatty acids (EFAs), psyllium husks plus other fibers, capsaicin, quercetin.

*Potential side effects:* *Panax ginseng is not recommended during pregnancy, unless under professional health care supervision. For all other natural choices, refer to specific chapters in this book.

### *Gout (an arthritic condition)*

*Pharmacological Drug Therapy:* Allopurinol, Colchicine.

*Potential side effects:* Diarrhea, abdominal pains, aplastic anemia, hair loss, liver damage, muscle aches, nausea, vomiting, skin rash, poor absorption of vitamin $B_{12}$.

*Natural Choices:* Organically grown and cold-pressed pure cherry juice, bromelain, celery seed extract, colchicum autuminale, devil's claw*, quercetin, vitamin E, folic acid, essential fatty acids.

*Potential side effects:* *Devil's claw is not recommended during pregnancy, unless under professional health care supervision. For all other natural choices, refer to specific chapters in this book.

***Hair: Graying, thinning, balding.*** See page 16.

***Headaches:*** See Migraine headaches.

### *High blood pressure*

*Pharmacological Drug Therapy:* ACE Inhibitors, Beta blockers (Atenolol), Calcium channel blockers (Nifedipine), Diuretics (Hydroflumethiazide, Hydrochlorothiazide), Diuretics that spare potassium, Loop diuretics (Furosemide).

*Potential side effects:* allergic reactions, diarrhea, loss of magnesium and potassium, higher cholesterol and triglyceride levels, increased uric acid levels, nausea, vomiting, decreased sex drive (libido), impotence, blurred vision.

*Natural Choices:* Garlic, grapefruit pectin, capiscum, celery, hawthorn, hops, valerian*, mistletoe*, pycnogenol, grape seed extract, B complex with extra vitamin $B_6$, vitamin C, vitamin E, coenzyme Q10, calcium, magnesium, potassium.

*Potential side effects:* Valerian and mistletoe are not recommended during pregnancy, unless under professional health care supervision. For all other natural choices, refer to specific chapters in this book.

### *High cholesterol*

*Pharmacological Drug Therapies:*

1) Bile acid sequestering resins (i.e. Questran)

*Potential side effects:* Abdominal pains, constipation, gastrointestinal bleeding, nausea, vomiting, deficiency of fat soluble vitamins A, D, E, and K.

2) HMG CoA Reductase inhibitors (i.e. Mevacor).

*Potential side effects:* Abdominal pain, diarrhea, flatulence, headaches, liver damage, destruction of muscle tissue, muscle pain, skin rash.

*Natural Choices:* Artichoke, garlic, grapefruit pectin, hawthorn, panax ginseng*, linden, pycnogenol, grape seed extract, chromium, omega 3 essential fatty acids, organically grown cold-pressed flax seed oil, gugulipid, reishi mushroom extract, B complex vitamin with extra $B_5$ and niacin**, the combination herbal product Provex CV™.

*Potential side effects:* *Panax ginseng is not recommended during pregnancy, unless under professional health care supervision. **Niacin over 100 mg can cause liver damage, stomach irritations, skin flushing, ulcers; try the 'no-flush' form Inositol Hexaniacinate. Provex CV™ should not be used by patients on blood thinners. For all other natural choices, refer to specific chapters in this book.

### Hypothyroidism

*Pharmacological Drug Therapy:* L-Thyroxine

*Potential side effects:* Diarrhea, insomnia, sweating.

*Natural Choices:* Kelp, gugulipid, L-tyrosine, vitamin A, vitamin E, zinc, B complex vitamin (with extra $B_2$, $B_3$ and $B_6$).

*Potential side effects:* For all natural choices, refer to specific chapters in this book.

### Infections

*Pharmacological Drug Therapy:* Penicillins, Ampicillin, Clindamycin, Cephalosporins, Chloramphenicol, Erythromycin, Kanamycin, Metronidazole, Neomycin, Puromycin, Streptomycin, Tetracyclines.

*Potential side effects:* Suppression of the immune system (results in recurring infections as well as fungal and yeast infections), abdominal pain, abdominal cramping, diarrhea, nausea, vomiting. Tetracycline may darken children's teeth.

*Natural Choices:* Echinacea*, angelica, astragalus, barberry, black seed extract, black walnut, fruit polyphenols, garlic, goldenseal*, grapefruit seed extract, grape seed extract, oak bark, onion, peppermint, propolis, pycnogenol, red clover, saw palmetto, sage, thyme, tea tree oil, turmeric, wormwood*, vitamin C.

*Potential side effects:* *Goldenseal and wormwood are not recommended during pregnancy, unless under professional health care supervision. Wormwood should not be used for long periods of time. Echinacea users who have an auto-immune disorder, should consult a physician or professionally trained health care professional. For all other natural choices, refer to specific chapters in this book.

***Insomnia:*** See Anxiety/Insomnia.

### *Menopausal symptoms*

*Pharmacological Drug Therapy:* Hormone replacement therapy (HRT) using estrogen (Premarin, C.E.S., Estradiol-17B, Estropipate); using synthetic progesterone (Provera, M.P.A.).

*Potential side effects:* Breast tenderness, increased risk of breast cancer, dizziness, heartburn, hypertension, loss of libido (desire for sex), migraine headaches, nausea, phlebitis – inflammation of the walls of a vein, pulmonary embolism – obstruction of pulmonary arteries carrying blood from the heart to the lungs, vomiting, weight gain.

*Natural Choices:* Black cohosh*, dong quai*, evening primrose oil, ginkgo biloba, licorice*, vitex*, red clover, cuddle fish, hesperidin, essential fatty acids, essential oil of clary sage, soybean proteins for their isoflavones, the homeopathic remedy Calendula, B complex with extra vitamin $B_6$, vitamin C, vitamin E, natural progesterone cream.

***Note:*** Dr. Alvin Pettle recommends a 3 percent progesterone cream which originates from wild yam. The treatment protocol is based on the work of Dr. John Lee, author of *What Your Doctor May Not Tell You About Menopause*. Dr. Pettle found that natural progesterone is the only hormone that can build new bone and it alone can treat two out of every three menopausal women's symptoms. In addition, based on Dr. Jonathon Wrights book, *Natural Hormonal Replacement*, if the patient is at high risk for cardiovascular disease and osteoporosis, Dr. Pettle adds 'tri-est'(short for three-estrogens) to the treatment, a compounding pharmacist's formulation using soy. He has found that 'tri-est', a combination of 80 percent estriol (the weakest and safest, of the three estrogens), 10 percent estradiol and 10 percent estrone, in a capsule or cream form, can protect the patient without the added risk of breast cancer. The combination of natural progesterone and 'tri-est' offers relief from menopausal symptoms as well as preventative measures for osteoporosis and cardiovascular disease, without the unacceptable side effects of drug therapy.

*Potential side effects:* *Black cohosh, dong quai, licorice and vitex are not recommended during pregnancy, unless under professional health care supervision. For all other natural choices, refer to specific chapters in this book.

### *Menstrual cramps*

*Pharmacological Drug Therapy:* Ibuprofen, Naproxen.

*Potential side effects:* Gastric and gastrointestinal bleeding.

*Natural Choices:* Blue cohosh*, chamomile, crampbark*, dong quai*, evening primrose oil, vitex, wild yam, the homeopathic remedy Calendula, essential fatty acids, clary sage essential oil.

*Potential side effects:* * Blue cohosh may cause abdominal pains. For all other natural choices refer to specific chapters in this book.

***Note:*** If you are trying to become pregnant or believe that you are pregnant, do not use Blue cohosh, crampbark, or dong quai unless under the direction of a health care professional

### *Migraine headaches*

*Pharmacological Drug Therapy:* 1) Amitriptyline (Elavil, Endep)

*Potential side effects:* Constipation, dry mouth, drowsiness, weight loss or gain.

*Pharmacological Drug Therapy:* 2) Ergotamine (Cafergot, Ergostat).

*Potential side effects:* Convulsions, diarrhea, dizziness, nausea, vomiting.

*Natural Choices:* Feverfew*, ginger, caffeine in some cases, white willow, essential fatty acids, B complex with extra vitamin $B_6$, magnesium.

*Additional Headache choices include:* Peppermint essential oil is great for headaches due to stress, lavender, linden, passionflower, rosemary, valerian, wood betony. Include fish in your diet, such as mackerel, salmon, sardines and tuna. Exclude from your diet foods that can trigger headaches: alcohol, artificial sweeteners, aspartame, baked goods, caffeine, cheese, chocolate, citrus fruits foods containing yeast, monosodium glutamate, nuts, sauerkraut, yogurt.

*Potential side effects:* *Feverfew is not recommended during pregnancy, unless under professional health care supervision. For all other natural choices, refer to specific chapters in this book.

### *Prostate enlargement (Benign prostatic hyperplasia, BPH)*

*Pharmacological Drug Therapy:* Finesteride (Proscar)

*Potential side effects:* Decreased libido (loss of sex drive), ejaculation problems, impotence.

*Natural Choices:* Saw palmetto, pygeum africanum, cerilton (flower pollen extract), stinging nettle, uva ursi, lycopene, pumpkin seed, essential fatty acids, flax seed oil, cypress essential oil, zinc, selenium, B complex with extra vitamin $B_6$, vitamin E, amino acids, especially alanine, taurine, glycine, glutamic acid.

*Potential side effects:* None known. For all other natural choices, refer to specific chapters in this book.

### Skin disorders:

Acne, Eczema, Psoriasis.

*Pharmacological Drug Therapies:*

***For Acne —***

*1)* Orally taken treatment with Tetracycline.

*Potential side effects:* loss of appetite, Candida albicans (yeast infection), colitis, diarrhea, nausea, vomiting, darkening teeth.

*2)* Orally taken treatment with Isotretinoin (Accutane)

*Potential side effects:* Skin (dry, peeling, itching), decreased sex drive (libido), thinning hair, higher cholesterol readings.

*3)* Topical (external application) treatments (Benzoyl peroxide, tetracycline, tretinoin).

*Potential side effects:* Allergic reaction, dry skin, peeling of skin, redness, tenderness.

***For Eczema and Psoriasis —***

cortisone creams, ointments and lotions to lessen inflammation.

*Potential side effects:* Acne-like eruptions, allergic reactions, excessive hair growth, irritation, dry skin, thinning skin, loss of pigmentation.

*Natural Choices for all three:* Chamomile extracts, calendula oil, burdock root, licorice extracts*, milk thistle extract, red clover, tea tree oil, yellow dock, selenium, sulfur (MSM), zinc, essential fatty acids, vitamin A, B complex vitamins, vitamin E.

For *Acne add:* chromium, potassium.

*For Psoriasis add:* cod liver oil, folic acid, chickweed, echinacea, evening primrose oil, flax seed oil, red clover, sarsaparilla, yellow dock.

*For Eczema add:* sarsaparilla, vitamin C and bioflavonoids, chickweed, goldenseal, nettles, red clover.

*Potential side effects:* *Licorice extract is not recommended during pregnancy, unless under professional health care supervision. Take as directed by your physician or a naturally orientated licensed heal care professional. For all other natural choices, refer to specific chapters in this book.

## *Naturopathic Doctor Elvis Ali's Prescription for You and Your Family's Daily Nutrient Supplementation*

These guidelines are for healthy individuals in the categories listed. They include daily suggestions plus quick references for some commonly experienced problems, to give you an idea of the extent to which natural remedies can be used.

Self-health care means incorporating vitamins and minerals along with soluble and insoluble fibers, clean water, digestive enzymes, protein (plant and/or animal sources), good fats and carbohydrates into your life, on a daily basis.

The supplements you choose should have no preservatives, no artificial colors, no artificial flavors, no added salt, no corn, no starch and be gluten free. When possible they should have digestive enzymes or you should supplement your diet with them. Enzymes make supplements more bio-available for the body.

The high-potency multiple vitamin should have natural vitamin E. The multi-mineral complex should be chelated, citrated or fructose compound bonded, which means your body will get many times more of the mineral than ones in a regular hard pill.

A broad spectrum whole green super food product, also called green power food drink, is recommended for its antioxidant and detoxification properties. At the very least it should have beta-carotene, vitamin C, vitamin E, selenium, L-glutathione, genistein and daidzein in the soy isoflavones, bilberry, ginkgo biloba, grape seed extract, lycopene, and lutein.

If you are taking any drugs or over-the-counter medications, consult with your nutritionally orientated health care provider, physician and/or pharmacist to avoid adverse drug interactions.

Always take your supplements with food, unless the label says otherwise. For example, amino acids are usually taken on an empty stomach, between meals, without protein.

The current Recommended Daily Allowances (RDAs) do not account for needs due to gender, lifestyle, occupation, illness, weight size and biochemical-metabolic individuality. Nor do they address supplementation for prevention for prevention of diseases that may take

lop, such as cancer and diabetes. About one third of these
e established RDAs. The RDAs are under revision, but it is
guidelines will fully address these points.

Dr. Ali's self-health care supplementation guidelines focus on the healthy individual's needs at various stages of life. The ranges given help maintain an optimal state of health. Lifestyle changes, illnesses and daily stresses change your nutrient needs. During stressful times for example, it is beneficial to increase your B-vitamin complex intake. For health problems or concerns, consult with a naturopath or nutritionally oriented health care professional about your supplementation program.

## *Dr. Ali's Daily Vitamin and Mineral Guidelines*

| **Nutrient Description** | **Teenagers** | **Adults** | **Seniors** |
|---|---|---|---|
| ***Fat Soluble Vitamins*** | | | |
| A | 5000 IU | 5000-10,000 IU | 10,000-15,000 IU |
| D | 400 IU | 400-600 IU | 400-600 IU |
| E | 10-100 IU | 400-800 IU | 400-800 IU |
| F | 1-3 teaspoons | 2-3 tablespoons | 2-3 tablespoons |
| ***Water-Soluble Vitamins*** | | | |
| $B_1$ | 5 mg | 50-100 mg | 100-150 mg |
| $B_2$ | 5 mg | 50-100 mg | 100-150 mg |
| $B_3$ (Niacinaminde) | 10 mg | 50-100 mg | 100-150 mg |
| $B_6$ | 5 mg | 50-100 mg | 100-150 mg |
| $B_{12}$ (Cyanocobalamin) | 250 mcg | 100-1000 mcg | 100-2000 mcg |
| PABA | 5 mg | 50-100 mg | 100-150 mg |
| Biotin (Vitamin H) | 10-100 mcg | 100-300 mcg | 100-300 mcg |
| Pantothenic Acid ($B_5$) | 5 mg | 50-100 mg | 100-200 mg |
| Folic Acid | 0.05 mg | 0.4-1 mg | 0.5-1 mg |
| Choline | 15 mg | 250-500 mg | 250-500 mg |
| Inositol | 15 mg | 75-100 mg | 100-200 mg |
| Vitamin C | 500-2000 mg | 2000-6000 mg | 2000-4000 mg |
| Beta-carotene | 15,000-30,000 IU | 20,000-40,000 IU | 20,000-40,000 IU |
| ***Minerals*** | | | |
| Calcium | 800-1500 mg | 500-1500 mg | 1000-1500 mg |
| Magnesium | 400-750 mg | 250-750 mg | 500-750 mg |
| Phosphorus | 1000-1200 mg | 1000-1500 mg | 800-1200 mg |
| Potassium | 1500-4500 mg | 1000-1500 mg | 1800-5500 mg |
| Sodium | 900-2500 mg | 1100-3000 mg | 1100-3000 mg |
| Iron | 15 mg | 15-30 mg | 15-20 mg |
| Copper | 2-3 mg | 2-5 mg | 2-3 mg |
| Manganese | 5-10 mg | 15-50 mg | 15-50 mg |
| Chromium | 50 mcg | 25-200 mcg | 50-200 mcg |
| Selenium | 50 mcg | 25-200 mcg | 50-200 mcg |
| Vanadium | 15-50 mcg | 10-100 mcg | 15-100 mcg |
| Molybdenum | 15-50 mcg | 10-100 mcg | 15-50 mcg |

## *Adult Females*

*Daily:* A full spectrum multi-vitamin and multi-mineral complex. For antioxidants and detoxification use a broad spectrum whole green super food product. For PMS tension, initially try dong quai, black cohosh, isoflavones from soy, evening primrose oil. For anemia, initially try spirulina, algae, vitamin $B_{12}$ and iron.

*Pregnant females:* Before and during pregnancy, supplementation may prevent health related problems in the mother or baby. Start with a multi-mineral complex and multi-vitamin that provides extra vitamin $B_{12}$, folic acid, iron, vitamin A (or beta-carotene), vitamin C, vitamin E, B complex and, to prevent swelling and nausea, take extra vitamin $B_6$.

## *Adult Males*

*Daily:* A full spectrum multi-vitamin and multi-mineral complex. For detoxification use whole green super food products.

*To maintain the male reproductive system:* Puncturevine, ginseng, flaxseed, pumpkin, saw palmetto, pygeum and zinc.

*Energy:* Calcium pyruvate and creatine.

*Muscles:* Soya protein powder and amino acids.

## *Seniors*

*Daily:* Chewable or liquid supplements are preferred. A full spectrum multivitamin and multi-mineral complex. Fiber is very important, along with green power food drinks for detoxification and general well-being.

*For bones:* Glucosamine, organic sulfur (MSM), and a calcium/magnesium complex.

*To enhance memory:* Lecithin, Phosphatidyl serine (PS-30), ginkgo biloba, soy lecithin granules.

*Energy and vitality:* Ginseng.

*Reproductive system support and enhancement:* Zinc, pumpkin seeds, saw palmetto, flax seed oil and pygeum.

## *Infants: Ages 1 to 4 years*

*Daily:* Check with your pediatrician first as to what vitamins to give your infant. We suggest you use a liquid one, or a good tasting chewable multiple vitamin, without artificial sweeteners or sugars, flavors, coloring or preservatives.

***Children: Ages 5 to 12 years***

*Daily:* These are the growth years. A good full spectrum multi-vitamin and multi-mineral complex with iron, calcium and magnesium to build bone strength. Make sure it has a full day's worth of the complete B-complex and vitamin C. The supplement should be without artificial sweeteners or sugars, flavorings, coloring or preservatives.

***Quick Tip:*** To discover how to get the most out of your supplements, refer to Chapter 9 *Price versus Value.*

For specific information about the benefits of specific vitamins, minerals, amino acids or herbs refer to the index at the back of the book. If you are interested in a nutrient's category, refer to the following specific chapters:

| | |
|---|---|
| chapter 11 | Vitamins |
| chapter 12 | Minerals |
| chapter 13 | Amino Acids & Protein |
| chapter 14 | Herbs |
| chapter 15 | Aromatherapy |
| chapter 16 | Homeopathy |
| chapter 17 | Flower Remedies |
| chapter 18 | Leading Edge Supplements: Nutraceuticals, Phytochemicals and Oldies but Goodies |

# chapter 11

# Vitamins

## Their specific roles and uses

## Tips on taking vitamins

## Quick Reference Chart of Benefits

***How do vitamins help your body deal with the many types of stresses you're exposed to?***

Your metabolism is regulated by vitamins that keep your body functioning at high performance levels. They reduce blood pressure. They are critical for immune system support, improved resistance to infection, protection against heart disease and prevention or cure of many other health problems.

Vitamins are essential nutrients for optimal health. They are referred to as micro-nutrients, because in comparison to carbohydrates, fats, proteins and water, they are used in comparatively small amounts to maintain and keep the body's biological chemistry functioning properly. Vitamins can act as coenzymes, drug therapies and become integrated into body parts such as blood, bones, cells, enzymes, hormones and muscles.

These biochemical reactions constantly occur in the body, keeping it fine tuned and ready to deal with the many assaults upon it, such as polluted air and water. Since vitamins occur naturally in animals and plants, they are called organic compounds. They function as coenzymes, acting as activators or catalysts to create a balanced biochemical state in your body. For example, vitamin $B_6$ is needed for the enzyme that triggers nerve impulses to your fingers. Without it, the enzyme could not work, and a deficiency could result in numbness to your fingers. The partnership between vitamins and enzymes is essential to your state of health. (For additional information about enzymes, refer to Chapter 4.)

Vitamins are either water or fat soluble. This means that they require fats or water to be absorbed into and transported throughout your body. Water-soluble vitamins stay in the body for a short time – two to four days. When you eat, or swallow vitamin pills, they go to work the moment your digestive system absorbs them, which can take many hours. Other methods of administering vitamins, such as injection into the body or liposomal sprays in the mouth, allow the body to access the vitamins much faster, since they are quickly absorbed and bypass the digestive tract. Excess amounts are usually excreted through urination, defecation or sweating. Since they are not stored in the body for a long time, they must be constantly replenished. The Food and Drug Administration (FDA) and Canada's Health Protection Branch have no record of a water-soluble vitamin or combination of them ever being the sole cause of death. Toxicity is virtually unknown.

Fat-soluble vitamins require fats to be assimilated into and carried throughout your body. Some are stored in the fat (lipid) tissue of the body and others in organs, especially the liver, and stay in the body for longer periods of time. Toxicity of fat-soluble vitamins generally is not a concern. Problems can occur, though, if fat-soluble vitamins are taken in large doses. Moderation is the key, when it comes to maintaining your health. Specific or life-threatening health problems may necessitate large doses of vitamins, which should be done in consultation with a health care practitioner trained in this area of healing. In these instances it may be wise to consult a naturopath and have a naturopath work in partnership with your traditional doctor.

***Note:*** Antibiotics are not as effective, when taken at the same time as supplements. It is recommended that you take your supplements a minimum of 1½ hours before, or 3 hours after, taking any prescription antibiotics.

***Vitamin A*** – See also Beta-Carotene.

Fat soluble. Vitamin A needs fat to be absorbed in the digestive tract.

*Nutrients that maximize the amount of Vitamin A the body can use:* B complex, choline, C, D, E (essential for proper functioning of vitamin A), F, calcium, magnesium, phosphorous, selenium and zinc.

*Foods, drugs, nutrients and conditions that prevent the maximum utilization of this vitamin by the body:* Alcohol, coffee, cortisone, excessive iron, mineral oil, polyunsaturated fatty acids with carotene, vitamin D deficiency.

*Drugs that can cause vitamin A deficiency:* Over-the-counter medications containing alcohol, such as cough syrups and elixirs (e.g Nyquil). Antacids such as Gelusil, Maalox, Rolaids, Tums. Anticoagulants such as Coumadin, Dicumarol and Panwarfin. Aspirin and drugs containing aspirin. Barbiturates such as Butisol, Phenobarbital, Seconal, Nembutal and Tuinal. Laxatives and lubricants such as castor oil and mineral oil. Other medications such as Chloramphenicol (Chlomycetin), Cholestyramine (Questran), Colchicine (Colbenemid).

***Note:*** For maximum absorption of vitamin A, avoid strenuous physical activity for five hours after taking it. Do not take high doses of vitamin A when taking broad spectrum antibiotics. When using isotretinoin (Accutane), the acne treatment drug, do not take vitamin A.

*Excellent natural sources:* yellow and dark green vegetables, yellow fruits, eggs, milk and dairy products, margarine, fish liver oil. Here are some foods and their approximate vitamin A content:

| | |
|---|---|
| Apricots (dried), 1 cup (250 ml) | 16,000 IU |
| Liver (beef), 1/4 pound (115 grams) | 50,000 IU |
| Spinach (cooked), 1 cup (250 ml) | 8,000 IU |
| Carrots (raw), 1 medium | 10,000 IU |

*Main body parts that vitamin A benefits:* Bones, eyes, hair, skin, soft tissue, teeth.

*Main body functions it supports:* Outer layers of body tissue and organ reparation and maintenance, antioxidant (counteracts free radical formation), immune system, resistance to respiratory infections, protection against cancer and cardiovascular disease, decreases duration of diseases, aids in reproduction and lactation, aids vaginal healing, helps slow the aging process, helps visual purple production which is needed for night vision.

*Symptoms of deficiency:* Allergies, loss of appetite, blemishes, dry hair, fatigue, itching eyes, burning eyes, loss of smell, night blindness, rough dry skin, sinus problems, soft tooth enamel, susceptibility to infections, xerophthalmia (excessive dryness of parts of the eye). Usually deficiencies are found in children under five years old, due to a lack of dietary intake. Deficiency of vitamin A can result in decreased levels of vitamin C.

*Helpful in treating these conditions:* Acne, alcoholism, allergies, arthritis, asthma, athlete's foot, boils, bronchitis, carbuncles, colds, cystitis, diabetes, eczema, emphysema, heart disease, hepatitis, hyperthyroidism, migraine headaches, open ulcers when externally applied, psoriasis, sinusitis, stress, tooth and gum problems.

*Suggested dosage ranges:* Teenagers 5000 IU; adults 5000-10,000 IU; and seniors 10,000-15,000 IU a day. The Recommended Daily Intake (RDI) is 5000 IU. Dosages over 20,000 IU should never be taken for more than a few days, for therapeutic purposes. As needed, the body converts beta-carotene into vitamin A. Since beta-carotene is not toxic, whereas vitamin A can be, substituting vitamin A supplementation, with beta-carotene is appropriate, unless your health care provider indicates otherwise. Instead, you can take 25,000 to 200,000 IU of beta-carotene.

*Toxicity:* Vitamin A can produce toxic affects in adults if more than 50,000 IU are taken daily for many months. In infants it can produce toxic affects if more than 18,500 IU are taken daily. Symptoms of toxic overload include bone pain, blurred vision, diarrhea, fatigue, hair loss, headaches, irregular menstruation, liver enlargement, nausea, rashes, scaly skin, vomiting. In patients getting megadoses for dermatological conditions, chronic hypervitaminosis A (a condition resulting from ingesting an excessive amount of a vitamin) can occur. A single massive dose may cause acute symptoms, which are reversible. Pregnant women should avoid large doses of vitamin A, particularly in the first trimester, since it may cause birth defects. Beta-carotene, which the body converts to vitamin A on an as-needed basis is the best choice for pregnant women.

Consult with your veterinarian before giving it to cats or dogs.

***Ascorbic acid*** – See vitamin C

***Beta-Carotene*** – See also Vitamin A.

Water soluble. Needs water to be absorbed in the digestive tract. Beta-carotene should be taken instead of vitamin A, since the body converts it to the amounts of vitamin A it needs.

*Suggested dosage ranges:* Teenagers, 15,000-30,000 IU; adults, 20,000-40,000 IU; and seniors 20,000-40,000 IU a day. Dosage ranges from 25,000 to 500,000 IU a day, may have therapeutic affects ranging from clearing up skin conditions, counteracting respiratory problems, HIV/AIDS, cancer prevention, improving immune system function, ulcers, and counteracting environmental air pollution levels. Consult with a nutritionally orientated health care practitioner when dealing with specific conditions.

*Toxicity:* High dosages show no symptoms of toxicity. A symptom of beta-carotene overload is a harmless yellowing of one's eyes and skin, hypercarotenemia, which can occur due to a too excessive intake of beta-carotene.

## *Vitamin B Complex*

Refers to a balanced combination of all the B vitamins. Taking B Complex vitamins is an effective approach to supplementing with the B family of vitamins. Water soluble. Needs water to be absorbed in the digestive tract.

*Nutrients that maximize the amount the body can use:* C, E, calcium, cobalt, copper, iron, magnesium, manganese, phosphorous, potassium, selenium, sodium, zinc.

*Foods, drugs, nutrients and conditions that prevent the maximum utilization of this vitamin by the body:* Alcohol, birth control pills, corticosteroids, coffee, estrogen, infections, sleeping pills, stress, excessive sugar, sulfa drugs, tobacco.

*Drugs that can cause B Complex vitamin deficiency:* Aspirin and medicines containing aspirin. Antacids such as Gelusil, Maalox, Rolaids, Tums. Diuretics such as Diuril, Hydrodiuril, Lasix, Serapes. Cholesterol lowering drugs.

*Excellent natural sources:* Brewer's yeast, liver, whole grains (rice, wheat, rye).

*Main body parts that it benefits:* Eyes, gastrointestinal tract, hair, lips, liver, mouth, nerves, skin.

*Main body functions it supports:* Energy, maintenance of muscle tone in the gastrointestinal tract, metabolism of carbohydrates, fats and proteins, nerves, red blood cells.

*Symptoms of deficiency:* Acne, anemia, constipation, high cholesterol, cracked lips, digestive disturbances, fatigue, dull and/or dry hair, hair falling out, insomnia, dry and/or rough skin.

*Helpful in treating these conditions:* alcoholic psychosis, allergies, anemia, baldness, barbiturate overdose, cystitis, heart abnormalities, hypoglycemia, hypersensitivity, Meniere's syndrome, menstrual difficulties, migraine headaches, overweight, postoperative nausea, stress.

*Suggested dosage ranges:* 50 to 300 milligrams (mg) in equal amounts of vitamin $B_1$, $B_2$, $B_3$, $B_6$, choline, inositol, and PABA and 50 to 300 micrograms (mcg) of $B_{12}$, folic acid, and biotin.

*Toxicity:* None reported for these water-soluble vitamins.

*Symptoms of toxic overload:* Jaundice, weight loss, abdominal cramps, diarrhea, vomiting.

***Warning:*** Consult with your veterinarian before giving vitamin A to cats or dogs.

## *Vitamin $B_1$ – Thiamine*

Water soluble. Needs water to be absorbed in the digestive tract. Amount is measured in milligrams (mg).

*Nutrients that maximize the amount the body can use:* B complex (essential for proper functioning, B vitamins work synergistically and are more potent together than separately), $B_2$, $B_6$, folic acid, niacin, C, E, manganese (essential for proper functioning), sulfur.

***Note:*** $B_1$, $B_2$ and $B_6$ should all be the same amount in terms of mg, to maximize their effectiveness.

*Foods, drugs, nutrients and conditions that prevent the maximum utilization of this vitamin by the body:* alcohol, antacids, baking soda, caffeine (in coffee, chocolates and soft drinks), fever, raw clams, raw fish, excessive sugar, stress, sulfa drugs, surgery, tobacco. Additionally, heat from cooking destroys this vitamin, as well as food processing.

*Drugs that can cause vitamin $B_1$ deficiency:* Over-the-counter medications containing alcohol such as cough syrups and elixirs (e.g. Nyquil). Caffeine and medicines containing caffeine. Tobacco. Other medications such as Cimetidine (Tagamet), Indomethacin (Indocin), diuretics, and tetracyclines.

*Excellent natural sources:* Blackstrap molasses, bran, brewer's yeast, brown rice, fish, lean pork, legumes, meat, milk, nuts, oatmeal, organ meats, potatoes, poultry, raisins, rice husks, many vegetables, wheat germ, whole grains (unrefined), whole wheat. Here are some foods and their approximate vitamin $B_1$ content:

| | |
|---|---|
| Brewers yeast, 2 tbsp (30 ml) | 3 mg |
| Peanuts, 1 1/4 cups (313 ml) | 1 mg |
| Sunflower seeds, 1 cup (250 ml) | 2 mg |
| Brazil nuts, 1 cup (250 ml) | 3 mg |

*Main body parts that it benefits:* Brain, ears, eyes, hair, heart, nervous system.

*Main body functions it supports:* Appetite stabilization, blood building, carbohydrate metabolism, cardiovascular, circulation, digestion (hydrochloric acid production), energy production, growth, learning capacity, mental attitude, muscle tone maintenance (heart, intestines, stomach), nervous system (neurological).

*Symptoms of deficiency:* Appetite loss, amnesia, beriberi disease, coma, digestive disturbances, fatigue, irritability, mental deterioration, nervousness, numbness of hands and feet, pain and noise sensitivity, pains around the heart, shortness of breath.

*Helpful in treating these conditions:* Airsickness, alcoholism, anemia, anxiety attacks (can be alleviated by above-average dosages), congestive heart failure, constipation, depression (can be alleviated by above-average dosages) diarrhea, diabetes, edema, herpes zoster, indigestion, mental illness, nausea, pain (particularly dental post-operative pain), rapid heart rate, restlessness, seasickness, stress.

*Suggested dosage ranges:* Teenagers, 5 mg; adults 50-100 mg; and seniors 100-150 mg a day. Vitamins $B_1$, $B_2$ and $B_6$ should all be the same amount in terms of mg, to maximize their effectiveness. Even more effective when teamed with folic acid, pantothenic acid and $B_{12}$. If you take birth control pills, are pregnant or nursing, your body needs more $B_1$. Drinkers, smokers, heavy users of sugar and those taking antacids should increase vitamin $B_1$ intake. All those with stress conditions, such as anxiety, disease, post surgical recovery and trauma, should take a B complex vitamin, since these vitamins are destroyed by sulfate drugs used during surgery.

*Toxicity:* None known. Excess amounts are excreted in the urine. Generally considered safe at all levels of intake. See below.

*Symptoms of vitamin $B_1$ overload:* When daily dosages are excessive, these symptoms may, but rarely, manifest themselves – allergies, anaphylactic shock, edema, herpes, nervousness, rapid heart rate, tremors. An overload can affect insulin production and thyroid functioning, as well as possibly cause a deficiency of $B_6$ and other B vitamins. Prolonged use of any single B vitamin can cause an imbalance which creates a significant deficiency of other B vitamins.

### *Vitamin $B_2$ – Riboflavin*

also known as Vitamin G

Water soluble. Needs water to be absorbed in the digestive tract. It is easily absorbed. Body does not store it. Protein loss can result when excessive amounts are excreted.

*Nutrients that maximize the amount the body can use:* B complex (essential for proper functioning, B vitamins work synergistically and are more potent together than separately), $B_6$, $B_3$ (niacin), C, phosphorous (essential for proper functioning).

***Note:*** $B_1$, $B_2$ and $B_6$ should all be the same amount in terms of mg, to maximize their effectiveness.

*Food, drugs, nutrients and conditions that prevent the maximum utilization of this vitamin by the body:* Alcohol, coffee, excessive intake of sugar and tobacco. Oral contraceptives and strenuous exercise increase the need for $B_2$.

*Drugs that can cause vitamin $B_2$ deficiency:* Over-the-counter medications containing alcohol such as cough syrups and elixirs (e.g. Nyquil). Oral contraceptives (for example Brevicon, Demulen, Enovid, Lo/Ovral, Norinyl, Ovral). Sulfonamides Systemic (for example Bactrim, Gantanol, Tantrisin, Septra). Tricyclic antidepressants.

*Excellent natural sources:* Cheeses, eggs, leafy green vegetables, blackstrap molasses, milk, nuts, organ meats (kidney and liver), yeast, whole grains, yogurt. Here are some foods and their approximate vitamin $B_2$ content:

| | |
|---|---|
| Almonds, 1 cup (250 ml) | 1 mg |
| Brussels sprouts, 1 cup (250 ml) | 2 mg |
| Brewer's yeast, 3 tbsp (45 ml) | 1 mg |
| Liver (beef), 1/4 lb (115 g) | 5 mg |

*Main body parts that it benefits:* Eyes, hair, nails, skin, soft body tissue.

*Main body functions it supports:* Cataract prevention, antibody and red blood cell formation, cell energy production, cell respiration, essential for metabolism of all nutrients (carbohydrates, fats, proteins), dandruff elimination, growth, reproduction, skin, nails, hair, absorption of vitamin $B_6$ and iron.

*Symptoms of deficiency:* Bloodshot eyes, cataracts, corner of mouth (cracks and sores), dermatitis (skin inflammations), difficulty of eyes adjusting to darkness, dizziness, inflammations, itching burning eyes, night blindness, poor digestion (gastritis, gastric ulcers, gallbladder, digestive problems), retarded growth, red sore tongue, sore throat, sties, vaginal itching. A deficiency of this vitamin is called ariboflavinosis, and affecting the – genitals, lips, mouth and resulting in skin lesions.

*Helpful in treating these conditions:* Acne, alcoholism, arthritis, athlete's foot, baldness, severe burns, cataracts, diabetes, diarrhea, indigestion, sore mouth, sore lips, sore tongue, stress, recent surgery.

*Suggested dosage ranges:* Teenagers, 5 mg; adults 50-100 mg; and seniors, 100-150 mg a day. Pregnant and nursing mothers usually require higher amounts and should ask their health care provider for the amount they should take. Increase when in stressful situations. One of the most commonly deficient vitamins. Low, medium and high potency ranges are 25 mg, 100 mg and 500 mg. $B_1$, $B_2$ and $B_6$ should all be the same amount in terms of mg, to maximize their effectiveness. Best when taken with all the B vitamins.

*Toxicity:* None known. Prolonged ingestion of just $B_2$ will cause an imbalance leading to substantial depletion of other B vitamins.

*Symptoms of possible minor excess are:* Itching, sensations of prickling or burning, numbness. Large doses can cause sensitivity to sunlight, which is best counteracted by taking antioxidants with it. Prolonged use of any single B vitamin can cause an imbalance which creates a significant deficiency of other B vitamins.

## *Vitamin $B_3$*

also known as niacin, nicotinic acid, niacinamide, nicotinamide

Vitamin $B_3$ is great against cholesterol. For additional information about 'no-flush niacin', refer to 'Inositol Hexaniacinate' at the end of this section on vitamin $B_3$.

Water soluble. Needs water to be absorbed in the digestive tract. Measured in milligrams (mg).

*Principal benefits:* Niacin is necessary for the nervous system to function properly, lowers triglycerides, synthesizes hormones.

*Nutrients that maximize the amount the body can use:* B complex (essential for proper functioning, B vitamins work synergistically and are more potent together than separately), $B_1$, $B_2$, C, phosphorous (essential for proper functioning).

**Note:** The amino acid tryptophan helps the body produce vitamin $B_3$ on its own. A deficiency of vitamins $B_1$, $B_2$ and $B_6$ will prevent this from happening.

*Foods, drugs, nutrients and conditions that prevent the maximum utilization of this vitamin by the body:* Alcohol, antibiotics, coffee, corn, estrogen, sleeping pills, excessive sugar and/ or starch intake, sulfa drugs, tobacco, water.

*Drugs that can cause vitamin $B_3$ deficiency:* Over-the-counter medications containing alcohol such as cough syrups and elixirs, (e.g. Nyquil). Caffeine and medicines containing caffeine. All forms of penicillin. Tobacco. Sulfa drugs.

*Excellent natural sources:* Avocados, brewer's yeast, dates, desiccated liver, eggs, figs, fish, kidney, lean meats, legumes, milk, milk products, peanuts (roasted with skin), poultry (white meat), prunes, wheat germ, whole wheat products. One of the few vitamins that lose little potency with cooking and storing. Relatively stable in foods. Here are some foods and their approximate vitamin $B_3$ content:

| | |
|---|---|
| Rhubarb (cooked), 1 cup (250 ml) | 80 mg |
| Chicken (breast fried), 1/2 lb (230 g) | 25 mg |
| Peanuts (roasted with skin), 1 cup (250 ml) | 40 mg |

*Main body parts and systems that it benefits:* Brain, cardiovascular system, liver, nerves, skin, soft tissue, tongue.

*Main body functions it supports:* Production of adrenal hormones, brain functioning, cancer prevention possibilities, cardiovascular system, circulation, cholesterol level reduction, cortisone production, energy production in conjunction with other B vitamins, growth, helpful for heart disease, improves circulation, maintains digestive system with hydrochloric acid production as well as normal secretion of bile and stomach fluids, insulin production – aids regulation of blood sugar levels, maintains nervous system, metabolism (carbohydrates, fats, proteins), sex hormone production (estrogen, progesterone, testosterone), healthier looking skin, thyroxine production.

*Symptoms of deficiency:* Appetite loss, canker sores, depression, severe dermatitis (skin inflammations), diarrhea, fatigue, gastrointestinal disturbances, halitosis, headaches, indigestion, insomnia, muscular weakness, nausea, negative personality changes, nervous disorders, skin eruptions – skin that becomes sensitive to sunlight, offers an early indication of deficiency, the disease pellagra, whose symptoms include depression, diarrhea and dementia.

*Helpful in treating these conditions:* Acne, baldness, canker sores, high cholesterol and triglyceride levels, depression, diarrhea, low energy, halitosis, high blood pressure, leg cramps, prevent or ease severity of migraine headaches, Meniere's syndrome, reduces symptoms of vertigo, pellagra (symptoms include depression, diarrhea and dementia), poor circulation, stress, tinnitus, tooth decay.

*Suggested dosage ranges:* Teenagers, 10 mg; adults, 50-100 mg; and seniors, 100-150 mg a day. While niacinamide and nicotinamide do not cause skin flushing, the niacin and niacinamide forms of $B_3$ can. If taking niacin, you can minimize the flushing and itching effects by taking it on a full stomach or with an equal amount of inositol.

*Toxicity:* Practically non-toxic. Dosages above 100 mg can cause side effects. Individual sensitivity may result in skin flushing and itching. Antibiotics commonly increase the severity of flushing, but it is not cause for alarm. Switch to the gentler niacinamide form of this vitamin. Prolonged use of any single B vitamin can cause an imbalance which creates a significant deficiency of other B vitamins.

*Symptoms of toxic overload:* None known in dosages of 2000 milligrams or less. If a person has a history of duodenal or gastric ulcers, niacin can worsen the pre-existing condition. People with a liver disorder and on high dosage niacin therapy should be monitored by their doctor. Jaundice.

***Note:*** Vitamin $B_3$ can cause flushing and itching of the skin. This usually happens when taking it in the nicotinic acid form of niacin. Using niacinamide generally minimizes the flushing and skin itching. Normally it takes about 20 to 30 minutes for this reaction to abate. Drink a glass of water, eat a meal, or take an aspirin before taking niacin, to help minimize these symptoms.

To produce cholesterol lowering results, with the minimum of side effects, the best combination is a chromium-niacin complex of 2 mg niacin bound with 200 mcg of chromium.

Vitamin $B_3$ can interfere with uric acid control, resulting in gout attacks for those prone to this disease.

***Tip:*** Inositol hexaniacinate (IHN) is a newer 'flush free' or 'no flush' form of niacin that seems to be much safer. You can take up to 1500 mg of capsules each day. See the end of this section.

***Warning***: Large amounts of niacin may interfere with the body's ability to utilize sugar. This may cause a problem with borderline diabetics, due to the loss of the body's glucose control, and it can result in diabetes. Niacin use should be closely watched by those suffering from severe diabetes, impaired liver function, glaucoma, peptic ulcers or gout. When taking higher dosages of niacin, using time- or sustained-release niacin, liver toxicity has been reported, even when under medical supervision. Persons with internal bleeding should not use free-flush or no-flush niacin.

Consult with your veterinarian before giving it to cats or dogs.

### *Inositol Hexaniacinate*

also known as Inositol hexanicotinate, IHN or 'no-flush' niacin

A form of vitamin $B_3$, niacin, it is a vasodilator, meaning it increases blood flow. It has properties that can help lower cholesterol levels; improve circulatory conditions; reduce high triglyceride, and high homocysteine levels. The net result is that it helps prevent heart disease and may improve memory. It offers all the benefits of niacin, without any of the side effects.

***Caution:*** Persons with internal bleeding should not use inositol hexaniacinate.

***Vitamin $B_5$*** – see Pantothenic Acid.

### *Vitamin $B_6$ – Pyridoxine*

Water soluble. Needs water to be absorbed in the digestive tract. The body excretes it within eight hours after consumption. Like other B vitamins it needs to be replaced by supplements or whole foods. Vitamin $B_6$ is a part of a group of closely related substances, that function synergistically – pyridoxine, pyridoxal and pyridoxamine.

*Nutrients that maximize the amount the body can use:* B complex (essential for proper functioning). B vitamins work synergistically (that is, they are more potent together than separately). $B_1$, $B_2$, pantothenic acid, C, magnesium, potassium, linoleic acid, sodium.

*Foods, drugs, nutrients and conditions that prevent the maximum utilization of this vitamin by the body:* Alcohol, birth control pills, canning, coffee, excessive doses of choline taken over a long time periods, estrogen, exposure to radiation, food processing, freezing vegetables and fruits, heavy protein consumption, long storage, stewing or roasting of meats, water, tobacco.

*Drugs that can cause vitamin $B_6$ deficiency:* Birth control pills (for example, Brevicon, Demulen, Enovid, Lo/Ovral, Norinyl, Ovral). Dilantin. Synthetic estrogens. Meprednisone (Betapar).

Penicillamine (Cuprimine). DES (Diethylstilbestrol). Inh and nydrazid (isoniazid). All forms of penicillin. Phenobarbital. Prednisone (e.g. Meticorten, Prednisolone, Orasone).

*Excellent natural sources:* Blackstrap molasses, brewer's yeast, cantaloupe, cabbage, desiccated liver, eggs, green leafy vegetables, lentils, meat, oats, organ meats – kidney and liver, peanuts, salt water fish, soy beans, unmilled rice, walnuts, wheat bran, wheat germ, whole grains. Here are some foods and their approximate vitamin $B_6$ content:

| | |
|---|---|
| Liver (beef), 1/4 lb (115 g) | 1 mg |
| Prunes (cooked), 1 cup (250 ml) | 2 mg |
| Brown rice, 1 cup (250 ml) | 2 mg |
| Peas, 1 cup (250 ml) | 2 mg |

***Note:*** Dairy products are a poor source of $B_6$.

*Main body parts that it benefits:* Blood, muscles, nerves, skin.

*Main body functions it supports:* Antibody formation, asthma, critical for normal brain function, conversion of the essential amino acid tryptophan into niacin, diabetes – may decrease insulin requirements (watch for low blood sugar reactions), digestion (hydrochloric acid production), diuretic, female hormone production, red blood cell production, utilization of carbohydrates, fat and protein utilization (weight control), maintains sodium/potassium balance for the nerves, heart disease – helps prevent homocysteine accumulation, magnesium production, PMS, menopause, perimenopause, inhibits oxalate kidney stones, $B_{12}$ absorption, immune system functioning, prevention of skin disorders, synthesis of anti-aging nucleic acids.

*Symptoms of deficiency:* Acne, anemia, arthritis, convulsions in babies, depression, dizziness, glossitis, hair loss, irritability, learning disabilities, seborrheic dermatitis, weakness.

*Helpful in treating these conditions:* Atherosclerosis, baldness, carpal tunnel syndrome, cholesterol, cystitis, dandruff, dermatitis, depression, epilepsy, facial oiliness, glossitis, hypoglycemia, mental retardation, mouth sores and cracks, muscular disorders (calf tenderness, charley horse, leg cramps, migraines, night cramps, spasms, muscle weakness, hand numbness and some types of neuritis in the extremities), nausea in pregnancy, nervous disorders, overweight, post operative nausea, urination and dry mouth problems caused by tricyclic antidepressants, stress, sun sensitivity, water retention.

*Suggested dosage ranges:* Teenagers, 5 mg; adults, 50-100 mg; and seniors, 100-150 mg a day. Vitamins $B_1$, $B_2$ and $B_6$ should all be the same amount in terms of mg, to maximize their effectiveness. Pregnant and lactating women should always check with their doctor before taking doses over 50 mg for long periods of time. It is an ingredient in many of the preparations prescribed by doctors to alleviate morning sickness (nausea). Speak to your health care provider about your needs. Parkinson's disease patients under L-dopa (levodopa) treatment should not take vitamin $B_6$.

*Toxicity:* Symptoms of nerve toxicity can be caused by prolonged or daily dosages over 2000 mg (2 grams). Daily dosages over 500 mg are not recommended except under your health care provider's direction. When supplementing with vitamin $B_3$ to correct a health condition, do so with the supervision of your naturally orientated health care practitioner or doctor. Prolonged use of any single B vitamin can cause an imbalance which creates a significant deficiency of other B vitamins.

*Symptoms of toxic overload include:* Night restlessness and dream recall that is too vivid.

***Warning:*** Parkinson's disease patients undergoing L-dopa treatment should NOT supplement with this vitamin. Your doctor can prescribe the drug Sinemet to prevent this adverse vitamin interaction.

### *Vitamin $B_{12}$*

also known as Cobalamin and Cyanocobalamin.

Water soluble. Needs water to be absorbed in the digestive tract.

*Nutrients that maximize the amount the body can use:* B complex (essential for proper functioning, B vitamins work synergistically and are more potent together than separately), $B_6$ (essential for proper functioning), choline, inositol, C, potassium, sodium.

*Foods, drugs, nutrients and conditions that prevent the maximum utilization of this vitamin by the body:* Alcohol, coffee, laxatives, tobacco.

*Drugs that can cause vitamin $B_{12}$ deficiency:* Birth control pills (for example Brevicon, Demulen, Enovid, Lo/Ovral, Norinyl, Ovral). Sulfonamides and topical steroids (for example Aerosporin, Cortisporin, Neosporin, Polysporin). Trifluoperazine (Stelazine), Other medications such as Colchicine (Colbenemid), Kanamycin (Kantrex).

*Excellent natural sources:* Cheese, fish, milk, milk products, organ meats. Here are some foods and their approximate vitamin $B_{12}$ content:

| | |
|---|---|
| Clams (steamed) 3 ounces | 84 mcg |
| Cottage cheese, 1 cup (250 ml) | 2 mcg |
| Liver (beef) 1/4 lb (115 g) | 90 mcg |
| Tuna fish (canned) 1/2 lb (230 g) | 5 mcg |
| Eggs, 1 medium | 1 mcg |
| Milk, 1 cup (250 ml) | 1 mcg |

*Main body parts that it benefits:* Blood, nerves.

*Main body functions it supports:* Appetite, blood cell formation, cell longevity, healthy nervous system, metabolism (carbohydrates, fats, proteins), mental functions.

*Symptoms of deficiency:* Anxiety, depression, general weakness, nervousness, pernicious anemia, difficulties in walking and speaking, physical and emotional stress.

*Helpful in treating these conditions:* Alcoholism, allergies, anemia, arthritis, bronchial asthma, bursitis, epilepsy, fatigue, hypoglycemia, insomnia, overweight, shingles, stress.

*Suggested dosage ranges:* Teenagers, 50 mcg; adults, 100-1000 mcg; and seniors 100-2000 mcg a day. Higher levels may be required to treat specific health conditions. Vegetarians can suffer from vitamin $B_{12}$ depletion.

*Toxicity:* None known.

***Caution:*** Individuals suffering from psychiatric conditions, should consult with their physicians prior to supplementing.

### *Vitamin $B_{13}$ – Orotic acid*

Some doctors have used orotic acid to lower high blood pressure.

### *Vitamin $B_{15}$*

also known as Dimethylglycine, DMG, Pangamic Acid

Water soluble. Needs water to be absorbed in the digestive tract. In the strict sense it is not a vitamin, yet it works similarly to vitamin E. Dietary guidelines have not been established for minimum daily requirements.

*Nutrients that maximize the amount the body can use:* A, B complex (essential for proper functioning), C, E.

*Foods, drugs, nutrients and conditions that prevent the maximum utilization of this vitamin by the body:* Alcohol, coffee.

***Note:*** Sunlight and water easily destroy it.

*Drugs that can cause vitamin $B_{15}$ deficiency:* Over-the-counter medications containing alcohol such as cough syrups and elixirs (e.g. Nyquil).

*Excellent natural sources:* Brewer's yeast, brown rice, meat (rare), seeds (sunflower, sesame, pumpkin), whole grains, organ meats.

*Principal benefit:* Antioxidant.

*Main body parts that it benefits:* Glands, heart, kidneys, nerves.

*Main body functions it supports:* Cell oxidation and respiration, stimulates immune response, increases cell lifespan, metabolism (fat, protein, sugar), can control blood sugar levels, glandular and nervous system stimulation, aids recovery from fatigue, lowers blood cholesterol levels, protects against pollutants, protects liver against cirrhosis.

*Symptoms of deficiency:* Heart disease, nervous and glandular disorders.

*Helpful in treating these conditions:* Alcoholism, angina, asthma, atherosclerosis, cholesterol (high), cravings, diabetes, eases hangovers, emphysema, heart disease, headaches, insomnia, poor circulation, premature aging, rheumatism, shortness of breath.

*Suggested dosage ranges:* 50 to 150 mgs daily.

*Toxicity:* None known. In some cases, people experience nausea when they start a $B_{15}$ supplement regime. The nausea can be alleviated by taking $B_{15}$ after the largest meal of the day. This symptom usually disappears after taking $B_{15}$ for a few days.

## *Vitamin $B_{17}$ – Laetrile*

This is a controversial vitamin because of its use as a cancer treatment by some doctors. The Food and Drug Administration has rejected it, based on its potentially poisonous chemical composition due to its cyanide content. It is composed of two sugar molecules, one benzaldehyde and one cyanide, and is called an amygdalin.

*Excellent natural sources:* Found in the whole kernels of apples, apricot, cherries, peaches, plums, nectarines.

*Main body functions it supports:* Supposedly prevents cancer and has cancer-controlling properties.

*Symptoms of deficiency:* Deficiency may result in lowered resistance to cancer.

*Suggested dosage ranges:* At this time, we do not endorse the use of this vitamin, until additional studies or information become available. Consult with a nutritionally orientated physician before starting any treatments or supplementation involving laetrile. Some suggest a dosage range between 0.25 to 1.0 gram per day. Do not ingest more than 1 gram at a time. Eat a maximum of 15 apricot kernels spread out over a day, not all at once, and this may be beneficial for cancer prevention.

*Toxicity:* Not established, but taking excessive amounts can be dangerous. Contains approximately 6 percent cyanide, extremely toxic.

## *Bioflavonoids – Vitamin P*

Water soluble. Needs water to be absorbed in the digestive tract.

*Nutrient that maximizes the amount the body can use:* Vitamin C.

*Foods, drugs, nutrients and conditions that prevent the maximum utilization of this vitamin by the body:* Antibiotics, aspirin, cortisone, high fever, stress, tobacco, nutrients which cause a tendency to bleed or bruise easily.

*Excellent natural sources:* fruit (skins and pulp) – apricots, cherries, grapes, grapefruit, lemons, plums.

*Main body parts that it benefits:* Blood, capillary walls, connective tissue (bones, gums, ligaments, skin), teeth.

*Main body functions it supports:* Blood vessel wall maintenance, bruising minimization, cold and flu prevention, strong capillary maintenance.

*Symptoms of deficiency:* Anemia, bleeding gums, capillary wall ruptures, bruise easily, dental cavities, low infection resistance (colds), nosebleeds, poor digestion.

*Helpful in treating these conditions:* Asthma, bleeding gums, colds, eczema, dizziness (caused by inner ear), hemorrhoids, high blood pressure, miscarriages, rheumatic fever, rheumatism, ulcers.

*Suggested dosage ranges:* For adult maintenance levels, we suggest 250 to 1000 mg a day, taken with an equal amount of vitamin C, to maximize health benefits. For prevention of various health conditions supplementation with specific flavonoids, at varying dosages, is recommended. Consult with a nutritionally orientated health care provider, if you are not sure. For specific flavonoids and their benefits, refer to sections on curcumin (turmeric), pycnogenol, proanthocyanidins, grape seed extract, rutin, hesperidin, genistein and quercetin.

### Vitamin C – Ascorbic Acid

Water soluble. Needs water to be absorbed in the digestive tract.

*Nutrients that maximize the amount the body can use:* All vitamins and minerals, bioflavonoids, calcium (essential to proper functioning), cobalt, copper, iron, magnesium (essential to proper functioning).

*Foods, drugs, nutrients and conditions that prevent the maximum utilization of this vitamin by the body:* Antibiotics, aspirin, cortisone, high fever, stress, tobacco.

*Drugs that can cause vitamin C deficiency:* Ammonium chloride in drugs such as Ambenyl, birth control pills (for example Brevicon, Demulen, Enovid, Lo/Ovral, Norinyl, Ovral), Decongestant Cough Syrup (Expectorant, P.V. Tussin Syrup and Triaminicol), Antihistamines such as Chlortrimeton and Pyribenzamine, Aspirin and drugs containing aspirin. Barbiturates such as Butisol, Phenobarbital, Seconal, Nembutal and Tuinal, Fluorides, Indomethacin (Indocid). Meprednisone (Betapar), Prednisone (e.g. Meticorten, Prednisolone, Orasone), Tobacco.

*Excellent natural sources:* citrus fruits, cantaloupe, berries, green peppers, leafy green vegetables, cauliflower, potatoes, tomatoes. Here are some foods and their approximate vitamin C content:

| | |
|---|---|
| Broccoli (cooked), 1 cup (250 ml) | 135 mg |
| Oranges, 1 medium | 100 mg |
| Peppers (green), 1 medium | 120 mg |
| Grapefruit, 1 medium | 100 mg |
| Papaya (raw), 1 large | 225 mg |
| Strawberries, 1 cup (250 ml) | 90 mg |

*Main body parts that it benefits:* Adrenal glands, blood, capillary walls, connective tissue (bones, ligaments, skin), gums, heart, teeth.

*Main body functions it supports:* Bone and tooth formation, collagen production, digestion, healing (burns and wounds), iodine conservation, red blood cell formation (prevention of hemorrhaging), shock and infection resistance (colds), vitamin protection by prevention of oxidation.

*Symptoms of deficiency:* Anemia, bleeding gums, capillary wall ruptures, bruise easily, dental cavities, low infection resistance (colds), nosebleeds, poor digestion.

*Helpful in treating these conditions:* Alcoholism, allergies, atherosclerosis, arthritis, baldness, cholesterol (high), colds, cystitis, hypoglycemia, heart disease, hepatitis, insect bites, overweight, prickly heat, sinusitis, stress, tooth decay.

*Suggested dosage ranges:* Teenagers, 500-2000 mg; adults, 2000-6000 mg; and seniors 2000-4000 mg a day. Use rose hips vitamin C since it contains bioflavonoids and enzymes, which make it easier for your system to absorb it. The most absorbable and best form of vitamin C contains citrus salts – bioflavonoids, rutin, hesperidin. If using a chewable vitamin C, make sure to brush your teeth afterwards, since it can destroy your tooth enamel. Higher dosages may be beneficial for allergies, asthma, cancer prevention, prevention of heart disease, improved immune function, reducing the effects of environmental and emotional stress, improves wound healing. Consult with your health care provider before increasing dosages when having medical or dental procedures.

***Note:*** Tell your doctor if you are taking megadoses of vitamin C. Heart patients and diabetics may need to reduce the dosage of their medications. Vitamin C enhances iron absorption which can cause iron deposits (hemochromatosis). Large dosages of vitamin C can effect the accuracy of lab tests for sugar in urine and blood. In addition to this, stool specimens may give false negative test results for blood. Large amounts reverse the anticoagulant properties of the blood thinner Warafin (Coumadin). High doses flush out vitamin $B_{12}$ and folic acid. Increase your levels of supplementation to compensate for this process.

Researchers at the Veterans Affairs Medical Center, reported in the March 1999 issue of Archives of Internal Medicine that there is no association between high vitamin C levels and the risk of developing kidney stones. Higher vitamin C levels correlated with a significantly lower risk of men developing kidney stones. The study involved 10,000 male and female participants aged 20 to 74 years. The researchers also discovered no correlation between vitamin $B_{12}$ deficiency and vitamin C levels in the blood. In women there was a correlation between high vitamin C levels and high iron (serum ferritin) levels, whereas in men there was no correlation.

### *Vitamin D*

Fat soluble. Needs fat to be absorbed in the digestive tract.

*Nutrients that maximize the amount the body can use:* A, choline, C, F, calcium, copper, magnesium, phosphorous, selenium and sodium.

*Food/nutrient product that prevents the maximum utilization of this vitamin by the body:* Mineral oil.

*Drugs that can cause vitamin D deficiency:* Barbiturates such as Butisol, Phenobarbital, Seconal, Nembutal and Tuinal. Laxatives and lubricants such as castor oil and mineral oil. Prednisone (e.g. Meticorten, Prednisolone, Orasone). Other medications such as Phenytoin (Dilantin), Chloramphenicol (Chlomycetin), Cholestyramine (Questran).

*Excellent natural sources:* egg yolks, organ meats, bone meal, sunlight. When your skin is exposed to sunlight, it produces vitamin D. Here are some foods and their approximate vitamin D content:

| | |
|---|---|
| Liver (beef), 1/4 lb (115 g) | 40 IU |
| Milk, 1 cup (250 ml) | 100 IU |
| Salmon (canned), 1/4 lb (115 g) | 300 IU |
| Tuna (canned), 1/4 lb (115 g) | 300 IU |

*Main body parts that it benefits:* Bones, heart, nerves, skin, teeth, thyroid gland.

*Main body functions it supports:* Calcium and phosphorous metabolism (bone formation), heart action, nervous system maintenance, normal blood clotting, skin respiration.

*Symptoms of deficiency:* Burning sensation (mouth and throat), possibly mild to moderate depression – seasonal affective disorder (SAD), diarrhea, insomnia, myopia, nervousness, poor metabolism, softening bones and teeth.

*Helpful in treating these conditions:* Acne, alcoholism, allergies, arthritis, cystitis, depression, eczema, high blood pressure, insomnia, osteoporosis, psoriasis, SADs, stress.

*Suggested dosage ranges:* Teenagers, 400 IU; adults, 400-600 IU; and seniors 400-600 IU a day. Individuals suffering from vitamin D malabsorption may be better served by taking a synthetic active form of vitamin D that is only available by prescription, since lower amounts may be used to more quickly reverse symptoms of deficiency.

*Toxicity:* Dosages over 25,000 IU.

*Symptoms of toxic overload include:* vomiting, nausea, loss of appetite, diarrhea, fatigue, headache, restlessness, dry mouth and dizziness.

***Warning:*** If you are suffering from a heart problem or are a heart patient, you should check with your physician, before taking vitamin D. High doses of vitamin D are contraindicated if you are taking the heart medication Digoxin, also known as Lanoxin. Excessive stored levels of vitamin D can cause excessive amounts of calcium accumulation in the blood, called hypercalcemia. Excess calcium can also be an indication of a para-thyroid problem. Milk and milk products containing high levels of synthetic vitamin D can deplete magnesium.

Consult with your veterinarian before giving vitamin D to cats or dogs.

### *Vitamin E – tocopherol, D-alpha tocopherol*

The natural form of vitamin E. Fat soluble. Needs fat to be absorbed in the digestive tract. Studies indicate the synthetic form of this vitamin is not as effective as the natural forms, which appear to be significantly more potent and absorbable – bio-available.

*Nutrients that maximize the amount the body can use:* A, B complex, $B_1$, inositol (essential for proper functioning), C, F, calcium, iron, manganese (essential for proper functioning), phosphorous (essential for proper functioning), potassium, selenium, and sodium.

*Foods, drugs, nutrients and conditions that prevent the maximum utilization of this vitamin by the body:* Birth control pills, chlorine – used in many municipal water systems, mineral water, rancid fats and oils, zinc deficiency.

*Drugs that can cause vitamin E deficiency:* Birth control pills (Brevicon, Demulen, Enovid, Lo/Ovral, Norinyl, Ovral). Chloramphenicol (Chlomycetin). Cholestyramine (Questran). Laxatives and lubricants such as castor oil and mineral oil.

*Excellent natural sources:* dark green vegetables, eggs, liver, organ meats, wheat germ, vegetable oils (preferably organically processed), desiccated liver. Here are some foods and their approximate vitamin E content:

| | |
|---|---|
| Oatmeal (cooked), 1 cup (250 ml) | 7 IU |
| Safflower oil, 1 tbsp (15 ml) | 20 IU |

| | |
|---|---|
| Vegetable oils, 1 tbsp (15 ml) | 12 IU |
| Peanuts (roasted with skin), 1 cup (250 ml) | 13 IU |
| Tomatoes, 2 medium | 3 IU |
| Wheat germ oil, 1 tbsp (15 ml) | 40 IU |

*Main body parts that it benefits:* Blood vessels, heart, lungs, nerves, pituitary gland, skin.

*Main body functions it supports:* Aging retardation, anti-clotting factor, antioxidant, blood cholesterol reduction, blood flow to the heart, capillary wall strengthening (antipollution), muscle and nerve maintenance.

*Symptoms of deficiency:* Dry, dull or falling hair, enlarged prostrate gland, gastrointestinal disease, heart disease, impotency, miscarriages, muscular wasting, sterility.

*Helpful in treating these conditions:* Allergies, arthritis, atherosclerosis, baldness, crossed eyes, cystitis, diabetes, headaches, heart disease (coronary thrombosis, angina pectoris, rheumatic heart disease), high cholesterol, menstrual problems, menopause, migraines, myopia, overweight, phlebitis, sinusitis, stress, thrombosis, varicose veins.

*External application to treat these conditions:* Burns, scars, warts, wrinkles, wounds.

*Suggested dosage ranges:* Teenagers, 10-100 IU; adults 400-800 IU; and seniors, 400-800 IU a day. Significantly higher than the recommended daily intake of 30 IU. Even high intakes are safe over prolonged periods of time. People on anticoagulants should avoid doses in excess of 400 IU, unless a medical professional recommends increased amounts. See Warning below.

*Toxicity:* Dosages over 3000 IU may cause toxicity.

*Symptoms* of toxic overload include flatulence, nausea, headaches, diarrhea, heart palpitations, fainting. Reducing your intake to lower levels, immediately reverses symptoms.

***Warning:*** Those suffering from rheumatic heart disease, diabetes, an overactive thyroid and high blood pressure, and wanting to supplement with vitamin E, should start cautiously, preferably under the guidance of a physician or nutritionally orientated practitioner. Those with rheumatic heart fever may suffer from an imbalance between the two sides of their heart. Large vitamin E doses can worsen this problem. While vitamin E can increase one's blood pressure, its diuretic properties can also reduce blood pressure levels. Diabetics may be able to decrease their insulin levels, under medical supervision.

In general, those with health conditions, should start vitamin E supplementation at a lower dosage of 100 IU, then slowly increase the dosage by 100 IU monthly, until you reach a range between 400 to 800 IU a day, without side effects. We suggest you have your physician or nutritionally orientated healer monitor you, until you find a suitable dosage. If you choose to decrease your dosage, do it gradually.

## *Vitamin F*

Unsaturated fatty acids also known as Essential Fatty Acids (EFAs).

*Nutrients that maximize the amount the body can use:* A, C, D, E, phosphorous.

*Foods, drugs, nutrients and conditions that prevent the maximum utilization of this vitamin by the body:* Radiation, x-rays, hydrogenated fats, trans-fatty acids.

*Excellent natural sources:* cold-pressed organic vegetable oils (safflower, soy, corn), sunflower seeds, wheat germ.

*Main body parts that it benefits:* Cells, adrenal and thyroid glands, hair, mucous membranes, nerves, skin.

*Main body functions it supports:* Artery hardening prevention, blood coagulation, blood pressure normalizer, cholesterol destroyer, glandular activity, growth, vital organ respiration.

*Symptoms of deficiency:* Acne, allergies, diarrhea, dry skin, dry brittle hair, eczema, gallstones, nail problems, underweight, varicose veins.

*Helpful in treating these conditions:* Allergies, baldness, bronchial asthma, eczema, high cholesterol, gallbladder problems or removal, heart disease, leg ulcers, psoriasis, rheumatoid arthritis, overweight, underweight.

*Suggested dosage ranges:* Teenagers, 1-3 teaspoons; adults 2-3 tablespoons; and seniors, 2-3 tablespoons a day. For additional information, see Chapter 5, Fats and Oils: The good, the bad & the ugly

***Vitamin G*** – see Vitamin $B_2$, also known as Riboflavin.

***Vitamin H*** – see Biotin, also known as Coenzyme R

## *Vitamin K*

Fat soluble.

*Drugs that can cause vitamin K deficiency:* Anticoagulants such as Coumadin, Dicumarol and Panwarfin. Caffeine and medicines containing caffeine. Laxatives and lubricants such as castor oil and mineral oil. All forms of penicillin. Sulfonamides, systemic (Bactrim, Gantanol, Tantrisin, Septra). Sulfonamides and topical steroids (Aerosporin, Cortisporin, Neosporin, Polysporin). Tetracyclines (Achromycin-V, Sumycin, Tetracyn). Other medications such as Chloramphenicol (Chlomycetin), Cholestyramine (Questran), Clofibrate (Atromid-S), Kanamycin (Kantrex), Propantheline (Pro-banthine).

*Excellent natural sources:* Spinach, broccoli, cabbage, liver and tomatoes. Yogurt with active bacterial cultures and probiotics, full spectrum good bacteria, help create vitamin K in the intestines.

*Main body parts that it benefits:* Blood system.

*Main body functions it supports:* Helps produce blood-clotting factors (coagulates) in the body. Morning sickness. May be beneficial for prevention of osteoporosis and behavioral problems. Anticoagulant drugs improve cancer patients' survival rates, since they reduce the spread of cancer (metastasis). Vitamin K's unusual anti-tumor (antineoplastic) properties appear to be beneficial in this regard, even when used during chemotherapy (radiation therapy). The literature indicates it increases anticoagulant therapy's antimetastatic capacity.

*Suggested dosage ranges:* Teenagers, 50-150 mcg; adults, 300-500 mcg; and seniors, 300-500 mcg a day; only supplement when doctor prescribes; foods usually supply enough for your needs.

***Caution:*** If on anticoagulants, consult with your physician or nutritionally orientated healer before starting supplementation with vitamin K. Conversely, Dicumarol prevents the natural vitamin K from being absorbed. Doctors use it to prevent hemorrhaging in newborns, when warranted.

*Toxicity:* Only vitamin K3, the synthetic form, has toxic affects. It is only available by prescription. Synthetic vitamin K3 can counteract the effectiveness of the blood thinner Dicumarol. The symptom of toxic overload is hemolytic anemia, red blood cells dying at a faster rate than that of replacement by the body. Excessive amounts of vitamin K may cause sweats and flushes.

## *Biotin*

part of B complex also known as Coenzyme R or Vitamin H

Water soluble. Needs water to be absorbed in the digestive tract. Intestinal bacteria can synthesize biotin. It is produced by the body and is abundant in foods.

*Nutrients that maximize the amount the body can use:* Vitamin A, B complex (B vitamins work synergistically, that is, are more potent together than separately, and are essential for proper functioning), particularly $B_2$, $B_6$, niacin, $B_{12}$, folic acid, pantothenic acid, C, sulfur.

*Foods, drugs, nutrients and conditions that prevent the maximum utilization of this vitamin by the body:* Alcohol and coffee. Anti-seizure medication. Raw egg whites (avidin) deactivate the body's biotin. Long term therapy with antibiotics or sulfa drugs that destroy the intestinal bacterial levels can cause biotin deficiency. Over-the-counter medications containing alcohol, such as cough syrups and elixirs (e.g. Nyquil). Caffeine and medicines containing caffeine.

*Excellent natural sources:* Brewer's yeast, egg yolks, legumes, whole grains, organ meats (liver), soybeans. Here are some foods and their approximate biotin content:

| | |
|---|---|
| Brewer's yeast, 1 tbsp (15 ml) | 20 mcg |
| Lentils, 1 cup (250 ml) | 25 mcg |
| Mungbean sprouts, 1 cup (250 ml) | 200 mcg |
| Egg yolk, 1 medium | 10 mcg |
| Liver (beef), 1/4 lb (115 g) | 112 mcg |
| Soybeans, 1 cup (250 ml) | 120 mcg |

*Main body parts that it benefits:* Hair, muscles, nails, skin.

*Main body functions it supports:* Cell growth, fatty acid production, needed for synthesis of vitamin C (ascorbic acid), metabolism (carbohydrates, fats, proteins), vitamin B utilization.

*Symptoms of possible deficiency:* Anorexia, alopecia, poor appetite, depression, seborrheic dermatitis – usually found in infants, dry skin, eczema of the face and body, fatigue, grayish skin color, hair loss, high cholesterol levels, impairment of fat metabolism, nausea, numbness, insomnia, muscular pain.

*Helpful in treating these conditions:* When taken orally it helps prevent hair from turning gray, baldness, athlete's foot, dermatitis, eczema, eases leg cramps and muscle pains.

*Suggested dosage ranges:* Teenagers, 10-100 mcg; adults, 100-300 mcg; and seniors 100-300 mcg a day. Rarely is there a need to only supplement with biotin. Sufficient amounts of it are usually found in most B-complex and multi-vitamin supplements. If you are on a long-term course of treatment with, or are using antibiotics or sulfa drugs, take a minimum of 25 mcg each day. For balding men or women with thinning hair, biotin may help keep hair longer and looking more youthful. During pregnancy, biotin levels fall; ask your doctor about supplementing with biotin, as this may help prevent you from feeling low.

*Toxicity:* Considered non-toxic. No known cases of adverse effects.

## Choline

Water soluble. Needs water to be absorbed in the digestive tract.

*Nutrients that maximize the amount the body can use:* A, B complex, $B_{12}$, folic acid, inositol (essential for proper functioning), linoleic acid.

*Foods, drugs, nutrients and conditions that prevent the maximum utilization of this vitamin by the body:* Alcohol, coffee, excessive sugar.

*Drugs that can cause choline deficiency:* Over-the-counter medications containing alcohol, such as cough syrups, elixirs and over-the-counter medications such as Nyquil.

*Excellent natural sources:* Brewer's yeast, fish, legumes, organ meats, soybeans, wheat germ, lecithin. Here are some foods and their approximate choline content:

| | |
|---|---|
| Liver (beef), 1/4 lb (115 gm) | 500 mg |
| Egg yolks, 1 medium | 250 mg |
| Peanuts (roasted with skin), 1/2 cup (125 ml) | 190 mg |

*Main body parts that it benefits:* Hair, kidneys, liver, thymus gland.

*Main body functions it supports:* Lecithin formation, gallbladder and liver regulation, metabolism (cholesterol, fats), nerve transmission.

*Symptoms of deficiency:* Bleeding stomach ulcers, growth problems, heart trouble, high blood pressure, impaired kidney and liver functioning, fat intolerance.

*Helpful in treating these conditions:* Alcoholism, atherosclerosis, baldness, cholesterol (high), constipation, dizziness, ear noises, hardening of the arteries, headaches, heart trouble, high blood pressure, hypoglycemia.

*Suggested dosage ranges:* Teenagers, 15 mg; adults 250-500 mg; and seniors, 250-500 mg a day.

***Note:*** During the depressive phase of manic-depression, choline is not recommended, as it may cause a deepening of this type of depression.

***Coenzyme R*** – see Biotin, also known as vitamin H

## *Folic Acid – folacin B complex*

Water soluble. Needs water to be absorbed in the digestive tract.

*Nutrients that maximize the amount the body can use:* B complex (essential for proper functioning), $B_{12}$ (essential for proper functioning), biotin, pantothenic acid, C.

*Foods, drugs, nutrients and conditions that prevent the maximum utilization of this vitamin by the body:* Alcohol, coffee, stress, tobacco.

*Drugs that can cause folic acid deficiency:* Alcohol and over-the-counter medications containing alcohol such as cough syrups and elixirs (e.g. Nyquil); Barbiturates such as Butisol, Phenobarbital, Seconal, Nembutal and Tuinal; Glutethimide (Doriden); Methotrexate (Mexate); Nitrofurantoin (e.g. Furadantin, Macrodantin); Oral contraceptives (e.g. Brevicon, Demulen, Enovid, Lo/Ovral, Norinyl, Ovral); Phenylbutazone (e.g. Azolid, Butazolidin); Phenytoin (Dilantin); Pyrimethamine (Daraprim); Sulfonamides, systemic (e.g. Bactrim, Gantanol, Tantrisin, Septra); Sulfonamides and topical steroids (e.g. Aerosporin, Cortisporin, Neosporin, Polysporin); Tobacco; Triamterene.

*Excellent natural sources:* Citrus fruits, beets, green leafy vegetables, milk, milk products, organ meats, oysters, salmon, whole grains. Here are some foods and their approximate folic acid content:

| | |
|---|---|
| Brewer's yeast, 1 tbsp (15 ml) | 200 mcg |
| Dates (dried), 1 medium | 2500 mcg |
| Spinach (steamed), 1 cup (250 ml) | 448 mcg |
| Tuna fish (canned), 1/4 lb (115 g) | 2250 mcg |

*Main body parts that it benefits:* Blood, glands, liver.

*Main body functions it supports:* Appetite, body growth and reduction, hydrochloric acid production, protein metabolism, red blood cell formation.

*Symptoms of deficiency:* Anemia, digestive disturbances, graying hair, growth problems.

*Helpful in treating these conditions:* Alcoholism, anemia, atherosclerosis, anxiety, baldness, cervical dysplasia, chemotherapy, depression, diarrhea, fatigue, gingivitis, HIV, menstrual problems, mental illness, stomach ulcers, stress.

*Suggested dosage ranges:* Teenagers, 0.05 mg; adults, 0.4-1 mg; and seniors, 0.5-1 mg a day. When trying to or being pregnant, ask your doctor or health care provider for their recommendations about supplementing with folic acid to prevent birth defects of the spine, arms, legs, heart, cleft palate, and cleft lip. For treatment of specific conditions, consult with your nutritionally orientated health care provider to determine the best levels for folic acid supplementation.

*Toxicity:* None known. Women taking oral contraceptives, should check their plasma zinc levels. Supplementation with zinc may be warranted. Check your vitamin $B_{12}$ levels when supplementing with folic acid.

**Note:** The anticonvulsant benefits of Dilantin (phenytoin) and the anti-convulsant phenotoin are decreased by folic acid. Do not supplement with folic acid when taking anticonvulsants. High doses of folic acid are not recommended for those with hormone related cancer. Excessive folic acid can hide pernicious anemia symptoms.

### *Inositol*

Water soluble. Needs water to be absorbed in the digestive tract.

*Nutrients that maximize the amount the body can use:* B complex (essential for proper functioning), $B_{12}$, choline (essential for proper functioning), linoleic acid.

*Foods, drugs, nutrients and conditions that prevent the maximum utilization of this vitamin by the body:* Alcohol, coffee, cola drinks, estrogen, processed foods, teas and water create a shortage of inositol.

*Drugs that can cause inositol deficiency:* Caffeine and medicines containing caffeine. Sulfa drugs. Estrogen supplementation.

*Excellent natural sources:* Blackstrap molasses, citrus fruits, brewer's yeast, meat, milk, peanuts, cabbage, cantaloupe, dried lima beans, grapefruit, whole grains, lecithin. Here are some foods and their approximate inositol content:

| | |
|---|---|
| Oranges (fresh), 1 medium | 400 mg |
| Grapefruit, 1 medium | 500 mg |
| Peanuts (roasted with skin), 1 cup (250 ml) | 400 mg |

*Main body parts that it benefits:* Brain, hair, heart, kidneys, liver, muscles.

*Main body functions it supports:* Artery hardening retardation, cholesterol reduction, hair growth, lecithin formation, metabolism (fats and cholesterol), prevents eczema, calms the mind. Helps maximize the effectiveness of vitamin E.

*Symptoms of deficiency:* Constipation, eczema, eye abnormalities, hair loss, high cholesterol.

*Helpful in treating these conditions:* Atherosclerosis, baldness, cholesterol (high), constipation, heart disease, overweight.

*Suggested dosage ranges:* Teenagers, 15 mg; adults, 75-100 mg; and seniors, 100-200 mg a day. Best taken with choline and a B-complex vitamin. Better yet, consume 1 to 2 tablespoons of soya lecithin granules each day, and get a wider range of beneficial nutrients.

*Toxicity:* None known.

***Note:*** People with chronic renal failure show elevated levels of inositol.

***Laetrile*** – see Vitamin $B_{17}$

***Niacin*** – see Vitamin $B_3$

***Niacinamide*** – see Vitamin $B_3$

***Nicotinamide*** – see Vitamin $B_3$

***Nicotinic Acid*** – see Vitamin $B_3$

***Orotic acid*** – Vitamin $B_{13}$

***Vitamin P*** – see Bioflavonoids

***Pangamic Acid*** – see Vitamin $B_{15}$

## *Pantothenic Acid – Vitamin $B_5$*

Water soluble. Needs water to be absorbed in the digestive tract.

*Nutrients that maximize the amount the body can use:* B complex (essential for proper functioning), $B_6$, $B_{12}$, biotin, folic acid, C.

*Foods, drugs, nutrients and conditions that prevent the maximum utilization of this vitamin by the body:* Alcohol, coffee.

*Excellent natural sources:* Brewer's yeast, legumes, organ meats, salmon, wheat germ, whole grains. Here are some foods and their approximate pantothenic acid content:

| | |
|---|---|
| Liver (beef), 1/4 lb (115 g) | 8 mg |
| Mushrooms (cooked), 1 cup (250 ml) | 25 mg |
| Elderberries (raw), 1 cup (250 ml) | 82 mg |
| Orange juice (fresh), 1 cup (250 ml) | 45 mg |

*Main body parts that it benefits:* Adrenal glands, digestive tract, nerves, skin.

*Main body functions it supports:* Antibody formation, energy conversion (of carbohydrates, fats and protein), growth stimulation, vitamin utilization.

*Symptoms of deficiency:* Diarrhea, duodenal ulcers, eczema, hypoglycemia, intestinal disorders, kidney trouble, loss of hair, muscle cramps, premature aging, respiratory infections, restlessness, nerve problems, sore feet, vomiting.

*Helpful in treating these conditions:* Allergies, arthritis, baldness, cystitis, digestive disorders, hypoglycemia, tooth decay, stress.

*Suggested dosage ranges:* Teenagers, 5 mg; adults, 50-100 mg; and seniors 100-200 mg a day.

## *Paraminobenzoic Acid*

also known as PABA, paba B complex

Water soluble. Needs water to be absorbed in the digestive tract.

*Nutrients that maximize the amount the body can use:* B complex (essential for proper functioning), folic acid, C.

*Foods, drugs, nutrients and conditions that prevent the maximum utilization of PABA by the body:* alcohol, coffee, sulfa drugs.

*Excellent natural sources:* Blackstrap molasses, brewer's yeast, kidney, liver, mushrooms, wheat germ.

*Main body parts that it benefits:* Glands, hair, intestines, skin.

*Main body functions it supports:* Blood cell formation, graying hair (color restoration), intestinal bacteria activity, protein metabolism.

*Symptoms of deficiency:* Constipation, depression, digestive disorders, fatigue, headaches, irritability.

*Helpful in treating these conditions:* baldness, graying hair, infertility, overactive thyroid gland, parasitic diseases, rheumatic fever, stress. Used externally to treat burns, dark skin spots, dry skin, sunburn, wrinkles.

*Suggested dosage ranges:* Teenagers, 5 mg; adults, 50-100 mg; and seniors 100-150 mg a day.

*Toxicity:* Contraindicated when taking the cancer fighting drug Mexate (methotrexate). High doses in the 8 to 48 gram range may result in general malaise, heart problems, liver disease, kidney problems, reduced white blood cell counts and fever.

### *Multi-Vitamin Complexes:*

Refer to Naturopathic Doctor Elvis Ali's Prescription for You and Your Family's Daily Nutrient Supplementation at the end of Chapter 10 and Whole Green Super Food Supplements in Chapter 18.

# chapter 12

# Minerals

## Their specific roles and uses

## Tips on taking minerals

## Quick Reference Chart of Mineral Interactions

***What can minerals do to help your body deal with the many types of stresses you're exposed to?***

Minerals are the body's batteries. They charge you up and keep you going. Vitamins need trace minerals to function. Here are some examples: Calcium builds muscles and strong bones. Zinc promotes healing. Chromium helps regulate blood sugars. Copper can improve your immune system's effectiveness. Selenium is an antioxidant. Iron fights disease. Vanadium can help reverse adult-onset diabetes type 2.

***What are minerals?***

About four per cent of your total body weight is made up of minerals. Minerals are inorganic chemical elements. That means they are not bound to carbon. Basically, they are found in the soil and come from broken up rocks, since plant and animal life cannot create them.

In terms of your body, minerals are needed in very small amounts. Calcium and magnesium are major minerals needed and measured in milligrams (mg). Trace minerals are measured in micrograms (mcg). A lack or imbalance of minerals can cause major health problems.

***What are the major roles of minerals?***

Vitamins need minerals to function properly. Trace minerals help regulate your hormones, amino acids, enzymes and your immune system. They aid in optimal brain functioning, maintain and build your body's structure, keep your sugar levels balanced and aid in maintaining your intestinal system's health. Minerals need vitamins to help absorption and utilization by the body.

## *How important are minerals?*

Minerals are essential for optimal health and healing. Calcium is necessary for maintenance and growth of your bones and helps prevent osteoporosis. It is also critical in helping muscles function properly. The heart, being a large muscle, needs calcium to function properly. The source of calcium is also important, plus its bio-availability for use by the body. Cow's milk and milk products are not good sources of calcium, compared to liver, almonds, non-dairy almond drinks, and tofu. Milk is a very poor source of calcium since the type of calcium in it is not easily absorbed and used by the body. The trace mineral boron is a component of vitamin $B_{12}$. Iron is a component of hemoglobin. Copper helps veins and arteries stay supple and pliable, rather than becoming stiff and rigid, thereby preventing brain aneurysms. Gray hair is a sign of copper deficiency or imbalance. Selenium has been found to have anticancer and numerous other benefits to one's health.

To be able to assimilate the minerals you ingest, it is important to maximize the benefits you derive from them. In that regard, it is important to know that certain minerals partner with others to make them more bio-available to your body. For example, zinc, which has been found to be very important in immune system functioning, teams up with copper in an optimum ratio of 10 to 15 parts zinc for each part of copper. This balanced ratio helps your body maximize the benefits of supplementation of these two minerals. For centuries, oysters have been reputed to be an aphrodisiac. According to Dr. Sheldon Hendler, of the University of California in San Diego, oysters are high in zinc, a mineral component important to the prostrate and semen. Men suffering from reduced sex drive and low sperm counts due to a severe to moderate zinc deficiency, may benefit from oysters. Other foods rich in zinc include wheat germ, whole-grain products, lean meat and seafood.

It is important to note that minute quantities of numerous other trace minerals are also required for long term health and healing. These interactions are subtle and critical to maintaining a balanced harmonious physical state of well-being. Too much of any mineral over an extended period of time, can create an imbalance that can imperil your well-being. This list is a partial indication of what the body requires. It is thought by some, that we need in excess of 60 trace minerals, to support our body's disease prevention abilities.

The critical factors for your body to use the minerals you consume are the amount of minerals available for your body to assimilate and, more importantly, the presence and proportion of other minerals.

***Important News Flash:*** Kelp is the most nutrient rich food, containing more minerals and vitamins than any other. It is a seaweed containing 23 minerals. Most prevalent are calcium, copper, iodine, iron, magnesium, manganese, phosphorus, potassium, sodium, sulfur, zinc. Kelp also contains vitamins $B_2$, niacin, choline, carotene and algenic acid. Kelp is a good source of easily absorbable minerals. The iodine content normalizes thyroid gland functioning. For example, if you are suffering from a thyroid problem, and you are thin, you might gain weight. If you are obese, you may lose weight. If you have thyroid problems or are on thyroid medications, speak to a nutritionally orientated health care provider or your doctor before supplementing with kelp. Your medication levels may have to be adjusted. It is important to know the underlying cause of the problem.

## *Too much or too little of a mineral can cause an excess or deficiency of another mineral.*

The following is a list of minerals known to interact with each other:

| *Mineral* | | *Interacts with* |
|---|---|---|
| **Boron** | – | calcium, magnesium, zinc |
| **Calcium** | – | boron, chromium, copper, iron, magnesium, manganese, phosphorus, silicon, strontium, zinc |
| **Chromium** | – | calcium, manganese, vanadium, zinc |
| **Cobalt** | – | iron, zinc |
| **Copper** | – | calcium, iron, manganese, molybdenum, nickel, phosphorus, selenium, |
| **Germanium** | – | zinc |
| **Iron** | – | calcium, cobalt, copper, magnesium, manganese, nickel, phosphorus, potassium, selenium, zinc |
| **Lithium** | – | sodium |
| **Magnesium** | – | boron, calcium, iron, manganese, phosphorus, potassium, strontium |
| **Manganese** | – | calcium, chromium, copper, iron, magnesium, phosphorus, zinc |
| **Molybdenum** | – | copper, nickel, phosphorus, silicon, zinc |

**Nickel** – copper, iron, molybdenum, zinc

**Phosphorus** – calcium, copper, iron, magnesium, manganese, molybdenum, zinc

**Potassium** – iron, magnesium, sodium

**Selenium** – copper, iron, zinc

**Silicon** – calcium, molybdenum, zinc

**Sodium** – lithium, potassium

**Strontium** – calcium, magnesium, zinc

**Tin** – zinc

**Vanadium** – chromium

**Zinc** – boron, calcium, chromium, cobalt, germanium, iron, manganese, molybdenum, nickel, phosphorus, selenium, silicon, strontium, tin

## Quick Reference Chart

## Mineral Interactions

Last Update
1999 - November



| | Boron | Calcium | Chromium | Cobalt | Copper | Germanium | Iron | Lithium | Magnesium | Manganese | Molybdenum | Nickel | Phosphorus | Potassium | Selenium | Silicon | Sodium | Strontium | Tin | Vanadium | Zinc |
|---|---|---|---|---|---|---|---|---|---|---|---|---|---|---|---|---|---|---|---|---|---|
| Boron | | ● | | | | | | | ● | | | | | | | | | | | | ● |
| Calcium | ● | | ● | | ● | | ● | | ● | ● | | | ● | | | ● | | ● | | | ● |
| Chromium | | ● | | | | | | | | ● | | | | | | | | | | ● | ● |
| Cobalt | | | | | | | ● | | | | | | | | | | | | | | ● |
| Copper | | ● | | | | | ● | | | ● | ● | ● | ● | | ● | | | | | | |
| Germanium | | | | | | | | | | | | | | | | | | | | | ● |
| Iron | | ● | | ● | ● | | | | ● | ● | | ● | ● | ● | ● | | | | | | ● |
| Lithium | | | | | | | | | | | | | | | | | ● | | | | |
| Magnesium | ● | ● | | | | | ● | | | ● | | | ● | ● | | | | ● | | | |
| Manganese | | ● | ● | | ● | | ● | | ● | | | | ● | | | | | | | | ● |
| Molybdenum | | | | | ● | | | | | | | ● | ● | | | ● | | | | | ● |
| Nickel | | | | | ● | | ● | | | | ● | | | | | | | | | | ● |
| Phosphorus | | ● | | | ● | | ● | | ● | ● | ● | | | | | | | | | | ● |
| Potassium | | | | | | | ● | | ● | | | | | | | | ● | | | | |
| Selenium | | | | | ● | | ● | | | | | | | | | | | | | | ● |
| Silicon | | ● | | | | | | | | | ● | | | | | | | | | | ● |
| Sodium | | | | | | | | ● | | | | | | ● | | | | | | | |
| Strontium | | ● | | | | | | | ● | | | | | | | | | | | | ● |
| Tin | | | | | | | | | | | | | | | | | | | | | ● |
| Vanadium | | | ● | | | | | | | | | | | | | | | | | | |
| Zinc | ● | ● | ● | ● | | ● | ● | | | ● | ● | ● | ● | | ● | ● | | ● | ● | | |

**Note:** Antibiotics are not as effective, when taken at the same time as supplements. It is recommended that you take your supplements a minimum of $1\frac{1}{2}$ hours before, or 3 hours after, taking any prescription antibiotics.

### *Aluminum – toxic*

*Sources:* Aluminum cookware, aluminum foil, antiperspirants, antacids, bleached flour, drugs, municipal water sources.

*Main body parts that it effects:* Brain, kidneys.

*Main body functions it negatively impacts on:* May cause Alzheimer's disease and seizures. Can impair kidney function.

*Protect yourself with these supplements:* Apple pectin, a balanced calcium and magnesium supplement, chlorophyll, garlic, kelp, lecithin, vitamin $B_6$ and $B_{12}$ in a multi-vitamin and mineral supplement, spirulina, whole green food combination supplements.

### *Boron*

A trace mineral, with health benefits that are just being explored.

*Main body parts that it benefits:* Bones, brain, muscle mass.

*Main body functions it supports:* Boron is a component of vitamin $B_{12}$. Prevents dimineralization and bone loss. Aids calcium, magnesium and phosphorus metabolism. Needed for vitamin D metabolism. Aids the muscle building process. Helps prevent post-menopausal osteoporosis. Lessens calcium loss in the body. Improves brain function. Fosters alertness. Helps balance the immune system.

*Symptoms of deficiency:* Osteoporosis maybe a sign of deficiency. Vitamin D deficiency may be linked to a boron deficiency. A lack of boron may impair growth. No deficiency symptoms have been verified yet.

*Natural sources:* Fruits and vegetables – apples, carrots, grapes, grains, green leafy vegetables, pears and nuts.

*Minerals boron interacts with:* Calcium, magnesium, zinc.

*Suggested dosage ranges:* Between 1.5 to 7 mg a day. Clinicians suggest up to 6 mg a day for those at high risk of developing osteoporosis, particularly post-menopausal women. For seniors wanting to improve calcium absorption, 2 to 3 mg a day is recommended.

*Toxicity:* Occurs at levels of 150 mg or more per liter of water.

*Symptoms of toxicity include:* diarrhea, fatigue and nausea.

## Cadmium

Very poorly absorbed by the body and can take a very long time before it reaches toxic levels. Even after exposure to cadmium has stopped for many years, high amounts can stay in the body. Each day you excrete only about 10 mcg per liter of urine, even though your body absorbs between 12 to 25 mcg a day.

*Some sources:* Fertilizers, fungicides, pesticides, tobacco smoke, urban air pollution. Particular attention should be paid to the air quality near zinc refineries.

*Main body parts or systems it impacts negatively:* Blood system, immune system, joints.

*Main body functions it negatively impacts:* Can cause anemia, cancer, hair loss, high blood pressure, joint tenderness, weakened immune system. High levels of cadmium in the liver and kidneys are associated with proteinuria, amino aciduria and anemia. High incidences of pulmonary emphysema have been associated with excessive exposure to copper-cadmium alloys.

*Protect yourself from cadmium toxicity with these supplements:* Alfalfa (organically produced), amino acids (L-cysteine, L-lysine, L-methionine), calcium and magnesium, vitamin E, essential fatty acids (EFAs – Omega 3 and Omega 6), garlic, lecithin, rutin, whole green food combination supplements, zinc.

***Caution:*** Excessive amounts of cadmium or copper can greatly affect zinc's health and healing benefits.

## Calcium

A new form of calcium, Hydroxyapatite, is beneficial because it is identical to the calcium found in our bones and is the most easily absorbable form of calcium. It is derived from ground up cow or ox bone.

*Main body parts that it benefits:* Blood, bones, gums, heart, skin, soft tissue, teeth.

*Main body functions it supports:* Bone and tooth formation, blood clotting, promotes normal blood pressure, maintains cell membrane permeability, helpful in preventing colon cancer, heart rhythm, assists hormonal functions, nerve tranquilization, nerve transmission, muscle growth and contraction, prevents cramping. Helps reduce irritability and tension. Promotes relaxation and helps muscles function properly. Maintains and strengthens bones. Prevents osteoporosis.

*Nutrients that maximize the amount the body can use:* A (essential for proper function), C (essential for proper function), D (essential for proper function), F, iron (essential for proper function), magnesium (always take 1 part magnesium to 1.5 parts calcium), manganese, phosphorus (essential for proper function).

*Minerals calcium interacts with:* Boron, chromium, copper, iron, magnesium, manganese, phosphorus, silicon, strontium, zinc.

*Foods, drugs, lifestyle choices and nutrients that prevent the maximum utilization of calcium by the body:* Lack of exercise, excessive stress. Diets high in fats lower calcium levels.

*Drugs that can cause calcium deficiency:* Aspirin and drugs containing aspirin. Barbiturates such as Butisol, Phenobarbital, Nembutal, Seconal and Tuinal. Caffeine and medicines containing caffeine can inhibit calcium assimilation. Laxatives and lubricants such as castor oil and mineral oil. Tetracyclines (for example Achromycin-V, Sumycin, Tetracyn). Tobacco.

*Excellent natural sources:* Non-dairy almond drinks, bone meal, dolomite, cheese*, milk*, molasses, salmon, tofu. Here are some foods and their approximate calcium content:

| | |
|---|---|
| Ricotta cheese*, 1/2 cup (125 ml) | 337 mg |
| Almonds, 1 cup (250 ml) | 325 mg |
| American cheese*, 1 slice | 200 mg |
| Liver (beef), 1/4 lb (115 g) | 500 mg |

* ***Information you need:*** Milk and cheese are promoted as good sources of vitamin C. Milk is fortified with vitamin D to increase the absorption of calcium by the body. Milk containing synthetic vitamin D may deplete the magnesium in your body. The Physicians for Responsible Medicine recommend you not drink milk. In the 1990s, researchers at The Hospital for Sick Children in Toronto, Canada, discovered a link between milk and children developing juvenile diabetes. Around twelve years of age, half the population develops an intolerance to lactose, the sugar in milk and milk products. In addition to these and other nutritional concerns about milk, are the lack of independent studies and information regarding the effects on humans of the hormones and drugs being used to help increase the cows' production of milk. Are cows being feed genetically altered food, which we indirectly consume by drinking milk or eating milk products? We do not know. We bring these concerns to your attention, so you may objectively decide

if milk is the best choice as a source of calcium for you and your family.

***Note:*** Foods with calcium such as fruits, legumes, nuts and vegetables, contain substances like oxalate phytate and fiber, which interfere with calcium absorption in the body. For example, the calcium in spinach binds to oxalate, preventing your body from using the calcium. The above recommendations take this into account.

*Symptoms of deficiency:* Heart palpitations, insomnia, muscle cramps, nervousness, arm and leg numbness, tooth decay.

*Helpful in treating these conditions:* Arthritis, aging symptoms (backaches, bone pain, finger tremors), foot/leg cramps, insomnia, menstrual cramps, menopause problems, nervousness, overweight, premenstrual tension, rheumatism.

*Suggested dosage ranges:* Adolescents in their growth stage need 1300 to 1500 mg, adults up to age 50 should get between 500 to 1000 mg, and adults over 50 need 1000 to 1500 mg a day. The most absorbable type of calcium is hydroxyapatite; the second most absorbable is calcium citrate, which is not made from animal bones.

***Note:*** Always take 2 parts magnesium to 3 parts calcium when supplementing, to maximize the benefits to your body and adsorbability. For prevention of bone density loss, magnesium appears to be as important as calcium is. Calcium may prevent tetracycline from being effective.

***Warning:*** High doses of calcium abscorbate are contraindicated if you are taking the heart medication Digoxin, also known as Lanoxin.

*Toxicity:* Bone meal, dolomite and oyster shells are good sources of calcium unfortunately they may contain toxic substances, such as lead and should be avoided as a source of calcium, if possible.

***Newsflash on calcium benefits:*** A study in the *New England Journal of Medicine* January 14, 1999, indicated supplementing with 1200 mg of calcium daily may help the colon by decreasing the odds of developing new adenomas (polyps), possible precursors to colon cancer. Aids muscle contraction and relaxation, which makes movement possible. Eases muscle fatigue. Heart, since it is the most important single muscle group in the body. Important for blood clotting, normal heartbeat, regulating blood pressure, wound healing, nerve functioning. If your diet lacks sufficient calcium, your body takes the calcium it needs from your bones. Over time, this leads to a bone density problem called osteoporosis.

### *Chlorine*

*Nutrients that maximize the amount the body can use:* Works in a compound form with potassium and sodium.

*Excellent natural sources:* Table salt (adequate sources already present in food), olives, kelp.

*Main body functions it supports:* Stimulates the digestive system production of hydrochloric acid. Aids the liver's body cleansing abilities. Helps joints and tendons stay agile. Aids distribution of hormones. With sodium, it helps regulate and maintain the pH (acid-alkaline) balance of the body.

*Symptoms of deficiency:* Loss of teeth or hair.

*Suggested dosage ranges:* Sufficient amounts in better multi-vitamin/mineral complexes. Added to many municipal water supplies.

*Toxicity:* Excessive amount over 15 grams can cause side effects.

*Symptoms of toxic overload:* Chlorinated water elevates LDL cholesterol levels, destroys vitamin E and the intestinal bacteria balance.

### *Chromium – a valuable trace mineral*

*Nutrients that maximize the amount the body can use:* When bound with niacin, it is more bio-available than in the picolinate form.

*Excellent natural sources:* Black pepper, brewer's yeast, cheese, clams, corn oil, calves liver, chicken, lean meat, whole grain cereals, thyme.

*Main body parts that it benefits:* Blood, circulatory system, insulin metabolism.

*Main body functions it supports:* maintains blood sugar levels, reducing arterial plaque, inhibits cholesterol formation in the liver, reducing blood cholesterol levels, glucose metabolism (energy), promotes fat loss, curbs sugar cravings, aids protein transportation to the appropriate areas.

*Symptoms of deficiency:* Atherosclerosis, glucose intolerance in diabetes, Type 2 adult onset diabetes.

*Helpful in treating these conditions:* Acne, diabetes, hypoglycemia.

*Minerals chromium interacts with:* Calcium, manganese, vanadium, zinc.

*Suggested dosage ranges:* Teenagers, 50 mcg; adults, 25-200 mcg; and seniors, 50-200 mcg a day.

*Toxicity:* Chromium picolinate should not be used for long periods of time, unless under medical supervision.

***Note:*** Chelated zinc aids bodies low in chromium, which is a condition affecting about 9 out of 10 adults. When combined with vanadium (vanadyl sulfate) in an appropriate program, under medical supervision, it has been reported that Type 2 diabetics have been able to reduce their insulin levels. When done gradually over a course of 6 to 12 months, some Type 2 diabetics have been weaned off insulin altogether, or restored their body's internal glucose tolerance levels to a normal range. As we age, our bodies are less able to retain chromium.

### *Cobalt*

*Nutrients that maximize the amount the body can use:* Usually ingested or injected as vitamin $B_{12}$. Cobalt is the biological twin of $B_{12}$.

*Foods, drugs, nutrients and conditions that prevent the maximum utilization of cobalt by the body:* Molybdenum antagonizes cobalt. Anything that is antagonistic to vitamin $B_{12}$.

*Excellent natural sources:* Animal glandulars, meats and shellfish.

*Main body part that it benefits:* Red blood cells.

*Main body functions it supports:* Enzyme activation, hemoglobin formation, helps immune system ward off infections, needed for synthesis of $B_{12}$, can stimulate red blood cell production.

*Minerals cobalt interacts with:* Iron, zinc.

*Suggested dosage ranges:* Rarely available as a supplement. Best obtained from food sources. Vegetarians or people who do not eat shellfish or meats can become deficient in cobalt.

***Caution:*** Too much cobalt can cause an enlargement of the thyroid. Toxic levels are unknown.

*Symptom of toxic overload:* unwanted enlargement of the thyroid gland.

### *Copper*

*Nutrients that maximize the amount the body can use:* Cobalt, iron, zinc.

*Foods, drugs, nutrients and conditions that prevent the maximum utilization of copper by the body:* High intakes of zinc. Lithium disrupts copper absorption. Long term use may lead to a copper deficiency. Molybdenum may affect copper's ability to be absorbed.

*Excellent natural sources:* Avocado, bananas and other fruit, bone meal, carrots (cooked), dried peas and other legumes, dark green leafy vegetables, fish, nuts, organ meats, poultry, seafood – especially oysters, shellfish, raisins, molasses, whole-grain cereals and breads. Here are some foods and their approximate copper content:

| | |
|---|---|
| Brazil nuts, 1 cup (250 ml) | 4 mg |
| Soybeans, 1 cup (250 ml) | 2 mg |

*Main body parts that it benefits:* Blood, bones, circulatory system, skin.

*Main body functions it supports:* Bone formation, prevention of cardiovascular diseases, constituent of many enzymes, hair and skin color, healing processes of the body, hemoglobin and red blood cell formation, healthy nerves and joints.

*Symptoms of deficiency:* General weakness, impaired respiration, skin sores.

*Helpful in treating these conditions:* Anemia, baldness, osteoarthritis, rheumatoid arthritis, sciatica.

*Suggested dosage ranges:* Teenagers, 2-3 mg; adults, 2-5 mg; and seniors, 2-3 mg a day. Ratio of 10 to 15 parts zinc for 1 part copper. Excessive amounts of copper or cadmium can greatly affect zinc's health and healing benefits.

*Toxicity:* 10 mg or more usually causes nausea. Over 3 grams can be lethal. People with Wilson's disease are susceptible to copper toxicity. Excessive copper ingestion or levels can cause iron, zinc and manganese losses as they compete with each other for absorption: this can result in an higher risk of infection or other diseases. Of these elements, zinc and copper compete the most for absorption.

*Symptoms of toxic overload include:* Nausea. Copper tends to accumulate in the blood, reducing the zinc supply to the brain.

### *Fluorine – toxic*

Originally a byproduct of Second World War weapons manufacturers, excessive amounts created a disposal problem. The idea of fluoridation of the water supply for prevention of cavities was a welcomed solution. What had cost money to dispose of, now became a solution and profit center for businesses. Fluorine is also used as a rat poison. Controversy around its effectiveness for cavity prevention is mounting. It is highly toxic and must be specially stored and monitored when used in municipal water supplies.

*Some sources:* Municipal water sources, fluoride toothpastes, processed foods using fluoridated water (cakes, breads, juices, et cetera).

*Main body parts that it effects:* Teeth and bones.

*Main body functions it negatively impacts:* Excess fluorine is believed to be responsible for molting, splotched discoloration of teeth in children and adults. In adults, it may be responsible for cancer, hip fractures and kidney stones.

*Protect yourself with these supplements:* A proper synergistic balance of calcium, phosphorus and magnesium help block absorption.

### *Germanium*

also known as GE 132

Organic germanium is a naturally occurring trace element found in foods and herbs. It enhances cellular oxygenation, and helps detoxify the body by ridding it of poisons and toxins. Inorganic germanium is different; it is a trace mineral used for commercial industrial purposes.

*Principal health related actions:* Used in Japan as part of an anticancer treatment. It may block the growth of cancerous cells and help relieve acute pain in some cancer patients. Organic germanium enhances immune system function by improving the natural disease killing B-cells and T-cells. Very effective in people having autoimmune diseases that cause their immune cells to attack their own body's immune system. Beneficial for rheumatoid arthritis. Effective against viral infections. Used to treat Epstein-Barr virus. Aids in clearing up yeast infections due to Candida albicans.

*Mineral germanium interacts with:* Zinc.

*Dosage:* During the course of active yeast, viral or other infections take 50 to 200 mg a day. In the case of some illnesses, such as rheumatoid arthritis, chronic viral infections, extreme food allergies, AIDS, long lasting and repeating candidiasis, take up to 300 mg a day. Cancer patients should consult with their medical professional. Diet is the best way to get organic germanium into your body. Eat lots of the following foods and herbs, as preventative and healing measures.

*Food sources:* Garlic, onions, shiitake mushroom.

*Herb sources:* Aloe vera, comfrey, ginseng, suma.

## *Iodine*

Critical for optimal thyroid function, a small amount is also needed in the rest of your body.

*Nutrients that maximize the amount the body can use:* None.

*Foods, drugs, nutrients and conditions that prevent the maximum utilization of iodine by the body:* Consuming large quantities of raw cabbage, cassava root, mustard, peaches, radishes, soybeans, spinach, strawberries, or turnip may block iodine absorption in people with low iodine intakes. Cooking usually inactivates the goitrogenic, iodine interfering properties of these chemicals. Cobalt antagonizes iodine.

*Substance that can cause iodine deficiency:* Goitrogens are substances that prevent the body's use of iodine, by interfering with and decreasing the production of thyroid hormones.

*Excellent natural sources:* Seafood, kelp tablets, seaweed, iodized salt.

*Main body parts that it benefits:* Breasts, hair, nails, skin, teeth, thyroid gland.

*Main body functions it supports:* Energy production, excess fat metabolism, physical and mental development, thyroid gland function, protects against harmful effects of electromagnetic radiation, breast cancer prevention.

*Symptoms of deficiency:* Cold hands and feet, dry hair, irritability, listlessness, lassitude, nervousness, obesity, sluggishness.

*Helpful in treating these conditions:* Atherosclerosis, hair problems, fibrocystic breasts, goiter (thyroid becomes enlarged), hyperthyroidism.

*Suggested dosage ranges:* 0 to 300 mcg. If you usually eat seaweed products or iodized salt, take up to 150 mcg. If you have a low iodine diet, check with a nutritionally orientated health practitioner in the area. The practitioner may suggest you ingest from 150 to 300 mcg. If you have a thyroid or other medical condition that iodine may effect, consult with your physician before supplementing. Some people are allergic to iodine and must avoid it.

*Toxicity:* Tincture of iodine, a topical antiseptic, is poisonous and should never be ingested. Iodine is considered safe up to 1000 mcg per day.

*Symptoms of toxic overload include:* Headaches, difficulty breathing, rash and a metallic taste in the mouth. Japanese who consume huge amounts of seaweed, resulting in large doses of 20,000 mcg per day or more, can suffer from 'iodide goiter'.

## *Iron*

*Nutrients that maximize the amount of iron the body can use:* $B_{12}$, folic acid, C (essential for proper functioning), calcium (essential for proper functioning), cobalt, copper (essential for proper functioning), phosphorus.

*Foods, drugs, nutrients and conditions that prevent the maximum utilization of iron by the body:* Coffee, low HCl (hydrochloric acid in the stomach), caffeine-loaded soft drinks, excessive amounts of caffeine, excess phosphorus, tea, zinc, phosphorus or magnesium carbonate. Magnesium carbonate is not a recommended form of supplement since it is not easily absorbed by the body. These herbs can interfere with iron absorption: bilberry, burdock, damiana, juniper, peppermint, white willow, sage, yarrow.

*Drugs that can cause iron deficiency:* Antacids. Caffeine and medicines containing caffeine inhibit iron assimilation. Tetracyclines (Achromycin V, Sumycin, Tetracyn).

*Excellent natural sources:* Apricots, blackstrap molasses, brewer's yeast, chickpeas, desiccated liver, duck, eggs, fish, kelp, lima beans, organ meats, parsley, poultry, shellfish, wheat germ. All of these are better sources than spinach. Here are some foods and their approximate iron content:

| | |
|---|---|
| Liver (beef), 1/4 lb (250 ml) | 200 mg |
| Shredded wheat, 1 biscuit | 30 mg |

*Main body parts that it benefits:* blood, bones, nails, skin, teeth.

*Main body functions it supports:* children's growth, myoglobin and hemoglobin production – oxygenation of red blood cells and blood-oxygen transportation, energy production, immune system, resistance to stress and disease.

*Symptoms of deficiency:* Breathing difficulties, brittle nails, constipation, female infertility, iron deficiency anemia (pale skin, fatigue).

*Helpful in treating these conditions:* Alcoholism, anemia, colitis, menstrual problems.

*Minerals iron interacts with:* Calcium, cobalt, copper, magnesium, manganese, nickel, phosphorus, potassium, selenium, zinc.

*Suggested dosage ranges:* Teenagers, 15 mg; adults: women, 15-30 mg; men, 10 to 25 mg; and seniors, 15-30 mg a day.

*Toxicity:* Excessive iron can result in higher risk of infection or other diseases.

*Symptoms of toxic overload include:* Excessive iron ingestion or levels can cause copper, zinc and manganese losses, since the minerals compete with each other for absorption. This can result in a higher risk of infection or other diseases.

***Special note:*** If using ferrous sulfate for your iron supplementation, you are causing a loss of vitamin E. Do not supplement with iron if you have hemochromatosis, sickle-cell anemia or thalassemia.

### *Lead – toxic*

It is stored in the liver and bones. Lead alters the body's cell membranes' permeability or destroys the cells. It can inhibit molecular components, in particular the sulfhydryl groups in molecules, which are vital for hemoglobin formation.

*Everyday sources of lead:* Insecticides, lead crystal, lead-based paints, lead solder, tobacco smoke, water and some foods – particularly plants grown in soil rich in lead.

*Important minerals that are negatively impacted by moderate to high lead levels in the body:* Calcium, copper, iron and zinc.

*Main body parts that it can negatively effect:* Heart, kidneys, liver, central nervous system. Even at low levels, with chronic exposure or sudden large levels of exposure, lead accumulation in infants and children can easily reach toxic levels. This is particularly important during their development, because of leads potential effect upon the central nervous systems. Lead poisoning may result in aggressive behavior, anemia, developmental delays, hyperactivity and learning disabilities.

*Main body functions it negatively impacts:* Destroys antioxidants. Causes metabolic poisoning.

*Protect yourself with these supplements:* apple pectin, amino acids (L-lysine, L-cysteine), vitamin C with bioflavonoids, a properly balanced calcium and magnesium supplement, essential fatty acids (EFAs – omega 3 and omega 6), garlic, selenium, zinc.

## *Lithium*

Lithium is used in the treatment of bipolar (manic/depressive) disorders. It should only be used under medical supervision. In ancient times, Greeks who felt low or depressed would drink from a lithium-rich pool of water. Lithium salts enhance moods, and alter an electrolyte balance in the brain. Long term use can affect the thyroid, liver and kidneys.

*Mineral lithium interacts with:* Sodium.

## *Magnesium*

*Principal benefit:* This is the anti-stress mineral. It is necessary for optimal nerve functioning.

*Nutrients that maximize the amount the body can use:* $B_6$ (essential to proper functioning), C, D, calcium, phosphorus. Milk usually contains a synthetic vitamin D, which may deplete the magnesium in your body.

*Foods, drugs, nutrients and conditions that prevent the maximum utilization of magnesium by the body:* Alcohol, coffee, chronic stress, sugar, tea. Milk containing synthetic vitamin D may deplete the magnesium in your body. Magnesium carbonate is not a recommended form of supplement since it is not easily absorbed by the body.

*Drugs that can cause magnesium deficiency:* Over-the-counter medications containing alcohol such as cough syrups and elixirs (e.g. Nyquil). Antibiotics. Diuretics such as Diuril, Hydrodiuril, Lasix, Ser-ap-es. Oral contraceptives. Tetracyclines (Achromycin V, Sumycin, Tetracyn).

*Drug interaction:* In 1999, Dr. Jay Seastrunk, of Texas, who runs a center for chronic fatigue patients, reported that patients using the medication Neurontin, an anti-convulsant and pain drug, have found it does not work well if taken when supplementing with magnesium or amino acid supplements.

*Excellent natural sources:* Almonds, bone meal, honey, green vegetables, kelp tablets, nuts, seafood, spinach, tofu, wheat bran. Here are some foods and their approximate magnesium content:

| | |
|---|---|
| Bran flakes, 1 cup (250 ml) | 90 mg |
| Peanuts (roasted with skin), 1 cup (250 ml) | 420 mg |
| Tuna fish (canned), 1/2 lb (230 g) | 150 mg |

*Main body parts that it benefits:* Arteries, bones, heart, muscles, nerves, stomach, teeth. It is called the 'gatekeeper of cellular activity', since it is involved in almost every essential body function.

*Main body functions it supports:* Acid/alkaline balance, blood sugar metabolism (energy), fat metabolism, metabolism of calcium and vitamin C, potassium and calcium uptake, nerve and muscle functions, muscle relaxation.

*Symptoms of deficiency:* Confusion, disorientation, easily aroused anger, nervousness, rapid pulse, tremors. Most Americans do not get enough magnesium. Post-menopausal women should pay particular attention to magnesium since it can prevent osteoporosis and blood clots that may lead to heart attacks. Pregnant women can develop toxemia, a potentially lethal form of high blood pressure due to magnesium deficiency. It may be a factor in PMS, premenstrual syndrome.

*Helpful in treating these conditions:* Angina, alcoholism, asthma, depression, diabetes, heart conditions, high blood pressure, high cholesterol, kidney stones, migraines, muscle weakness and twitching, nervousness, osteoporosis, PMS, prostrate problems, sensitivity to noise, stomach acidity, tooth decay, overweight.

*Minerals magnesium interacts with:* Boron, calcium, iron, manganese, phosphorus, potassium, strontium.

*Suggested dosage ranges:* Teenagers, 400-750 mg; adults 250-750 mg; and seniors, 500-750 mg a day. For each 100 mg of magnesium, take 200 mg of calcium. This ratio increases the amount of magnesium your body can use. Individuals with kidney problems should not exceed 3000 mg of magnesium a day.

## Manganese

*Principal benefit:* Aids in reducing nervous irritability.

*Nutrients that maximize the amount the body can use:* None.

*Foods, drugs, nutrients and conditions that prevent the maximum utilization of manganese by the body:* Excessive calcium/phosphorus intake.

*Excellent natural sources:* Bananas, bran, celery, cereals, egg yolks, green leafy vegetables, legumes, liver, milk, nuts, pineapples, shellfish, whole grains.

***Note:*** Vegetables grown in manganese-rich soils usually have high levels of beta-carotene and vitamin C.

*Main body parts that it benefits:* brain, mammary glands, muscles, nerves.

*Main body functions it supports:* Needed for cartilage formation and bone growth, supports the central nervous system and the immune system, energy production, enzyme activator, glucose metabolism, reproduction and growth, sex hormone production, tissue respiration, vitamin $B_1$ metabolism, vitamin E utilization.

*Symptoms of deficiency:* Ataxia (muscle coordination failure), dizziness, ear noises, loss of hearing.

*Helpful in treating these conditions:* Allergies, asthma, diabetes, epilepsy, fatigue, inflammations, sprains, strains.

*Minerals manganese interacts with:* Calcium, chromium, copper, iron, magnesium, phosphorus, zinc.

*Suggested dosage ranges:* Adult maintenance dosage is 5 to 10 mg a day. Heavy meat eaters and milk drinkers may need to supplement up to 30 mg a day, as well as those who suffer from dizziness or memory problems.

*Toxicity:* Excessive manganese dosage may cause weakness and motor problems.

*Symptoms of toxic overload:* Excessive manganese ingestion or levels can cause copper, zinc and iron losses, since these minerals compete with each other for absorption. This can result in a higher risk of infection or other diseases.

## *Mercury – highly toxic*

At room temperature it is somewhat volatile, which means it can easily become a gas vapor. The danger is that we readily absorb mercury fumes when we breath. It is attracted to, and alters the sulfhydryl groups of proteins which can have far reaching effects since they play a critical role in hemoglobin, hormones, enzymes and antibodies.

*Symptoms of mercury inhalation poisoning:* Initially acute gastrointestinal inflammation, thirst, nausea, a metallic taste in the mouth, abdominal pain. Bloody diarrhea follows. If mercury or any heavy metal poisoning is suspected, immediately drink milk. The mercury affects the milk protein rather than the digestive tract. Then to get rid of the mercury, induce vomiting. Always call an emergency poison control center, even after you have dealt with the immediate emergency.

*Symptoms of long-term exposure to mercury:* Key symptoms include fever, loss of memory, chills, loosening of teeth, chest pain, renal damage and weakness. Secondary symptoms include irritability, nervousness, loss of libido (sexual drive) and lack of ambition. Zinc and cadmium can accelerate mercury retention in mitochondria tissue when mercury is present in the environment.

*Some sources:* Amalgam dental fillings, fungicides, pesticides, plastics, solvents.

*Main body parts that it can negatively effect:* Retained in the brain and nervous system. Fifty percent of absorbed mercury is stored in the kidneys, the rest in blood, bone marrow, brain, liver, myocardium, muscles, salivary glands, skin, and spleen.

*Main body functions it negatively impacts:* Destroys antioxidants, can cause metabolic poisoning, arthritis, candidiasis, chronic fatigue, hyperactivity, mental and emotional dysfunction.

*Protect yourself with these supplements:* Vitamin A, apple pectin, amino acids (glutathione, L-methionine, L-cysteine), B complex, vitamin C with rutin, vitamin E. Drink lots of clean water, since our bodies rid themselves of mercury mainly through our urine and feces, than through exhalation, sweating, hair and breast milk.

***Caution:*** The fetus is very sensitive to mercury which can result in damage to its developing neurological system. So if you are trying to get pregnant or have succeeded, consult with your health care provider about checking the levels of mercury in your body.

***Note:*** Dental mercury amalgams are banned in many European countries. In extreme cases of mercury poisoning, consult your dentist. Make sure that dental amalgams are removed without allowing additional mercury gases to escape into your body.

## ***Molybdenum***

*Nutrients that maximize the amount the body can use:* Should be taken with 1.5 to 3 mg of copper as part of a balanced mineral and vitamin formulation, to maximize molybdenum's bio-availability for the body.

*Nutrient that prevents the maximum utilization of molybdenum by the body:* Copper.

*Excellent natural sources:* Beans, blue-green algae, dark green leafy vegetables, legumes, milk, peas, soybeans, whole grains. Hard water can supply up to 40 percent of your daily needs. Foods grown in soils depleted of molybdenum have been found to contain over 400 times lower molybdenum levels.

*Main body parts that it benefits:* Three enzyme systems that are responsible for metabolizing carbohydrates, fats and proteins.

*Main body functions it supports:* Alcohol detoxification. Reduces incidents of esophageal cancer. Mobilizes iron in the body. Nitrogen metabolism. Prevents male sexual impotence. Sulfite and uric acid metabolism. Reduces incidence of tooth decay.

*Symptoms of deficiency:* Age related cataracts. Anemia – molybdenum is needed for the metabolism of iron. Cancers of the esophagus and mouth. Decreased life expectancy. Stunted growth.

*Possible causes of deficiency aside from insufficient nutrient intake:* An high ratio of copper to molybdenum can create a deficiency of molybdenum and vice versa. Excess sulfur may result in a molybdenum deficiency.

*Helpful in treating this condition:* Wilson's disease.

*Minerals molybdenum interacts with:* Copper, nickel, silicon, zinc.

*Suggested dosage ranges:* Rarely is there a need to supplement with molybdenum. Your food should supply enough. If molybdenum poor soil used for your food, for young adults and adults take 50 to 250 mcg per day.

*Symptoms of toxicity:* Amounts in excess of 5 mg are considered toxic. Vary with age and the form and amount of molybdenum eaten, consult your health care provider.

## *Nickel – a trace mineral*

Nickel is needed by your body in very small amounts, but a small excess can become toxic. It is found in our RNA (genetic code carriers). Nickel may benefit enzyme production. It may help maintain cell membranes. Believed to have a role in the generation of liver arginase.

*Minerals nickel interacts with:* Copper, iron, zinc.

*Natural sources:* Beans (lentils, split and green peas, soybeans) and oats.

*Symptoms of possible toxic overload include:* Cancer, heart disease, skin problems and thyroid malfunctioning.

***Caution:*** A deficiency of nickel can harm the liver, other organs and body tissues.

***Note:*** Nickel is essential for animals. A lack of it in animals can cause retarded growth, poor reproductive success rate, dermatitis, poor liver function, inappropriate use of zinc, iron and vitamin $B_{12}$ by the body. Speak to your veterinarian about testing for low nickel levels if your pet or animal has these problems.

## *Phosphorus*

*Nutrients that maximize the amount the body can use:* A, D (essential for proper functioning), F, need twice as much calcium as phosphorus (two parts calcium to one part phosphorus). Diets high in fats cause increased phosphorus absorption by the body.

*Foods, drugs, nutrients and conditions that prevent the maximum utilization of phosphorus by the body:* aluminum, iron, excessive intake of magnesium, excessive intake of meats, excessive intake of soft drinks, excessive intake of sugar.

*Drugs that can cause phosphorus deficiency:* Laxatives and lubricants such as castor oil and mineral oil.

*Excellent natural sources:* Eggs, fish, grains, glandular meats, meat, nuts, poultry, seeds, yellow cheese, whole grains. Here are some foods and their approximate phosphorus content:

| | |
|---|---|
| Calf liver, 1/4 lb (115 g) | 600 mg |
| Milk/yogurt, 1 cup (250 ml) | 230 mg |
| Eggs (cooked), 1 medium | 110 mg |

*Main body parts that it benefits:* Bones, brain nerves, teeth.

*Main body functions it supports:* Participates in almost all chemical reactions in the body, bone and teeth formation, cell growth and repair, energy production and release, healthy gums, heart muscle contraction, kidney function, metabolism of sugar, fats, starches and calcium, nerve and muscle activity, vitamin utilization.

*Symptoms of deficiency:* Loss of appetite, fatigue, irregular breathing, nervous disorders, overweight, pyorrhea, rickets, weight loss.

*Helpful in treating these conditions:* Arthritis, stunted growth in children, stress, tooth and gum disorders.

*Minerals phosphorus interacts with:* Calcium, copper, iron, magnesium, manganese, molybdenum, zinc.

*Suggested dosage ranges:* Teenagers, 1000-1200 mg; adults, 1000-1500 mg; and seniors, 800-1200 mg a day. Pregnant and lactating women require higher amounts. Consult with your health care provider. Enough phosphorus is usually obtained through diet. If using bonemeal as the source of supplemental phosphorus, make sure vitamin D is added to make it more bio-available. A healthy body balance includes one part of phosphorus to two parts of calcium. After age 40, our bodies are less able to deal with excess phosphorus, since our kidneys are less able to excrete it. Be aware of the many ways we ingest phosphorus containing foods, such as soft drinks.

*Toxicity:* None known.

**Note:** Excessive phosphorus can decrease calcium levels. Too much phosphorus can lead to a loss of calcium, which can result in osteoporosis.

## *Potassium*

*Nutrients that maximize the amount the body can use:* $B_6$, sodium (equal dosage required, one part potassium with one part sodium).

*Foods, drugs, nutrients and conditions that prevent the maximum utilization of potassium by the body:* Alcohol, coffee, cortisone, diuretics, laxatives, excessive salt and sugar intake, stress.

*Drugs that can cause potassium deficiency:* Aspirin and drugs containing aspirin. Barbiturates such as Butisol, Phenobarbital, Seconal, Nembutal and Tuinal. Diuretics such as Diuril, Hydrodiuril, Lasix, Ser-ap-es. Caffeine and medicines containing caffeine. Chloramphenicol (Chlomycetin). Cholestyramine (Questran). Colchicine (Colbenemid). Meprednisone (Betapar). Prednisone (Meticorten, Prednisolone, Orasone).

*Excellent natural sources:* Bananas, blackstrap molasses, cantaloupe, citrus fruits, dates, figs, peaches, tomato juice, peanuts, raisins, seafood, sunflower seeds, tomatoes, watercress. Here are some foods and their approximate potassium content:

| | |
|---|---|
| Apricots (dried), 1 cup (250 ml) | 1450 mg |
| Bananas, 1 medium | 500 mg |
| Flounder (baked), 1/4 lb (115 g) | 650 mg |
| Potatoes (baked), 1 medium | 500 mg |
| Sunflower seeds, 1 cup (250 ml) | 900 mg |

*Main body parts that it benefits:* Adrenal gland, blood, heart, kidneys, muscles, nerves, skin.

*Main body functions it supports:* Acne prevention, adrenal function, blood pressure regulation, fluid balance in the cells, heartbeat, kidney function, glucose to glycogen conversion, rapid growth, hormone secretion, maintains proper pH balance (body's acid/alkalinity balance), muscle contraction, nerve tranquilization, nerve transmission to the heart.

*Symptoms of deficiency:* Acne, continuous thirst, dry skin, constipation, edema, general weakness, hypoglycemia, insomnia, muscle damage, nervousness, slow irregular heartbeat, weak reflexes.

*Helpful in treating these conditions:* Acne, alcoholism, allergies, burns, colic in infants, diabetes, high blood pressure, heart disease (angina pectoris, congestive heart failure, myocardial infarction).

*Minerals potassium interacts with:* Iron, magnesium, sodium.

*Suggested dosage ranges:* Teenagers, 1500-4500 mg; adults, 1000-1500 mg; and seniors, 1800-5500 mg.

*Toxicity:* 18 grams or more can be toxic. In cases of kidney disease, seek medical advice before supplementing with potassium.

## Selenium

Studies in China, the American National Cancer Institute and elsewhere have repeatedly shown selenium to have anticancer benefits, from skin cancer to colon, lung and prostate cancer. This trace mineral is a powerful preventative when it comes to cancer and strokes.

*Nutrient that prevents the maximum utilization of selenium by the body:* Copper, believed by some to be an antagonist to selenium, probably competing for absorption.

*Excellent natural sources:* Broccoli, brewer's yeast, cabbage, celery, cucumbers, garlic, fish, mushrooms, onions, poultry, red grapes, whole grains. Selenium levels in soil have been greatly depleted in America, causing plants to have levels that are too low for minimal, let alone maximum, nutritional benefit. In addition, modern food processing methods significantly reduce or destroy the selenium content of foods. Organically grown foods are a better source.

*Main body parts that it benefits:* Concentrated in the eyes, heart, brain, kidneys, liver, pancreas, skin, thyroid, testes. Present in all tissues.

*Main body functions it supports:* Slows the aging process, antioxidant critical for production of the body's main antioxidant glutathione peroxidase, aids action of vitamin E, powerful anticancer properties, antagonistic to heavy metal toxicity, prevents cataracts, improves immune system function, protects heart against disease, improves mental well-being, stroke prevention, healing and tissue repair, promotes a healthy heart and liver.

*Helpful in treating these conditions:* Allergies, eczema, psoriasis, Multiple Sclerosis (MS), prostrate enlargement (BPH), rheumatoid arthritis, thyroid function.

*Minerals selenium interacts with:* Copper, iron, zinc.

*Suggested dosage ranges:* Teenagers, 50 mcg; adults, 25-200 mcg; and seniors, 50-200 mcg. a day. When treating diseases such as arthritis, cancer, heart disease and mercury toxicity, consult with a naturally orientated physician or health care practitioner before deciding how much and what to use. Interactions with other natural remedies and supplements can enhance or reduce the benefits of selenium supplementation. The most absorbable and least toxic form of selenium appears to be selenomethionine, which is derived from ocean plants or selenium rich yeast.

*Nutrients that maximize the amount the body can use:* More beneficial when taken with vitamin E and even more so with vitamin C and zinc. For adults, we recommend a synergistic blend of beta-carotene, vitamin C, vitamin E and selenium.

*Toxicity:* High selenium content soils have caused animal poisonings. The Food and Nutrition Board says that humans ingesting 2400 mcg or more daily, for prolonged periods, may suffer from selenium toxicity.

*Symptoms of toxic overload:* Possibly a garlic odor in a person's breath, sweat and urine. Its teratogenic (monster producing) effect in certain animals, indicates that excessively high levels of selenium may cause human birth defects.

## *Silicon*

One of the earth's most abundant minerals. Every day we consume grams of it. The purpose and role it plays in our well-being is not well understood by traditional doctors and researchers. Low calcium intake may result in an increased need for silicon.

*Excellent natural sources:* Cereals, unrefined grains, root vegetables.

*Main body parts that it benefits:* Aorta (a part of the heart), bones, connective tissue, hair, heart, lungs, lymph nodes, nails, skin, tendons, trachea.

*Main body functions it supports:* Slows the aging process, maintains flexibility of arteries, enhances healing process, supports health of bones, hair, heart, nails, skin and connective tissue, prevents cardiovascular disease.

*Symptoms of deficiency:* As we age, the aorta, skin and thymus have a marked reduction in their amounts of silicon.

*Minerals silicon interacts with:* Calcium, molybdenum, zinc.

*Suggested dosage ranges:* 5 to 20 mg. These minerals aid the utilization of silicon: boron, calcium, magnesium, manganese and potassium

**Note:** Silicosis is the respiratory disease miners suffer when silicon fibers stimulate fibrosis of lungs and other tissues. This results in healthy lung tissue being replaced by an overabundance of collagen, which causes connective tissue patches to form, and can result in malignant tumors.

## *Silver*

According to many sources, silver in suspension, also known as colloidal silver, is a powerful antiviral and antibacterial trace mineral. At this time, insufficient information prevents us from describing the full-range of this trace mineral's healing properties.

*Main body parts that it benefits:* Eyes, skin, digestive system.

*Main body functions it supports:* Digestive aid, eye ointment for newborns, sterilizer.

*Helpful in treating these conditions:* Acne, eczema, digestive system, insect bites, psoriasis, rashes.

*Suggested dosage ranges:* Depends on the application. It is available in creams, ointments, also in colloidal water or concentrated trace mineral suspensions.

## *Sodium*

*Nutrients that maximize the amount the body can use:* Vitamin D, potassium (equal dosage required).

*Foods, drugs, nutrients and conditions that prevent the maximum utilization of sodium by the body:* Lack of chlorine and/or potassium.

*Minerals sodium interacts with:* Lithium, potassium.

*Excellent natural sources:* Sea salt, salt, milk, cheese, seafood.

*Main body parts that it benefits:* Blood, lymph system, muscles, nerves.

*Main body functions it supports:* Normal cellular fluid level, proper muscle contraction.

*Suggested dosage ranges:* Teenagers, 900-2500 mg; adults, 1100-3000 mg; and seniors, 1100-3000 mg a day. Rarely need to supplement with sodium.

*Symptoms of deficiency:* Appetite loss, intestinal gas, muscle shrinkage, vomiting, weight loss.

*Helpful in treating these conditions:* Dehydration, fever, heat stroke.

***Note:*** Excessive sodium can result in a loss of potassium. Too much perspiration may lead to a loss of sodium.

### *Strontium – can be toxic*

In the 1950s and 1960s radioactive fallout was responsible for bringing awareness of the potentially damaging side effects of strontium.

*Minerals strontium interacts with:* Calcium, magnesium, zinc.

### *Sulfur*

*Nutrients that maximize the amount the body can use:* B complex, $B_1$, biotin, pantothenic acid. With silicon, sulfur helps slow the aging process.

*Foods, drugs, nutrients and conditions that prevent the maximum utilization of sulfur by the body:* None

*Excellent natural sources:* Bran, cheese, clams, eggs, fish, garlic, nuts, onion, wheat germ.

*Main body parts that it benefits:* Hair, nails, nerves, skin.

*Main body functions it supports:* Stimulates bile secretion, disinfects blood, aids resistance to bacteria, protects cells against toxins, synthesizes collagen, aids oxidation processes, body tissue formation, helps heal skin problems.

*Symptoms of deficiency:* Not known.

*Helpful in treating these conditions:* Arthritis. External applications help these skin disorders – eczema, dermatitis and psoriasis.

*Suggested dosage ranges:* 400 to 1000 mg.

### *Tin – can be toxic*

Rats need it for normal growth. In humans, it may be toxic. Our bodies do not easily absorb tin.

Old styles of canning and storing food in uncoated tin containers were a major health problem. Technological advances have resulted in coated tin cans which do not cause tin toxicity. Unfortunately, recent research finds that the plastic coatings currently in use may represent a health problem. Caution should be exercised when consuming canned foods outside of North America. Some processed foods use stabilizers and preservatives that are partially composed of tin.

*Mineral tin interacts with:* Zinc.

Excess tin can interfere with glutathione production by the body. Glutathione is a powerful antioxidant. Overexposure may block the body's ability to absorb copper, iron and zinc.

## *Vanadium*

This trace mineral copies the biological action of insulin hormones. It is stored in our fat, liver, kidneys and bones. One of the best biologically active forms of vanadium is vanadyl sulfate. In partnership with a progressive alternatively orientated doctor or naturally orientated trained healer, it may be possible using vanadium, to better control blood sugar levels and insulin resistance, or Type 2 adult onset diabetes. Utilizing the trace minerals chromium and vanadium can be even more beneficial for diabetics or those prone to developing it.

*Mineral vanadium interacts with:* Chromium.

*Drug that prevents the maximum utilization of vanadium by the body:* Tobacco.

*Excellent natural sources:* Black pepper, dill seeds, olives, radishes, whole grains.

*Main body parts that it benefits:* Blood, bones, heart, nervous system, pancreas.

*Main body functions it may support:* Aids mineralization of bones and teeth. Anticarcinogenic properties. Inhibits cholesterol formation in the blood and nervous system. Improves the action of insulin by controlling blood sugar levels in diabetics – makes insulin work more efficiently. Aids cellular metabolism. Prevents cardiovascular disease. Involved in growth and reproduction. Stimulates cell division. Possibly increases and builds muscle strength and definition. Vanadium may affect thyroid function, since it may be involved in the formation of erythrocytes.

*Symptoms of deficiency:* Type 2 adult onset diabetes, cardiovascular problems, kidney disease, infant mortality. In laboratory tests on animals a vanadium deficiency has had the following results:

reduced overall growth, retention of fluids, changes to the thyroid, impaired growth of bones, teeth and cartilage. It can reduce lactation in lab animals and increase infant mortality.

*Helpful in treating these conditions:* A combination of vanadium and chromium, may help Type 2 adult onset diabetics wean themselves from insulin. This process should only be undertaken and monitored by your doctor. In experiments, vanadium exhibits anticarcinogenic activity.

*Suggested dosage ranges:* Teenagers, 15-50 mcg; adults, 10-100 mcg; and seniors, 15-100 mcg per day. Usually vanadium is not necessary as a supplement. If needed, use Vandyl sulfate, the more biologically absorbable form of vanadium. Body builders should take their dosage 30 minutes before working out. Diabetics should have their doctor closely monitor their blood sugar levels, until they are in the normal range. Under the doctor's care, diabetics can start at 6 mg per day and increase the amounts until they notice results or are taking 100 mg per day. Once they find a dosage that gets results, take it for a period of three weeks, then slowly taper down to 6 mg per day.

***Warning:*** Lithium reacts with vanadium. If taking lithium, speak to your medical professional before supplementing with vanadium. If you are using it for diabetes, ask your doctor or natural health care provider to monitor your levels and progress.

*Toxicity:* Do not exceed daily recommended dosages, as high levels of this trace mineral may be toxic. Only 5 percent of vanadium eaten is absorbed by the digestive system; however, the lungs readily absorb vanadium dust. The only toxic cases of vanadium poisoning reported are due to inhalation of vanadium dust.

## *Zinc*

*Principal benefits:* Aids healing. Helps optimize brain function and promotes mental alertness.

*Nutrients that maximize the amount the body can use:* Vitamin A or beta-carotene (high intake), calcium, copper, phosphorus.

*Foods, drugs, nutrients and conditions that prevent the maximum utilization of zinc by the body:* Alcohol, high intake of calcium, lack of phosphorus.

*Drugs that can cause zinc deficiency:* Diuretics such as Diuril, Hydrodiuril, Lasix, Ser-ap-es. Caffeine and medicines containing caffeine. Meprednisone (Betapar). Prednisone (Meticorten, Prednisolone, Orasone).

*Excellent natural sources:* Brewer's yeast, liver, meat, mushrooms, seafood (particularly oysters), soybeans, spinach, sunflower seeds, tofu, whole grains.

*Main body parts that it benefits:* Blood, eyes, heart, nails, prostrate gland, skin.

*Main body functions it supports:* Antioxidant, prevents acne, burn and wound healing, carbohydrate digestion, eyes, essential for many enzyme and body functions, immune system function, needed for healthy nails and skin, prostrate gland function, reproductive organ growth and development, sex organ growth and maturity, vitamin $B_1$, phosphorus and protein metabolism.

*Symptoms of deficiency:* Delayed sexual maturity, fatigue, poor appetite, prolonged wound healing, retarded growth, loss of smell, sterility, loss of taste.

*Helpful in treating these conditions:* Alcoholism, Alzheimer's disease, atherosclerosis, baldness, cirrhosis, colds (reduces severity and duration from 7.3 days to 4.4 days), diabetes, high cholesterol (eliminates deposits), infertility, internal and external injury and wound healing, reduced sex drive, Wilson's disease.

*Minerals zinc interacts with:* Boron, calcium, chromium, cobalt, germanium, iron, manganese, molybdenum, nickel, phosphorus, selenium, silicon, strontium, tin.

*Suggested dosage ranges:* 15 to 45 mg. A ratio of 10 to 15 parts zinc to one part copper provides for the best absorption rate by the body.

*Toxicity:* Excessive zinc ingestion or levels can cause copper, iron and manganese losses since they compete with each other for absorption. This can result in a higher risk of infection or other diseases.

*Symptoms of toxic overload include:* Excessive zinc levels or intake, may result in iron and copper deficiencies.

# chapter 13

# Amino Acids & Proteins — A team effort

## Keeping the body's systems in balance

Amino acids are popularly called 'the building blocks', or chemical components of proteins. They are the nitrogenous organic acids that form proteins necessary for all life. Twenty-six of the more than 100 naturally occurring amino acids are used by the body to create the proteins necessary for it to function optimally. Eight amino acids are essential for adults: isoleucine, leucine, lysine, methionine, phenylalanine, threonine, tryptophan and valine. Ten amino acids are essential when we are born, the extra two are histidine and arginine. "Essential" means the body cannot manufacture or produce a substance on its own from the available materials in the body and must get it from an external source, such as breast milk, other foods, or supplements. All amino acids are necessary; the non-essential ones can be manufactured by the body. When we reach adulthood, our body's chemistry has developed such that only eight amino acids remain essential.

The liver produces about 80 percent of our body's amino acid needs, the other 20 percent must come from our diet. When an essential amino acid is missing, or even just low, the ability of all the other amino acids is proportionately reduced. The amino acids are the building blocks of peptides, polypeptides and proteins in our bodies.

Protein is the second most abundant material, next to water, that makes up the human body. Proteins are part of your muscles, tendons, ligaments, glands, organs, nails, hair and body fluids critical to bone growth. The process of protein digestion also creates amino acids as an end product.

Essential to life, proteins are linked chains of amino acids held together by peptide bonds. Each type of protein is unique in its chemical sequencing. Each protein fills a specific need in the body and is not interchangeable with another protein. Proteins in the body are not directly derived from food. Dietary protein is broken down into its amino acid components in the body, then reconstituted as the specific proteins your body needs, at that time. This is why the amino acids are considered essential nutrients. The following lists some of the functions amino acids are involved in:

act as neurotransmitters or precursors to them; some are needed for the brain to send and receive messages.

some can pass through the blood-brain barrier; this barrier exists to maintain the health of the brain, its chemistry and processes.

aid in communication with nerve cells in other parts of the body.

empower vitamins and minerals to do their jobs right.

The following are some of the functions proteins are involved in:

bone growth.

brain function.

enzymes and hormones are proteins that catalyze and regulate all the body's processes.

disease and illness prevention.

maintenance of correct internal pH and water balance.

aids in nutrient exchange between the tissues, blood and lymph with intercellular fluids.

part of the structural basis of chromosomes.

Some amino acids stimulate the body's ability to produce human growth hormone (somatotrophin or STH). The pituitary gland stores this hormone, releasing it into the body from activities such as exercise, reduced food intake and sleep. As we age, the levels of growth hormone decrease until we finally stop producing it around age 50. You can stimulate your body's ability to produce growth hormone and return to levels you had as a young adult, using supplementation.

The release of human growth hormone from the pituitary is regulated by these hormones originating from the hypothalamus; somatostatin the growth hormone-inhibiting hormone (GH-IH) and growth-hormone releasing hormone (GH-RT). Other biochemical factors influencing the production of human growth hormone include hormones from other sources (e.g. thyroid, adrenal, gonads) and nutrient levels in the blood. The following are the principal health related actions of human growth hormone:

Have anti-aging properties.

Aid in fat burning by converting fat into muscle and energy, which aids weight loss.

Improve protein synthesis for building muscles.

Speed wound healing, also regenerates heart, kidneys, liver and lungs.

Restores hair growth and color.

Helps tissue repair.

Sharper vision.

Reduces wrinkles, improves skin elasticity and texture.

Reduce levels of urea in urine and blood.

Improve the quality of the body's connective tissue, which in turn strengthens ligaments and tendons.

Stronger bones, also restores bone and muscle mass. Growth hormone increases calcium osteocalcin and collagen levels.

Increases energy and endurance during exercise and body building.

Has an antidepressant action on the brain, elevates mood and increases concentration.

Strengthens the immune system through anti-body production and the thymus gland, which is responsible for T-cell production.

Increases oxygen intake and the ability to exercise.

Improves sleep.

Reduces blood pressure and cholesterol.

Greater cardiac output.

Powerful aphrodisiac for men and women.

Alleviates PMS and eliminates vaginal dryness.

Studies have shown that taking growth hormone directly for up to six months can be beneficial, but after that period it is no longer advisable, since it appears to negatively affect some adults. A better option is to help your body release growth hormones naturally using supplementation with amino acids and other nutrients. The amino acids are arginine, glutamine, glycine, ornithine, tryptophan and tyrosine. Their human growth hormone releasing properties are significantly enhanced when taken with vitamin $B_6$, vitamin C, niacinamide, calcium, magnesium, potassium, and zinc. Homeopathic remedies to stimulate an increase in the amount of human growth hormone, are now in the marketplace. To find out more about homeopathy, refer to Chapter 16.

***Note:*** Drug interaction with amino acids: In 1999, Dr. Jay Seastrunk, who runs a chronic fatigue center, reported that patients using the medication Neurontin, an anti-convulsant and pain drug, have found it does not work well if taken when supplementing with magnesium or amino acid.

The following is a list of key amino acids. Those marked with an asterisk (*) are the essential amino acids:

| | | | |
|---|---|---|---|
| alanine | asparagine | aspartic acid | carnitine |
| citrulline | cysteine | cystine | gamma-aminobutyric acid |
| glutamic acid | glutamine | glycine | isoleucine* |
| leucine* | lysine* | methionine* | ornithine |
| phenylalanine* | proline | serine | taurine |
| threonine* | tryptophan* | tyrosine | valine* |
| arginine* (in babies and children) | | histidine* (in babies and children) | |

An 'L-' used before an amino acid indicates a natural form that is easily absorbable by the body. For example, 'L-alanine' is the amino acid 'alanine' in a more biologically absorbable form.

A 'D-' before an amino acid indicates a synthetic variation of the amino acid.

## *Alanine*

A nonessential amino acid that the body can produce if the necessary materials are available. Beta-alanine, a form of alanine, is a component of coenzyme A and vitamin $B_5$ (pantothenic acid). Coenzyme A is an important catalyst in the body.

*Principal benefits:* Improves immune system. Helps metabolize glucose, a source energy for the body, and alleviates hypoglycemia. Reduces benign prostatic hyperplasia (BPH). Decreases risk of kidney stones. Excessive levels of alanine and low levels of phenylalanine and tyrosine are associated with the Epstein-Barr virus and chronic fatigue.

*Food sources:* Meat, poultry, fish, eggs.

*Non-food source(s):* Beta-alanine is found in vitamin $B_5$ (pantothenic acid) as well as coenzyme A, a vital catalyst.

### *Arginine*

(only essential for babies and children, nonessential for adults who can produce it from within, until about age 30)

***Important notice:*** After 30 years of age, the adult pituitary gland stops producing arginine. Supplementation may be needed.

*Principal benefits:* Needed for optimal functioning of the pituitary gland. Along with other amino acids, arginine aids the pituitary gland's production and release of growth hormone. Utilized in numerous other hormone and enzyme activities. For example, it is a component of vasopressin, a pituitary hormone, that helps the pancreas release insulin. It is found in high amounts in the skin, collagen and the body's connective tissue. This means it is important for repairing and healing damaged tissues, as is the case with arthritis, connective tissue problems, damaged tendons and building new bone. Increases sperm count. A lack of this component of protein can lead to male infertility, since this amino acid makes up to 80 percent of the protein needed in seminal fluid. Boosts the immune system, which can then slow the growth of cancers and tumors. Accelerates and aids in healing wounds. Tones muscles and metabolizes body fat. Vital for balancing nitrogen levels. Helps improve liver function by healing fatty liver and cirrhosis of the liver. Detoxifies the liver, by neutralizing ammonia. Fosters mental alertness. Promotes physical readiness. Boosts thymus gland function and size, which results in more production of the vital immune system component called T-cells (T lymphocytes). If you have suffered physical traumas, eat more arginine rich foods. Under medical supervision you may want to combine L-arginine and L-ornithine to stimulate weight loss.

*Food sources:* Brown rice, carob, chocolate, coconut, dairy products, gelatin desserts, nuts, oatmeal, popcorn, all protein-rich foods, raisins, sesame seeds, sunflower seeds, walnuts, white flour, wheat, wheat germ, whole wheat bread.

*Possible signs of deficiency:* Impaired liver lipid (fat) metabolism. Glucose intolerance. Improper insulin production and utilization.

*Dosages:* Use L-arginine. It is available in powder and tablet forms. Take 2000 mg (2 grams) with water or juice on an empty stomach just before going to bed. Body builders and those wanting to tone up their muscles can take 2000 mg (2 grams) one hour before vigorous exercise, on an empty stomach. To enhance male sexual performance take 3000 to 6000 mg (3 to 6 grams) on an empty stomach, an hour before sex.

***Warning:*** Do not give arginine to infants or growing children, since it may cause giantism. If dwarfism is the infant's or child's problem, discuss the options with your health care provider before using any amino acid supplements. Do not give to those with schizophrenic problems. Individuals with herpes should not use supplements or eat foods rich in this amino acid, as it is believed to trigger the herpes virus. To counteract this reaction, and still be able to take L-argnine, try taking 500 mg of L-lysine, which may inhibit an herpes virus outbreak. Excessively large dosages of 20 or more grams can cause bone and joint deformities. If you take too much arginine over a period of several weeks, your skin can become course or thicken. Reduce your arginine intake to allow the problem to rectify itself.

### *Asparagine*

A nonessential amino acid that the body can produce from within, if the necessary materials are available.

*Principal benefits:* Maintains and balances central nervous system by helping to prevent extreme conditions of over- or under-stimulation from affecting it. Helps the liver's ability to transform an amino acid from one type to another one that the body requires.

*Food source:* Mainly meats.

### *Aspartic acid*

A nonessential amino acid that the body can produce from within, if the necessary materials are available.

*Possible signs of deficiency:* Chronic fatigue and reduced stamina.

*Principal benefits:* Useful for brain and neural disorders. Aids functioning of all the cells and the carriers of our genetic codes, RNA and DNA. Protects the liver by helping to removing excess ammonia, which is very important for athletes and critical protection for the central nervous system; ammonia becomes very toxic once in the circulatory system. Boosts endurance and stamina. Improves immune system function. Aids metabolism. Increases stamina. Helps removes toxins, such as ammonia, from the bloodstream.

*Food source:* An excellent source is the plant protein found in sprouting seeds.

*Dosage:* Aspartic acid salts increase athletic endurance and stamina. The natural and best form is L-aspartic acid. It is available in tablets. Usually it is taken in 500 mg dosages, one to three times a day with water or juice, on an empty stomach, and at least a half hour before meals. Do not take protein at the same time, as it interferes with the body's ability to utilize aspartic acid.

### *Carnitine*

A nonessential amino acid that the body can produce from within, if the necessary materials are available. The body needs enough of the amino acids lysine and methionine, plus thiamine (vitamin $B_1$), pyridoxine (vitamin $B_6$), ascorbic acid (vitamin C) and iron to make carnitine. Neither lysine or methionine are available in large enough amounts from vegetable sources, which makes it very important for vegetarians to get sufficient amounts. Carnitine improves the benefits of vitamin C and E, two powerful antioxidants.

The form most easily used by the body is called L-carnitine. It is a vitamin-like nutrient found mainly in the brain, heart and skeletal muscles. It plays a vital role in delivering fatty acids to mitochondria, which supply the power for the cell and, in turn, the skeletal and heart cells. The cells are better able to utilize oxygen. Italian researchers have discovered it improves the potency of sperm in men with fertility problems.

*Possible signs of deficiency:* Confusion, heart pain, muscular dystrophy, muscle weakness, obesity.

*Principal benefit(s):* Aids conversion of fat to energy in the body. Improves cholesterol metabolism. Can help lower blood triglyceride levels. Helps improve fat metabolism problems due to diabetes and fatty liver caused by alcohol consumption. Beneficial for controlling hypoglycemia and diabetes. Needed for a healthy heart. Reduces frequency of angina attacks. Aids treatment for coronary artery disease. Reduces surgical cardiac damage to the heart. Helpful in treatment of kidney and liver diseases. Increases athletes' endurance time. Supports the skeletal muscular system and improves poor muscle tone as well as neuromuscular problems. Helps alleviate high cholesterol and/or triglycerides. Aids male infertility, caused by weak sperm. May be helpful in treating Alzheimer's disease patients, by slowing, preventing or even reversing the disease.

*Food sources:* Dairy products, meats, tempeh, soy-based products and grains fortified with lysine, such as cornmeal.

*Dosage:* Only take L-carnitine products, not D-carnitine, since it is more easily used by the body. On average, take 250 mg three times a day, at least an hour before, or two hours after, a meal. Take up to 1500 mg of tablets a day. There is no recommended daily intake amount for this amino acid. Men need more than women because of their greater muscle mass.

***Caution:*** L-carnitine has no side effects; it is safe. D-carnitine may have toxic side effects. Always consult your health care provider before taking supplements for existing heart conditions. If you take over 1 gram (1000 mg) a day, you may develop a fishy odor. This odor does not occur very often, is not dangerous and quickly disappears as soon as the dose is reduced. Vegetarians may become deficient in carnitine and may consider supplementation, since it is not found in vegetable proteins.

## *Citrulline*

A nonessential amino acid that the body can produce from within, if the necessary materials are available.

*Principal benefits:* Supports energy production. Increases immune system function. Can be transformed into L-arginine, which detoxifies the liver, by neutralizing ammonia (nitrocen in the blood).

*Food source:* Liver is the richest source of citrulline.

## *Cysteine (N-acetyl-L-cysteine)*

– see also Cystine

A quasi-essential amino acid because it is sometimes synthesized from methionine or phenylalanine. Cysteine is found in alpha-keratin. Two joined molecules of cysteine make up their close amino acid relative, cystine. Cysteine is not stable and easily converts to L-cystine. L-cystine in turn, easily converts to cysteine. Your body does this on an as-needed basis. Cysteine is more soluble than cystine, which means it is easier for your body to use. That is why cysteine is the preferred form of these two amino acids when used to treat most illnesses. Both of these amino acids contain sulfur. The body's stores of L-methionine form cysteine.

*Principal benefits:* Powerful antioxidant. Major metal and liver detoxifier. Detoxifies harmful toxins. Chelates, binds with heavy metals, thereby helping remove them from the body. Recommended for treating rheumatoid arthritis, mutogenic disorders like cancer and hardening of the arteries. Anti-aging properties exemplified through the reduction of age spots and prevention of baldness. Beneficial with respiratory tract problems and the treatment of mucus producing illnesses such as emphysema, bronchitis and tuberculosis. Beneficial for respiratory diseases such as asthma, bronchitis and emphysema. May improve allergy and sinusitis conditions. Keeps fingernails, toenails and hair in good condition. Important for collagen production which benefits the texture and elasticity of your skin. Alleviates psoriasis.

People with chronic diseases may need to supplement with cysteine. Important in the activity of the disease-fighting white blood cells. Promotes healing of severe burns and surgical wounds. Protects the brain and liver from alcohol and drug damage. Aids the body's fat burning mechanism. Helps build muscle. Aids in the absorption of iron. Protects against cigarette smoke's toxic compounds. Precursor to glutathione, a key detoxifier of the liver. Helps increase glutathione levels in bone marrow, kidneys, liver and lungs. Found in many digestive enzymes and other proteins in the body. Protects against radiation damage.

*Vitamin and mineral co-factors and other benefits:* Selenium and vitamin E improve cysteine's free radical fighting properties. Vitamin $B_6$ is needed to synthesize cysteine. You may use cystine or N-acetylcysteine instead of cysteine for supplementation. N-acetylcysteine and cysteine are beneficial in reducing or preventing side effects from radiation therapy (X-rays, nuclear radiation) and chemotherapy. N-acetylcysteine is a better booster of glutathione levels than cystine or even glutathione supplementation.

*Food source:* The body synthesizes it.

*Dosage:* People with chronic diseases may need larger amounts of cysteine supplements, up to 1000 mg, three times a day, for 30-day periods. For drinkers and smokers it is very beneficial to combine three parts vitamin C with one part cysteine.

***Caution:*** It is recommended that diabetics only use cysteine/cystine under medical supervision. When used alone or in combination with vitamins C and B, it can interfere with and deactivate insulin. Persons suffering the rare genetic illness cystinuria, that causes the formation of cystine kidney stones, should not supplement with the amino acid cysteine. Discontinue use if nausea, vomiting, diarrhea or stomach cramps occur, and consult with your physician or naturally oriented healer.

## *Cystine*

– see also Cysteine

Cystine is a nonessential amino acid that the body can produce from within, if the necessary materials are available.

*Principal benefits:* Stable form of the amino acid cysteine. When metabolized, cystine produces sulfuric acid which helps detoxify the body. It offers effective protection against copper toxicity. Useful for prevention of side effects from radiation therapy and chemotherapy. Aids in prevention of free radical damage due to smoking and alcohol. Helps in eliminating age spots.

## *DL-Phenylalanine (DLPA)*

– see also Phenylalanine

DL-Phenylalanine is not a naturally occurring amino acid. DLPA is another form of phenylalanine combined with equal amounts of synthetic D- and natural L-phenylalanine. This helps produce and activate endorphins, the body's natural pain killers. They are more powerful than opium derivatives and morphine. Endorphins are constantly destroyed by certain enzyme systems in the body; DLPA may inhibit these enzyme systems from functioning, better enabling the endorphins to do their job. Selective in its pain reducing qualities, DLPA can help people with chronic pain, since it does not interfere with the natural short term acute pain defense mechanisms of the body for injuries such as cuts, burns and scrapes.

*Principal benefits:* Alleviates lower back pain, muscle and leg cramps, migraines, osteoarthritis, postoperative pain, rheumatoid arthritis and whiplash. Powerful anti-depressant. Pain relief that gets more effective the longer used, and you do not build up a tolerance to it if taken for up to one month, without additional drugs. Curbs addictive cravings. Sexual stimulant. Has no known adverse interactions with other therapies and drugs and can increase pain killing benefits.

*Dosage:* The experience of pain is very personal. Individuals who have not achieved pain relief with traditional prescription medications may want to consider DLPA; it works when prescription drugs fail. Finding the best dosage, depends on the condition. In conjunction with your health care provider, start at 375 mg to 750 mg, taken three times a day, half an hour before each meal. Pain relief may occur within four to twenty-one days. After that period, if no relief has occurred, you may want to double the dosage for another twenty-one days. Once you have found a workable dosage, reduce your intake until you get to the minimal amount you need.

*Toxicity:* None known.

***Warning:*** DL-phenylalanine should not be used by pregnant women. DLPA elevates blood pressure and is not recommended for individuals with hypertension or heart conditions, unless under medical supervision, in which case it is usually prescribed to be taken after meals. DLPA is contraindicated for those with phenylketonuria, an inherited inability to oxidize a metabolic product of phenylalanine and exhibiting severe mental retardation. Persons with malignant melanoma and using anti-depressants containing monoamine oxidase inhibitors, should not use phenylalanine.

## *Dimethylglycine (DMG)*

– see also Glycine

Dimethylglycine is derived from the simplest of amino acids, glycine. It is also known as vitamin $B_{15}$ and pangamic acid, although, technically, DMG is not really a vitamin. It is a building block for other amino acids, DNA, hormones, and neurotransmitters. There are no known symptoms of deficiency.

*Principal benefits:* Supports and improves the immune system (e.g. flu virus, salmonella). Aids function of many organs. Increases mental alertness. Improves behavior of ADD and autistic individuals. Helps maintain suitable blood pressure levels. Helps the body sustain high energy levels. Normalizes glucose blood levels. Beneficial in lowering high blood cholesterol and triglyceride levels. May help curb or lessen the effects of epileptic seizures.

*Dosage, toxicity:* see Vitamin $B_{15}$ (pangamic acid).

## *Gamma-aminobutyric acid (GABA)*

A nonessential amino acid, that the body can produce with the necessary materials. It is formed from glutamic acid, another amino acid. In the central nervous system, it acts as a neurotransmitter. It depresses neuron activity. Prevents nerve cells from overworking. Combined with inositol and niacinamide, it helps stop stress and anxiety messages from reaching the brain's motor centers by occupying the stress and anxiety receptor sites in the brain.

*Principal benefits:* Vital for efficient brain function and proper metabolism. Analgesic effects. Beneficial for treating attention deficit disorder (ADD) and epilepsy. Works like the prescription tranquilizers Valium (diazepam) and Librium (chlordiazepoxide) to calm the body, without the need for concern about addiction. The benefits of being relaxed mean it may improve a depressed or inhibited sex drive. Beneficial for treating hypertension. Helps regulate sex hormones, so it is useful for treating enlarged prostrate glands.

***Warning:*** Excessive amount of GABA may increase anxiety. It can lead to shortness of breath or very shallow breathing. Too much can result in tingling extremities and numbness around the mouth.

### Glutamic acid

A nonessential amino acid that the body can produce from within, if the required materials are there. It becomes glutamine or gamma-aminobutyric acid (GABA) when needed. It fires the neurons in the central nervous system, brain and spinal cord. Helps the movement of potassium through the brain-blood barrier. The brain uses it as fuel.

*Principal benefits:* Aids brain functioning. Elevates mood. Converts excess ammonia, which inhibits brain function, into the buffer, glutamine, which is the only amino acid able to detoxify ammonia in the brain. Reduces fatigue. Aids in metabolism of fats and sugars. Reduces cravings for sugar. Beneficial in treating alcoholism, muscular dystrophy, personality disorders (such as schizophrenia), epilepsy, and the diabetic complication caused by insulin, hypoglycemic coma. Treats behavioral disorders in children. Speeds healing of ulcers and prostatic hyperplasia.

*Dosage:* see Glutamine.

***Warning:*** When used for treating children, always do it under proper medical supervision. Individuals with a sensitivity to monosodium glutamate (MSG), even though it is not the same as glutamic acid or glutamine, may experience an allergic reaction to them. Before taking these supplements, consult with a doctor.

### Glutamine

Parois de l'intestin

The natural form is known as L-glutamine.

*Principal benefits:* Glutamine helps produce higher levels of glutamic acid, which benefits brain functioning. It is known as 'brain fuel' since it can pass through the brain-blood barrier. Beneficial in treatments of senility, schizophrenia, epilepsy and developmental disabilities.

Glutamine aids the pituitary gland's production and release of growth hormone. Reduces recovery time and possibility of infection for cancer patients undergoing bone marrow transplant treatments. Reduces fatigue. It is the most abundant free-form acid found in the muscles. Helps build muscle mass in people who exercise. It may help reduce sugar cravings, which means it can help dieters. Elevates mood. Aids in controlling alcoholism. Reduces time it takes ulcers to heal. Promotes wound and burn healing. Aids in muscle-wasting prevention, particularly important for those who are bed ridden or chronically ill. Beneficial in treatments for impotence.

Thomas Welbourne of Louisiana State University College of Medicine discovered glutamine raised human growth hormone levels to four times their pretest levels. The results occurred regardless of age, in female and male test subjects ranging in age from 30 to 64.

*Dosage:* L-glutamine is usually taken in divided daily dosages totaling between 1000 to 4000 mg (1 to 4 grams). Best taken 30 minutes before, or 2 hours after, a meal or at bedtime. When used to treat depression, impotence, fatigue, alcoholism, senility and schizophrenia, seek the guidance of your health care provider.

***Warning:*** When used for treating children, always do it under proper medical supervision. Individuals with a sensitivity to monosodium glutamate (MSG), though different from glutamic acid and glutamine, may experience an allergic reaction. Before taking these supplements, speak to a doctor. Do not take if you have any of these conditions: kidney problems, cirrhosis of the liver or Reye's syndrome.

## *Glutathione*

Not an amino acid. It is a tripeptide. The amino acids cysteine, glycine and glutamic acid are involved in the production of glutathione. The liver produces this very powerful antioxidant, which helps detoxify the body, excreting toxins from the body. It is also found in the intestinal tract and lungs. It may have anti-aging properties. As we age, our stores of it decrease, and in turn the aging process accelerates. To counteract this, the least expensive and currently most effective way to increase your glutathione levels is to supplement with the amino acids glycine, glutamic acid and cysteine. For more information on glutathione, refer to Chapter 18.

## *Glycine*

– see also Dimethylglycine (DMG)

Glycine is a nonessential amino acid that the body can produce from within, if the necessary materials are there. It is used to build RNA and DNA, our genetic code carriers. It is essential for the production of bile acids and nucleic acids and for the synthesis of some nonessential amino acids. Glycine is found in muscle, skin and connective tissues. When needed, it converts to serine, another nonessential amino acid.

*Principal benefits:* Aids in treating certain types of low pH in the blood (acidemia), in particular those due to an imbalance of leucine, which manifests itself as bad breath and body odor. Improves low pituitary gland function. Critical for a healthy prostate. Vital for proper central nervous system functioning. Its neurotransmitter dampening affect can be beneficial in treating epileptic seizures. Useful in treating hyperactivity and manic-depressive disorder, also called bipolar disorder. Aids in the treatment of muscular dystrophy, due to its ability to produce creatine, which is vital for muscle function. Used in treatment of gastric hyperacidity, glycine is also a component of some gastric antacid drugs. Used in the treatment of hypoglycemia, since it stimulates glucagon production, which activate and release glycogen into the blood stream as glucose.

***Caution:*** While the right amount increases energy, excess amounts may cause fatigue.

## *Histidine*

A semi-essential amino acid, meaning external sources are needed to replenish its levels in the body. It is essential that babies and children get it through food or, if medically prescribed, supplementation. It is vital for the growth, maintenance and repair of tissues. Beneficial for maintaining proper red and white blood cell levels. Protects the nerve cells by maintaining their myelin sheathing, that is, their outer protective layers. Prevents radiation damage to the body. Helps remove potentially toxic heavy metals from the body.

Histidine is important in the production of the immune system chemical, histamine, which improves one's ability to experience sexual arousal and pleasure. To increase histamine levels, combine histidine with niacin (vitamin $B_3$) and pyridoxine (vitamin $B_6$).

*Principal benefits:* Improves rheumatoid arthritic conditions. Helps improve libido, sex drive. Alleviates stress and allergies. Beneficial for indigestion, since it increases gastric juice levels. May help prevent AIDS.

*Food sources:* Wheat, rye, rice, fish, poultry, pork, cheese.

***Caution:*** Excessive levels of histidine may result in psychological problems, such as schizophrenia and anxiety. Methionine can be used to lower histidine levels. Insufficient levels are associated with nerve deafness. Low levels may result in rheumatoid arthritis. Do not take histidine if you have manic-depressive disorder (bipolar disorder) unless a deficiency has been discovered.

## *Isoleucine*

An essential amino acid, meaning external sources are needed to replenish its levels in the body. Important for regulating and maintaining energy and blood sugar levels. Vital for hemoglobin formation. Isoleucine is metabolized in the muscles.

*Symptoms of deficiency:* May exhibit similar symptoms to hypoglycemia. Deficiencies are found in some physical and mental disorders.

*Principal benefits:* Increases endurance and enhances energy levels. Helps repair and heal muscles.

*Food sources:* Almonds, chicken, chickpeas, cashews, fish, eggs, lentils, meat, liver, rye, soy protein.

*Dosage:* Take it in a combination supplement. Since it is a three-branched chain amino acid, it should be taken with a two-branched chain amino acid, to maintain a proper balance. Use the most bio-available form, identified by 'L-'. The best ratio in a combination supplement is 1 part L-isoleucine, 2 parts L-leucine and 2 parts L-valine.

## *Leucine*

An essential amino acid, meaning external sources are needed to replenish its levels in the body. It is one of the three-branched chain amino acids.

*Principal benefits:* Helps protect muscles. Fuels muscles. Can reduce elevated blood sugar levels. Beneficial for bone, muscle and skin healing. Promotes faster recovery from surgery. Can increase human growth hormone levels.

*Food sources:* Beans, brown rice, nuts, meat, soy flour, whole wheat.

*Dosage:* Always take in a combination supplement with the following ratio: 1 part L-isoleucine, 2 parts L-leucine and 2 parts L-valine.

**Caution:** Moderately excessive amounts may result in symptoms of hypoglycemia. Very high levels may result in more ammonia being present in the body and may induce pellagra.

## *Lysine*

An essential amino acid, meaning external sources are needed to replenish its levels in the body. It is necessary for growth and tissue repair. Lysine is a vital building block for body proteins. It maintains an appropriate level of nitrogen in adults. It plays a key role in the production of antibodies, enzymes and hormones.

*Principal health benefits:* Vital for optimal growth and bone formation in children. Promotes efficient use of fatty acids needed for energy production. May be beneficial for menopausal women, who are at risk of getting osteoporosis, since lysine helps the body use calcium more effectively. Possibly helpful in resolving some fertility problems. Improves concentration. May reduce or prevent the incidence of herpes simplex infection – cold sores and fever blisters.

Studies indicate lysine is beneficial for patients suffering from chest pain (angina); patients were given 6 grams a day and improved enough that they could stop taking their sublingual (under the tongue) nitroglycerin tablets within four weeks, and were able to increase their exercise levels, allowing their hearts to heal faster. Lysine can lower high serum triglyceride levels and high blood pressure.

Lysine is also a beauty aid that keeps skin looking young and vibrant; it does this by encouraging collagen formation, the underlying tissue that supports the surface layer of skin, which is vital for preventing wrinkles and sagging skin, as well as tissue repair. Improves recovery time from sports injuries and surgery.

*Symptoms of lysine deficiency may include:* Anemia, proneness to bloodshot eyes, poor concentration, dizziness, hair loss, nausea, fatigue, enzyme disorders, irritability, poor appetite, reproductive problems, weight loss and retarded growth. Older people need more lysine, particularly males.

*Food sources:* Cheese, milk, eggs, fish, lima beans, red meat, potatoes, soy products, yeast, all protein-rich foods.

*Dosage:* To improve your skin and strengthen your bones, take 500 mg of L-lysine tablets or capsules 1 or 2 times a day, 30 minutes before meals. For an individual having an outbreak of herpes, take 3000 to 6000 mg (3 to 6 grams) a day and eat the lysine-rich foods mentioned above. To prevent recurrence, take 500 to 1000 mg a day. Speak to your health care provider concerning this form of treatment.

***Caution:*** When supplementing for heart conditions, always do so in consultation with your doctor or naturally oriented healer.

### *Methionine*

aussi s. nerveux/dépression

An essential amino acid, meaning external sources are needed to replenish its levels in the body. This amino acid contains sulfur. It breaks down fats and inhibits the buildup of fats in arteries and in the liver. It is a powerful antioxidant. Methionine is needed for the production of collagen and nucleic acids, and is vital for protein synthesis.

*Principal benefits:* Helps lower cholesterol. Aids the digestive system. Beneficial in treating Parkinson's disease and schizophrenia. In schizophrenics, it is beneficial since it lowers histamine levels in the blood; histamine may cause the wrong messages to be relayed in the brain. Helps detoxify the system of heavy metals and prevents chemical allergies. The more toxic materials in the body, the more you need methionine. Protects and helps neutralize toxins in the liver. Possible tumor prevention properties. Keeps hair supple. It contains sulfur, which kills infections and obliterates free radicals. Protects against the effects of radiation. Beneficial for treating rheumatic fever. Helps lessen pregnant toxemia. Promotes estrogen excretion, which is helpful for women on oral contraceptives. Methionine is needed for the production of cysteine and taurine.

*Deficiency symptoms:* The body's failure to break down urine, resulting in edema, the retention of fluids that causes swelling, and increased chances of infection. Possible connection with atherosclerosis and cholesterol deposits. A liver disorder called Gilbert's syndrome. Possible connection with hair loss.

*Food sources:* Beans, eggs, fish, garlic, lentils, lecithin granules, meats, onions, seeds, soybeans, yogurt.

*Dosages:* A combination that offers protection against some tumors is methionine with folic acid and choline. Supplement with lecithin (high in choline) or choline directly, since methionine is derived from them. Choline is an excellent 'brain food'. Consult with your health care provider if you want to try this.

**Note:** Nutritionally oriented health care practitioners have reported positive results in treating cancerous cells with a blend of methionine, grape seed oil and a combination of other nutrients. In one case, a patient with lung cancer showed no signs of the cancer or any scarring, three weeks after treatments started. The product called 'C-Gone' is available from LifeStar, 2175 East Francisco Blvd., San Rafael, CA 94901 (415) 457-1400 or (800) 858-7477. This is neither an endorsement of their products, nor a guarantee of its effectiveness.

## *Ornithine*

A nonessential amino acid, synthesized from arginine, which is a precursor of glutamic acid, proline and citrulline. It is found mainly in the connective tissue and skin. Ornithine promotes the discharge of human growth hormone and helps the liver regenerate by ridding the body of ammonia.

*Principal benefits:* Helps repair damaged tissues and promotes healing. Aids in building muscles. Increases the levels, benefits and potency of the amino acid, arginine. In fact, this is a circular system where arginine is produced from ornithine and ornithine is released by arginine. Releases growth hormone while you sleep which, in turn helps you slim down. Aids insulin secretion and insulin's work as a muscle building (anabolic) hormone.

*Food sources:* Brown rice, carob, chocolate, gelatin desserts, nuts, oatmeal, popcorn, all protein-rich foods, raisins, sesame seeds, sunflower seeds, whole wheat bread.

*Dosages:* Most effective when taken with arginine just before bed. Ingest on an empty stomach, in a glass of water or juice, without any protein, which interferes with utilization. It is available in powder and tablet forms. Take 2000 mg (2 grams). Body builders and those wanting to tone their muscles can take 2000 mg (2 grams) on an empty stomach, one hour before vigorous exercise.

***Warning:*** Since ornithine and arginine are best taken together and are so closely related, the following approach is prudent: Supplementation is not recommended for pregnant or nursing mothers, unless medically warranted and suggested by your doctor. Do not give to infants or growing children, since arginine may cause giantism. If dwarfism is the infant's or child's problem, discuss the options with your health care provider before using any amino acid supplements. Do not give to those with schizophrenic problems. Individuals with herpes should not use supplements or eat foods rich in arginine. Excessively large dosages of 20 or more grams can cause bone and joint deformities. If you take too much arginine, over a period of several weeks, your skin can become course or thicken. Reduce your arginine intake to allow the problem to rectify itself.

### *Phenylalanine*

– see also DL-Phenylalanine (DLPA)

An essential amino acid, meaning external sources are needed to replenish its levels in the body. Phenylalanine becomes tyrosine, another amino acid. It is intimately involved with the central nervous system. Tyrosine becomes two vital neurotransmitters, norepinephrine and dopamine, that promote alertness.

*Principal benefits:* Critical to alleviating depression, phenylalanine enables the brain to release the antidepressants norepinephrine and dopamine. Increases libido (sex drive). Helps memory and mental alertness. Aids in appetite suppression. Used to treat menstrual cramps, migraines, obesity, schizophrenia, arthritis and Parkinson's disease. In some forms it relieves pain.

*Food sources:* Almonds, cottage cheese, lima beans, peanuts, protein rich foods, pumpkin seeds, powdered skim milk, sesame seeds, soy products.

*Dosage:* Tablets are available in 250 and 500 mg sizes. Not addictive. To increase vitality and alertness, take between meals with juice or water, but not protein. To control appetite, take one hour before meals with water or juice, but not protein. Note: Phenylalanine is not metabolized if you are deficient in vitamin C.

***Caution:*** Do not supplement with phenylalanine during pregnancy or if you have skin cancer (contraindicated for people with pigmented malignant melanomas) or phenylketonuria (PKU). If suffering from high blood pressure or a heart condition, consult with your doctor before using this supplement as it may increase blood pressure. If your doctor okays its use, it is advisable to take it half an hour after meals. Do not take with antidepressants, MAO inhibitors, St. John's wort and Licorice root.

***Note:*** DL-Phenylalanine or DLPA is another form of phenylalanine combined with equal amount of synthetic D- and natural L-phenylalanine. This produces and activates endorphins, the body's natural pain-killer. They are more powerful than opium derivatives and morphine. Selective in its pain reducing qualities, it can help chronic pain sufferers since it does not interfere with the natural short-term acute pain defense mechanisms of the body for injuries such as cuts, burns and scrapes.

*DL-Phenylalanine is beneficial in the following conditions:* lower back pain, muscle and leg cramps, migraines, osteoarthritis, postoperative pain, rheumatoid arthritis, whiplash. Powerful anti-depressant. Pain relief that gets more effective the longer used and you do not build up a tolerance to it – up to one month without using additional drugs. When used in conjunction with other therapies and drugs, it has no known adverse interactions and can increase the pain killing benefits. It is non-toxic.

## *Proline*

A nonessential amino acid, which means the body can produce it on its own.

*Principal benefits:* Increases ability to learn. Promotes wound recovery by healing cartilage and strengthening tendons, joints and the heart muscle. Acts synergistically with vitamin C, in keeping the connective tissue healthy. Aids the body's ability to produce collagen, which keeps the skin youthful and vibrant.

*Food sources:* Primarily meat.

## *Serine*

A nonessential amino acid, which means the body can produce it on its own. It can be made from glycine in the body. Serine helps diminish pain. It can mimic the actions of a natural antipsychotic. It is required for efficient metabolism of fatty acids and fats and for proper muscle growth. It facilitates production of antibodies and immunoglobulins, and helps maintain the immune system.

## *Taurine*

A nonessential amino acid, which means the body can produce it on its own, if given the needed materials. It is also known as the 'brain amino acid'. It is found primarily in heart tissues, the central nervous system, white blood cells and skeletal muscles. It is a building block for other amino acids.

Taurine can improve heart function. Japanese doctors use it to treat congestive heart failure and lower blood pressure. Reduces enlarged prostrate. Helps detoxify and alleviate liver congestion. Protects the brain. It utilizes choline which promotes one's ability to think and maintains neurotransmitters. May help in the treatment of brain malfunctions, such as epilepsy and anxiety. It is associated with zinc utilization for the eyes. Vital for fat-soluble vitamin absorption and creation of bile salts in the gallbladder, which are needed for proper digestion of fats. Critical for proper absorption of potassium, sodium, magnesium and calcium. Helps control serum cholesterol levels. Helpful in treating diabetes. Possibly beneficial for eye health and prevention of macular degeneration. It is a useful anti-aging supplement.

*Food sources:* Eggs, fish, milk, meat. It is not in vegetable proteins, but if there is enough vitamin $B_6$ in the body, as well as either cysteine or methionine, taurine can be synthesized.

*Drugs it may be an alternative for:* Phenobarbital and other chemotherapeutic drugs.

*Substances and problems that can lead to taurine deficiency:* Genetic or metabolic disorders. Excessive consumption of alcohol prevents the body from fully using taurine. Emotional stress, yeast infections (Candida albicans), cardiac arrhythmias, zinc deficiency, diabetes, intestinal problems, improper platelet formation.

*Diseases it may help treat:* Heart disease, cardiac arrhythmias, Down syndrome, epilepsy, anxiety, hyperactivity, seizures, hypertension, hypoglycemia, edema, diabetes, macular degeneration, muscular dystrophy.

*Dosage:* Take up to 1500 mg of capsules daily, with water or juice, on an empty stomach at least half an hour before meals. Diabetics should be monitored by their doctor or natural health care professional since they usually need more taurine. Taken with cystine, it may reduce the need for insulin.

***Caution:*** Taurine is a depressant. Large doses may result in loss of short-term memory.

### *Threonine*

An essential amino acid, meaning the body cannot manufacture it on its own and must receive it from an outside source. It is vital for the production of purines, which break down uric acid, itself a by product of protein digestion. An excess of uric acid may be responsible for gout, a form of arthritis, and other health problems. Threonine is also vital for the production of the nonessential amino acid, glycine.

Threonine is found mainly in the heart, skeletal muscles and central nervous system. It is vital for collagen and elastin formation. When threonine is combined with methionine and aspartic acid, it aids lipotropic and liver function. It is very helpful for prevention of fatty buildup in the liver. It boosts production of antibodies, which in turn improves the immune system. Vital for protein utilization in one's diet, as well as maintaining the appropriate protein balance.

***Caution:*** Vegetarians tend to be deficient in threonine, since their principle food sources, such as grains, are very low in it.

### *Tryptophan*

– also called L-tryptophan

It is an essential amino acid, meaning the body cannot manufacture it and needs to get it from an outside source. It is vital for the production of niacin (vitamin $B_3$). Tryptophan is the precursor to serotonin, which is important for sleep, appetite levels, stable moods and pain sensitivity.

The U.S. Food and Drug Administration (FDA), temporarily banned tryptophan in 1989 due to 26 deaths and hundreds of cases of reported illness in New Mexico, supposedly due to tryptophan. It was later discovered to be a problem at the Japanese manufacturer's plant. A toxic chemical accidentally contaminated batch of L-tryptophan. According to the Atlanta Center for Disease Control, no one has died or become ill due to properly processed L-Tryptophan.

*Principal benefits:* Anti-depressant qualities. Alleviates some alcohol-related chemical body problems. Helps control alcoholism. Reduces nicotine cravings. Natural tranquilizer reducing anxiety and tension. Best utilized with vitamins $B_6$ (pyridoxine) and $B_3$ (niacin) and the trace mineral magnesium to help the brain synthesize serotonin. Magnesium and tryptophan may prevent coronary artery spasms. Promotes sleep naturally. Alleviates migraines. Beneficial for treating hyperactivity. Promotes the release of human growth hormone.

*Food sources:* Bananas, brown rice, cottage cheese, dried dates, fish, milk, meat, peanuts, turkey and protein rich-foods.

*Dosage:* L-tryptophan is available through your doctor. When taking it, you should also take a balanced and complete B-complex vitamin formula that has at least 50 to 100 mg of $B_1$, $B_2$ and $B_6$ with your first or last meal of the day. To induce sleep, take 500 mg of tryptophan a half hour before bed with vitamin $B_6$ (100 mg), niacinamide (100 mg) and chelated or citrated magnesium (120 to 130 mg). Take it with juice or water, but not protein. As a relaxant, take between meals, during the day, with water or juice, but not protein nor milk. Single dosages over 2000 mg (2 grams) are not recommended.

## *Tyrosine*

A quasi-essential amino acid sometimes synthesized from methionine or phenylalanine.

*Principal benefits:* Can help suppress appetite. Critical neurotransmitter as it stimulates and modifies brain activity. The mood elevator phenylalanine must first be converted to tyrosine, without which norepinephrine will not be made in the brain, and this would result in depression. Acts as a mood elevator by aiding in neural brain activity by increasing the rate neurons produce the antidepressants norepinephrine and dopamine. Used to control medication resistant depression. Used to reduce the amount of amphetamine a patient is taking. Helps reduce the side effects of cocaine withdrawal such as depression, irritability and fatigue. Improves libido (sex drive). Alleviates stress.

*Dosage:* The use of tyrosine to alleviate cocaine withdrawal symptoms is more effective when combined with vitamins $B_1$, $B_2$, C, niacin, and the enzyme tyrosine hydroxylase, in a glass of orange juice.

***Caution:*** Contraindicated for people with pigmented malignant melanomas. May increase blood pressure. Not to be taken with antidepressants and MAO inhibitors, St. John's Wort or Licorice root.

## *Valine*

An essential amino acid, meaning the body cannot manufacture it and must get it from an outside source. It is a branched-chain amino acid, which is important for supplying energy to muscles. One key role is its stimulating effect. It aids muscle metabolism and is concentrated in the muscles. Balances the body's nitrogen levels.

*Principal benefits:* Aids tissue repair. Helps correct drug addiction-induced amino acid deficiencies.

*Food sources:* Grains, dairy products (especially cottage cheese), mushrooms, meats, peanuts, soy proteins.

*Valine deficiency:* May negatively affect the myelin covering of nerves.

*Dosage:* Always take in a balanced combination supplement having the following ratio: 2 parts L-valine, 1 part L-isoleucine and 2 parts L-leucine. For example, 2 mg L-valine, 1 mg L-isoleucine, 2 mg L-leucine.

***Caution:*** Very high dosages can result in a crawling sensation on the skin, and could even lead to hallucinations. If any symptoms occur, stop taking the supplement and see your health care provider.

# chapter 14

# Herbal Medicines

## Why, when and how to safely use herbs

## Terms and methods of use

## Quick Reference List of Common Uses of Herbs

### *Why use herbal medicines?*

Herbal medicine, also called Phytotherapy, is the science of using substances from plants to treat illness. It is the primary method of medical intervention used around the world, and is being rediscovered by North Americans. Phytotherapy is often a safer way to treat illness and maintain health. Vast amounts of research, studies and reports from doctors, principally in European and Far Eastern countries, have shown the incredible power of these natural herbal remedies.

Herbal medicines are made from the leaves, roots, seeds and/or stems of medicinal plants, which usually contain buffers or natural factors, which protect the body against the possible toxic effects of these medicinal plant products. The active ingredients are known as phytopharmaceuticals because of their beneficial physiological effects.

Humanity and plant life evolved in partnership. When we breath, we inhale oxygen and exhale a waste product called carbon dioxide. In turn, trees and plants need carbon dioxide and release oxygen. Sciences such as evolutionary biology and environmental studies examine these intimate and vital processes that govern life on our planet.

Pharmaceutical drugs are often synthetic versions, based on the benefits of herbal medicines. These drugs can be very toxic due to their chemical nature. As with any toxin, the body does not recognize the natural healing properties of these synthetic drugs and seeks to expel them from the body. The result can be damage to healthy body parts, particularly the kidneys and liver, plus undesirable side effects and chemical, as well as physiological, stress.

Growing interest from the public and health care professionals is leading to research into the potentially safer and more effective herbal remedies. Though this research remains in its infancy in North America, numerous studies are available from German, British, Chinese, Indian and Australian medical and pharmacological publications. These form the basis of the following information.

It should be noted that correct choices and dosages may vary with each medical condition, the individual's sex, age, physical and emotional states. Herbal product regulations tend to increase costs and make these inexpensive complementary alternatives much more expensive. It is possible that over-regulation, using a pharmacologically based system, may drive the cost so high that fewer and fewer consumers will be able to afford them.

## *A Unique Perspective — Chinese health care principles*

The foundation of Chinese health care is the grand principle of yin and yang. All things are seen as having these qualities: dynamic, polar and cyclic. The universe is guided by cycles, on micro and macro levels.

Yin is the energy gathering, assimilation and storing part of the cycle. Often associated with sensitivity, calm and rest. Yin herbs are described as cool. It is the essence of life and all functioning.

Yang is the energy use part of the cycle, which manifests action. Often associated with activity and expansion. Yang herbs are described as warm. It is the essential working part of any process.

Yin and yang co-exist. Their natures create balance and harmony in the universe. If one's health is not optimal, it is seen as an imbalance in these critical life forces. Chinese medicinal herbs are prescribed which restore the natural yin-yang balance.

## *How to safely and effectively use herbs*

### *Key definitions describing the health benefits of herbs*

Alteratives – purify blood.

Analgesics – relieve pain.

Antacids – counteract excess stomach and intestinal acidity.

Antiabortives – reduce abortive tendencies.

Antiasthmatics – alleviate asthma symptoms.

Antibiotics – inhibit growth and/or destroy amoebas, bacteria and viruses.

Anticatarrhals – counteract or eliminate mucus formation.

Antipyretics – reduce or prevent fever.

Antiseptics – stop and prevent bacterial growth on the skin.

Antispasmodics – prevent muscle spasms; muscle relaxants.

Aphrodisiacs – increase or improve libido, sexual power and potency.

Astringents – cause body tissues to constrict or bind; reduce swelling.

Carminatives – alleviate gas and severe bowel pain.

Cholagogues – increase bile flow and discharge into small intestines.

Demulcents – protective substances that sooth inflamed or damaged tissues.

Diaphoretics – induce sweat.

Diuretics – reduce retained water by promoting urine flow.

Emetics – stomach-emptying and vomit-inducing herbs.

Emmenagogues – promote menstruation, may increase blood flow and hasten monthly onset of menses.

Emollients – soothing, softening and protective substances for the skin.

Expectorants – help lungs and throat rid themselves of mucus.

Galactogogues – increase lactation and mother's milk flow.

Hemostatics – stop hemorrhaging.

Laxatives – promote bowel movements.

Lithotriptics – eliminate and/or dissolve stones and gravel in the kidneys, bladder and gallbladder.

Nervines – balances the nervous system and calms nervous tension; also known as tonics, since they render the nervous system more adaptive.

Oxytocics – hormone-like substances that provoke uterine contractions.

Parasiticides – destroy parasites either internally or topically (on the skin).

Purgatives – promote bowel movements.

Rubefacients – draw blood away from congestion and inflammations from deeper sources, toward the surface of the skin; cause blushing, flushing or redness of the skin.

Sedatives – powerful nervous system calmers.

Sialagogues – benefit digestion of starches and stimulates saliva flow.

Stimulants – increase activity of body systems or parts.

Stomachics – tonics that provide a general positive effect on the stomach and the digestive system and aid their adaptability by improving their function.

Tonics – aid body systems' adaptability, by improving their function; provide a general positive effect on a part or all of the body.

Vulneraries – encourage cell growth and repair of wounds.

## *Key words defined for using herbs*

*Bolus* – a large pill.

*Bulk herbs* – as developed in nature. In the grocery store you find them as ginger root, garlic bulbs, dillweed, peppermint leaves and basil. Bulk herbs vary in strength and quality. They are unpredictable and unreliable in effectively delivering the active ingredients.

*Infusion* – preparation of an herbal tea. Pour 2 cups (946 ml) of boiling water over an ounce (59 ml) of bulk herb (roots, bark, seeds and/or stems). Two tablespoonsful is the usual infusion dose.

*Decoction* – a method of preparing an herbal remedy. To one ounce of the herbs' plant parts, add twenty-four ounces (3 cups, 1420 ml) of cold water; boil for thirty minutes; let the liquid cool down; then strain it. One tablespoon is the usual decoction dose.

*Extracts* – whole herbs in concentrated forms, such as tinctures, fluid extracts and solid extracts. All three forms provide effective means of delivering the therapeutic benefits of herbs.

*Fluid extracts* – use the process of evaporation to create a 1:1 concentration, which means one part of herbal matter to one part of solvent. They are usually five times stronger than the same amount of tincture, by volume. This is a good way to use herbs therapeutically.

*Gelatin capsule* – contains the bulk herb(s) ground into powder. Gelatin bulk herb capsules vary in strength and quality, and are an unpredictable and unreliable way of receiving the active ingredients in an effective dosage.

*Solid extracts* – remove the solvent, thereby producing the most concentrated form of the three types of extracts. They are measured it terms of the amount of grams of an herb per gram of the extract. A 5:1 concentration indicates that 5 grams of the herb were used to make 1 gram of the extract. That means 100 mg of a powder extract has the equivalent of 500 mg of herb. Of the three extract methods, this is an excellent choice, since it offers the greatest chemical stability.

*Standardization* – the key to product reliability. Herbal products are standardized if they have been scientifically analyzed, containing a guaranteed percentage of the active constituent or component, within a specific narrow range of variance. Consistent levels of herbal matter are in the product. Many standardized preparations have a lot of active ingredients that act synergistically with each other. Those that insure a range of therapeutic components of a herb are better than those that isolate and guarantee only one active ingredient.

*Tablets* – the bulk herb(s) are ground into powder, then formed into tablets. Bulk herb tablets vary in strength and quality. This is an unpredictable and unreliable way of receiving the active ingredients in an effective dosage.

*Tinctures* – least concentrated of the three forms of extract. The herb is soaked in a solvent, like alcohol or water, for a set time, after which the solution is pressed out. The strength of a tincture is measured as a concentration. Usually a tincture is in a 1 to 5 (1:5) concentration, which means 5 parts of solvent for 1 part of herbal matter. This is a good way to use herbs therapeutically.

## *Safeguards and quality control checklist for herbs*

Wildcrafted herbs are found in nature. They may be effective, but it is better to use cultivated, organically grown herbs. Environmental issues and the threat to our ecosystem of losing valuable plant life, make even more pressing that herbs and plants growing wild be left alone.

Cultivated and organically grown herbs do not vary as much genetically as wildcrafted herbs, since they are grown in controlled conditions without harmful pesticides. This nets a more consistent final product.

At a minimum, any herbal product should be analyzed for its identity, any impurities, and potency. Read the labels and check the following:

Does the amount of active ingredient in the product give you the dosage you require?

Is it a standardized herb product? Standardized whole herb products are preferred.

What is the product's expiration date?

Are the directions for dosages and safety clearly indicated?

## *Herbs are versatile. Discover how plus a list of symptoms and what herbs to use*

The following uses are for dried bulk herbs. For prepackaged herbs, follow label directions. For herbs as stress busters:

### *For emotional stress use:*

Hops for relaxation. Mix 1/2 teaspoon in 1/2 cup of distilled water. Drink daily.

Passionflower is great for times of acute anxiety. Mix 15 to 60 drops of extract in a liquid. Drink daily. Not recommended during pregnancy

Valerian is known as mother nature's tranquilizer. Take one to three capsules daily, or ten drops of extract in liquid.

Skullcap is a very old remedy for stress. Make a home-brewed tea with 1 teaspoon of dried herb in one cup of hot water or mix three to twelve drops of extract in liquid. Take daily. Another alternative is to take one capsule three times daily.

### *Insomnia a problem?*

Stress can interfere with the ability to fall asleep. Try an herbal sleep formula in teas, tinctures, extracts or capsules. They're available in most health food stores. The preferred one combines balm, hops, chamomile, oats, passionflower and valerian.

Valerian, is one of the best herbs for sleep. It reduces activity in the central nervous system.

Hops is a sedative and digestive tonic, which may also help you relax. You can get dried hop flowers; put them in an air permeable bag and place under your pillow.

Siberian ginseng is known as one of the best herbal tonics. It also may cure insomnia.

***Fatigue become a source of stress?***

Use herbs to reenergize. Try these:

Cayenne's mildly stimulating properties may help. Try a cup of cayenne tea.

American, Panax or Siberian ginsengs, if taken consistently can help eliminate fatigue. They're available in capsules, extracts, whole green food formulae and teas.

Schizandra is a Chinese herb believed to increase stamina and energy.

Ma huang (Ephedra) is a long acting stimulant. A cup of ma huang tea is said to perk you up.

## *More mood enhancers*

The mood elevator *Ginkgo biloba* contains active ingredients that increase oxygen uptake and blood flow. Alleviates stress-producing symptoms by improving memory loss, depression, brain function, as well as cerebral and peripheral circulation. It may take a few days to weeks before sufficient amounts of the active ingredients, ginkgolides and heterosides, accumulate in your body to cause the wanted results. Suddenly, you may realize symptoms have been alleviated or disappeared altogether.

Some conditions it may help include: Alzheimer's disease, impotence, poor memory, asthma, tinnitus, heart and kidney disorders. It may improve your body's ability to utilize glucose.

What outsells Prozac, one of North America's top selling antidepressants, by more than 20 to 1 in Europe? According to the highly respected investigative TV show *60 Minutes*, St. John's Wort (Hypericum perforatum) is used by psychiatrists and other mental health care practitioners throughout Europe, more than any other antidepressant. It is a perennial with regular flowers which bloom during the summer.

St. John's Wort contains many active ingredients including pseudohypericin, hypericin, xanthrones and flavonoids. Xanthrones and hypericin contain monoamine oxidase (MAO) inhibitors that slow the breakdown of the neurotransmitters norepinephrine and serotonin in the brain. Too much serotonin makes people obsessive and anxious, while too little is thought to be a major cause of depression.

Clinical trials with hypericin extract show improved alleviation of stressful depressive symptoms, such as anxiety, apathy and insomnia. Add to that the healing and anti-inflammatory properties that current research into flavonoids indicates and the possible antiviral properties of hypericin and pseudohypericin, and you have a powerful healing plant. One of the greatest benefits of St. John's Wort, is that it appears to have none of the side effects of pharmaceutical drugs.

### *How to use this quick reference section*

First, look up the condition or problem.

Then check for the herbs you can use.

Next, refer to the information about that specific herb and see if it is the best choice for your situation.

***Tip:*** For a comprehensive list of all the remedies in this book, refer to the index for pages covering the condition or problem you looked up.

| ***Condition*** | ***Herbs you can use*** |
|---|---|
| Allergies | Nettles, Echinacea, Golden Seal, Bee Pollen. |
| Antibacterial | Angelica, Barberry, Echinacea, Garlic, Tea Tree Oil. |
| Anticarcinogenic | Rosemary. |
| Anticatarrhal | Elder, Goldenseal, Hyssop, Sandalwood. |
| Antidepressant | Damiana, Lavender, Licorice, Oats, Rosemary, St. John's Wort, Schizandra. |
| Antifungal | Black Walnut, Cinnamon, Garlic, Propolis, Tea Tree Oil. |
| Anti-inflammatory | Devil's Claw, Oak Bark, Passionflower, Plantain, White Willow, Tea Tree Oil. |
| Antiseptic | Black Walnut, Oak Bark, Peppermint, Propolis, Sage, Tea Tree Oil, Thyme. |

| | |
|---|---|
| Antispasmodic | Camomile, Catnip, Motherwort, Passionflower, Peppermint, Red Clover, Rosemary, Thyme, Valerian. |
| Antiviral | Astragalus, Echinacea, Garlic, St. John's Wort, Tea Tree Oil. |
| Aphrodisiac | Cinnamon, Damiana, Ginseng, Puncturevine, Schizandra. |
| Arthritis /Rheumatism | Alfalfa, Black Cohosh, Devil's Claw, Glucosamine, Sarsaparilla, Tea Tree, White Willow, Wild Yam. |
| Asthma | Blessed Thistle, Blue Cohosh, Coltsfoot, Elecampane, Ginkgo Biloba, Goldenseal, Horehound, Licorice, Mullein, Platycodon, Wild Cherry. |
| Astringent | Goldenseal, Nettles, Oak Bark, Plantain, Red Raspberry, Rhubarb, Sage, Tea Tree Oil, True Unicorn, Wild Cherry, Wood Betony, Yellow Dock. |
| Anxiety | Chamomile, Kava Kava, St. John's Wort (used more specifically for mild to moderate depression). |
| Bladder/Kidney | Alismatis Plantago, Birch, Cranberry, Eucommia Ulmoides, Goldenseal, Marshmallow, Nettle Leaves, Poria Cocos, Sarsaparilla, Uva Ursi |
| Blood Purifiers | Blessed Thistle, Burdock, Milk Thistle (used more specifically to detoxify the liver), Red Clover, Sarsaparilla. |
| Bronchial Support | Coltsfoot, Elecampane, Fenugreek, Goldenseal, Horehound, Hyssop, Licorice, Mullein, Myrrh, Platycodon, Schizandra, Thyme. |
| Cardiovascular | Fo-Ti, Butcher's Broom, Hawthorn, Ginkgo Biloba, Lily of the Valley, Mistletoe, Motherwort, Oats, Reishi. |
| Cholesterol | Garlic, Gugulipid, Hawthorn, Linden, Reishi. |
| Chronic Fatigue Syndrome | Licorice Root. |
| Circulatory | Bioflavonoids, Capsicum, Garlic, Ginger, Ginkgo Biloba, Gotu Kola, Hawthorn, Prickly Ash. |

| | |
|---|---|
| Colds/Flu | Boneset, Catnip, Echinacea, Elder, Goldenseal, Peppermint, Platycodon, Tea Tree Oil, Zinc Lozenge. |
| Cough | Coltsfoot, Horehound, Licorice (daytime usage), Platycodon, Slippery Elm, Wild Cherry Bark. |
| Depression (mild) | Kava Kava, Licorice, St. John's Wort. Recent studies indicate St. John's Wort is also effective in treating some moderate to deep depressions. |
| Diarrhea | Chamomile, Golden Seal, Nettles, Oak Bark, Plantain, Red Raspberry, Rhubarb, Sage, Tea Tree, Thyme, True Unicorn, Wild Cherry, Wood Betony, Yellow Dock. |
| Digestive Aids | Barberry, True Unicorn, Wild Cherry Bark, Wood Betony, Yellow Dock. |
| Diuretics | Buchu, Corn Silk, Couch Grass, Dandelion, Parsley, Rosehips, Uva Ursi, Sandalwood. |
| Ear Ache | Garlic, Mullein Oil, Sage (swab in and around the ear), Tea Tree Oil. |
| Eczema | Burdock, Chickweed, Goldenseal, Nettles, Red Clover, Tea Tree Oil. |
| Expectorant | Elecampane, Fenugreek, Garlic, Horehound, Hyssop, Licorice, Mullein, Plantain, Platycodon, Sage, Thyme. |
| Eyes | Bilberry, Eyebright, Camomile – for eye wash. |
| Fever | Echinacea, Nettles, Sage, Tea Tree Oil, Thyme, White Willow, Wild Indigo, Yarrow. |
| Flatulence | Fennel, Ginger, Peppermint, Sage. |
| Flu/Colds | Boneset, Catnip, Echinacea, Elder, Goldenseal, Peppermint, Platycodon, Tea Tree Oil, Zinc Lozenge. |
| Hair | For baldness prevention and regrowth of hair; Fo-Ti, Saw Palmetto. To restore graying or gray hair to its natural color, Fo-Ti. |
| Hay Fever | Echinacea, Nettles. See allergies for additional possibilities. |

| | |
|---|---|
| Headache | Ginger, Lavender, Linden, Passionflower, Peppermint, Rosemary, Valerian, White Willow, Wood Betony. |
| High Blood Pressure | Coenzyme Q10, Garlic, Hawthorn, Mistletoe, Yarrow. |
| Immune System Support | Astragalus, Cat's Claw, Echinacea, Garlic, Nettles, Pau D'Arco, Propolis, Reishi, Schizandra, Shiitake. |
| Impotency | Damiana, Ginseng, Oats, Sarsaparilla. |
| Kidney/Bladder | Couch Grass, Cranberry, Meadowsweet, Uva Ursi. |
| Laxative | Aloe Vera, Cascara Sagrada, Rhubarb (don't forget prunes and prune juice). |
| Liver | Barberry, Blessed Thistle, Boneset, Fo-Ti, Lipoic Acid, Milk Thistle, Yellow Dock. |
| Lymphatics | Echinacea, Poke Weed, Red Clover. |
| Male Hormonals | Damiana, Ginseng, Oats, Puncture Vine, Sarsaparilla, Saw Palmetto. |
| Menopause | Black Cohosh, Dong Quai, Evening Primrose Oil, Licorice, Wild Yam, Soya (Isoflavones). |
| Mental Alertness | Ginkgo Biloba, Gotu Kola, Periwinkle (good for senility), Rosemary. |
| Migraine | Feverfew, Caffeine (in some cases), Ginger, White Willow<br>See Headache for other non-migraine choices. |
| Mouthwash | Chlorophyll, Oak Bark, Myrrh Gum, Tea Tree Oil. |
| Nausea | Ginger, Peppermint, Red Raspberry. |
| Nervines | Chamomile, Hops, Kava Kava, Linden, Oats, Passionflower, Reishi, Rosemary, Skullcap, Valerian. |
| Oral Mouthwash and Antiseptic | Chlorophyll, Oak Bark, Myrrh Gum, Tea Tree Oil. |
| Pain | Hops, Valerian, White Willow. (You may also want to add an Immune System Support herb, depending on the cause and nature of the pain.) |

| | |
|---|---|
| Peptic Ulcers (gastric, duodenal) | Aloe Vera, DGL (Deglycyrrhizinated Licorice), Goldenseal, Chamomile. Use Bismuth with the herbals (the main ingredient in Pepto Bismol is bismuth). |
| Premenstrual Syndrome | Black Cohosh, Dong Quai, Evening Primrose Oil, Licorice. |
| Prostate | Flax Seed, Lycopene, Pumpkin Seed, Pygeum Africanum, Saw Palmetto, Stinging Nettle, Uva Ursi. |
| Psoriasis | Burdock, Chickweed, Echinacea, Evening Primrose Oil, Flax Seed Oil, Red Clover, Sarsaparilla, Yellow Dock. |
| Respiratory | Astragalus, Elecampane, Goldenseal, Horehound, Mullein, Myrrh, Platycodon. |
| Rheumatism /Arthritis | Alfalfa, Black Cohosh, Devil's Claw, Glucosamine, Sarsaparilla, Tea Tree Oil, White Willow, Wild Yam. |
| Senility | Periwinkle. |
| Shingles | Echinacea, Oats, Passionflower. (In addition, proper nutrition and stress support are very important.) |
| Sore Throat | Echinacea, Platycodon, Red Raspberry, Sage, Slippery Elm, Tea Tree Oil, Wild Indigo. |
| Stomachics | Chamomile, Fennel, Ginger, Peppermint. |
| Tonics | Fo-Ti, Ginseng, Gotu Kola, Nettles, Oat, Platycodon, Reishi, Schizandra. |

## *The Top 100 plus Western, European, Indian and Chinese Herbs*

### *Aconite (Aconitum carmichaeli)*

Also known as ***Fu tzu***. In the Chinese healing system, aconite is a warm herb considered the most 'Yang' of all Chinese herbs.

*Source:* Root.

*Principal body systems and parts it benefits:* Circulation, heart, nervous system, small intestine, spleen, urinary tract system.

*Principal health related actions:* Analgesic, antispasmodic, diaphoretic, diuretic, stimulant, tonic.

*Suggested uses:* Stimulates sexual potency. Reduces flatulence. Alleviates uncomfortable and painful conditions such as arthritis, neuralgia, numbness, coldness, pain, sciatica.

*Dosage:* Used in liniments. Orally it is always used in combination with other herbs appropriate to the condition. Never use dosages higher than 2 grams. See Caution.

***Caution:*** Only use under the supervision of a naturopath or Chinese medicine doctor. Excessive oral or topical use can be toxic. Should not be used by individuals who are considered to have a Yang condition. Not for use by hypertensives – people with high blood pressure.

### *Alfalfa (Medicago sativa)*

*Source:* Leaves and flowers.

*Principal health related actions:* Diuretic, tonic.

*Suggested uses:* Improves appetite. Increases lactation in nursing mothers. Thins blood. Cleanses kidneys. Relieves bowel and urinary problems such as cystitis and inflammation of the bladder. Boosts energy and endurance. Relieves constipation. May reduce inflammation and swelling due to rheumatism. Helps stomach ailments including peptic ulcers. Eliminates retained water. Very good source of nutrients since it contains trace minerals, eight digestive enzymes, eight essential amino acids, vitamins and vitamin U for peptic ulcers.

*Suggested dosage:* Use fresh alfalfa sprouts in salads and as a condiment with foods. As a dried herb use 1 to 1 1/2 tablespoons with 8 ounces (1 cup) of warm water and drink daily. Take tablets or capsules as per instructions or 2 to 6 each day.

***Caution:*** This is a deep rooted plant. When supplementing with it we only recommend organically sourced and certified alfalfa. If you have an autoimmune disorder, such as lupus or SLE, do not use this herb. Do not use if taking blood thinners.

### *Aloe Vera (Aloe barbadensis)*

A hardy succulent plant that is easy to grow indoors. Its Chinese name is ***Lu Hui***. It is a good air cleaner for pollutants in homes and offices.

Nutrient dense, aloe vera is filled with health promoting aloin, amino acids, minerals, polysaccharides and vitamins.

*Source:* Leaves.

*Principal health related actions:* Emollient, heals burns and wounds, laxative, purgative.

*Suggested uses:* Air purifier. When taken orally it helps rid adults with bronchial asthma of waste material in the lungs, soothes and heals stomach. For use as a laxative, the amount you drink depends on the product's concentration and label directions. With most products you can drink up to 1 cup (8 ounces) before bed time. Aloe vera juice is an excellent laxative. Externally aloe vera as a gel may be used as needed. It is beneficial for bug bites, burns, skin irritations, minor cuts and scratches.

*Dosage:* Orally in juice or gel forms, take as per instructions. Usually, 1 tablespoon (15 ml) 3 times a day. In capsules, take 1 capsule three times a day. As a laxative, drink up to 1 cup (8 ounces) before bed time. Do not use for more than a few days as a laxative, as this could cause the bowels to become lazy and weak. Switch to prune juice, a delicious and safe laxative.

***Caution:*** Children, pregnant women and elderly should not take aloe vera juice internally. Make sure the aloe product you use lists aloe as the first or second ingredient or states that it is 95 percent or more pure aloe vera. Adulterated, watered down or diluted products are usually not effective for health-related uses. It is very important to check the label, to ensure you get what you want. Be sure burn treatments with aloe vera do not contain lanolin since lanolin intensifies burns.

***Note:*** There are many varieties of aloe vera plants. These succulents are easy to grow in the home, requiring sunlight, sandy soil and the occasional watering. When needed, snap off a leaf and spread the gel on the affected area. An excellent alternative to aloe vera gel, for external use, is tea tree oil which is analgesic (pain killing) and six times more powerful than aloe vera gel in bactericidal properties. (*The Tea Tree Oil Bible* is an excellent guide to hundreds of ways to use tea tree oil for health, home and pet care. To order your copy, refer to the back of this book.)

### *Angelica (Angelica archangelica)*

For Chinese Angelica, see Dong Quai.

*Source:* Mainly the root.

*Principal health related actions:* Carminative, diaphoretic, emmenagogue, expectorant, stimulant.

*Principal body parts it benefits:* Blood, intestines, lungs and stomach.

*Suggested uses:* To help reduce feelings of cold in the extremities due to anemia or in people who get cold easily, as it aids blood flow to hands and feet. Expectorant for those with asthma and bronchitis, eliminates phlegm buildup; soothes stomach upset and indigestion. Eases painful menstrual cramps. May relieve swelling and pain from rheumatism when applied externally. Beneficial for reducing the itching caused by lice and helps eliminate them.

*Dosage:* Internally, you can take between 10 to 30 drops of a liquid tincture or extract, up to three times daily. Externally, rub the liquid onto the affected area.

***Caution:*** Do not exceed recommended dosages unless otherwise directed by your health care provider since large doses can affect your heart, blood pressure and breathing. Should be avoided by diabetics as it may increase blood sugar levels. Pregnant and lactating women should not use it. Avoid during prolonged exposure to sun and if taking blood thinners.

### *Anise (Umbelliferae)*
### *Aniseed (Pimpinella anisum)*

*Source:* Seeds.

*Principal body parts it benefits:* Kidney, liver, lungs, stomach.

*Principal health related actions:* Antispasmodic, carminative, diaphoretic, emmenagogue, expectorant, stimulant.

*Suggested uses:* alleviates abdominal pains, gas, nausea, colds and coughs. Targets several cold symptoms including a stuffy nose and tight chest. Clears phlegm.

### *Apricot seed (Prunus armeniaca)*

Also known as ***Ku xing ren*** in the Chinese healing system, apricot seed is a warm herb. In Chinese medicine it is not recognized or used for its purported anticancer properties.

*Source:* Kernel.

*Principal body parts it benefits:* Large intestines, lungs.

*Principal health related actions:* Demulcent, expectorant, lung tonic.

*Suggested uses:* Beneficial as a tonic which nourishes the lungs and helps eliminate toxic substances in the respiratory system.

*Dosage:* Only use under the supervision of a doctor of Chinese medicine, naturopath or nutritionally orientated physician.

**Caution:** Apricot kernels are the source of laetrile, an herb purported to be anticarcinogenic, which is banned in some states in the United States.

### *Arnica (Arnica montana)*

*Source:* Flower heads.

*Principal body system and part it benefits:* Blood, circulation.

*Principal health related actions:* Analgesic, stimulant.

*Suggested uses:* Externally as a liniment or oil for painful injuries and bruises. Sesquiterpene lactone helenalin is the main component in arnica, and accounts for its anti-inflammatory effect. Internally only use when a minute amount is prescribed by a naturally orientated health practitioner or in a homeopathic remedy.

### *Artichoke (Cynara scolymus)*

*Source:* Flower heads, roots and leaves.

*Principal health related actions:* Antidiarrhea, appetizing, choleretic, cleansing, diuretic, hypoglycemic, tonic.

*Suggested uses:* Helps the liver eliminate cholesterol from the blood. Its blood purifying abilities, by stimulating the liver, are so powerful that French doctors developed 'cynotherapy', exclusively using artichoke extract, to deal with many hepatobiliary conditions.

**Caution:** Individuals suffering from or prone to colitis, ileitis, chronic diarrhea, gallstones, stomach burns, stomach ulcers, or hepatitis should not stimulate their liver. Not recommended for pregnant or lactating women.

### *Asafoetida (Ferula assafoetida)*

Main ingredient in the Indian ayurvedic digestive formula ***hinga-shtak***. Taken as a pill or, more typically, a powder sprinkled on or blended with food to improve digestion and prevent gas, energy loss and mood swings that accompany consumption of some foods. Favored over garlic as a food flavoring in India and China, as it does not stay on the breath. A key ingredient in Worcestershire sauce.

*Source:* Gum resin.

*Principal body systems and parts it benefits:* Digestion, liver, stomach.

*Principal health related actions:* Antispasmodic, aromatic, carminative, digestant, expectorant.

*Suggested uses:* Colds and coughs, Candida albicans overgrowth, poor digestion, emotional swings (hysteria), food allergies or sensitivities, gas, hypoglycemia.

*Dosage:* Mix between 100 mg and 1 gram of the powdered gum with food or steep in boiling water.

### ***Ashwagandha (Withania somnifera)***

Also known as ***Indian ginseng***.

*Source:* Leaves and roots of *Withania somnifera* shrub.

*Principal health related actions:* Anti-inflammatory. Boosts immunity. Used in the Indian Ayurvedic medicinal system to treat arthritis, impotence, infertility and stress. Its range of beneficial affects has earned it a reputation as a tonic, reputed to increase physical and mental abilities. Called an adaptogen, due to its ability to help the body adapt to, and deal with, highly stressful situations.

*Suggested uses:* A reputed aphrodisiac, ashwagandha may enhance sex and treat infertility and impotence. Relieves arthritis and increases blood flow to urinary-genital region. May relieve stress. For sexually-related conditions, it is usually combined with puncturevine (tribulus). When combined with zinc, it may have powerful anti-inflammatory properties.

***Caution:*** Do not take ashwagandha during pregnancy, it can cause an abortion.

### ***Asparagus (Asparagus officinalis)***

The Indian Ayurvedic system uses asparagus, ***shatavari***, to promote fertility, alleviate menstrual pains, improve and increase milk production, generally acting as a tonic and aiding the female reproductive system. Chinese herbalists believe the root increases feelings of love and compassion, fostering patience in others.

*Source:* Root and sprouts.

*Principal body parts it benefits:* Kidneys and lungs.

*Principal health related actions:* Cardiac tonic, diuretic, demulcent tonic, laxative, mild sedative, nutrient tonic.

*Suggested uses:* The sprouts and shoots are used for bladder infections. The root is used for AIDS, consumption, fatigue and exhaustion, female hormones, gynecology, throat and lung dryness, TB (tuberculosis), and to improve emotional states of patience, love and compassion.

**Caution:** The root is contraindicated for those with the following problems: edema or obesity, unless combined with balancing spices, such as ginger and pepper.

*Dosage:* 5 to 15 grams of the root in a tea, decoction.

### *Astragalus (Astragalus membranaceus)*

Also known as ***huang chi*** in the Chinese healing system. A key Chinese medicinal herb that has a balancing affect upon the body's organs, internal systems and when used with other herbs.

*Source:* Root.

*Principal body parts it benefits:* Blood, kidneys, lungs, spleen.

*Principal health related actions:* Diuretic, stimulant, tonic.

*Suggested uses:* Increases energy, mildly stimulates. Improves and strengthens the immune system. For cancer patients, it may restore the immune system to normal levels of function. Builds resistance to disease and weakness. Supports and improves the benefits derived from other herbs. Improves digestion. Diuretic that reduces blood pressure by eliminating excess water in the body. Neutralizes fevers. Balances energy of internal organs.

*Dosage:* For tea, use a ball strainer with 4 to 18 grams a day. Take one to three 400 mg capsules each day or as directed.

**Caution:** If undergoing chemotherapy, first consult with a doctor who is knowledgeable about astragalus or any herbs, medications or supplements you want to use.

### *Barberry (Berberis vulgaris)*

*Source:* Root, bark.

*Principal body parts it benefits:* Gallbladder, kidneys.

*Suggested uses:* Improves appetite by increasing bile secretion. Beneficial for high blood pressure since it dilates the blood vessels. In a tea it is used as a mouthwash. The heart muscle is stimulated with low doses of barberry. When used with an equal amount of wild yam, it eliminates gas. Helps relieve constipation and purifies blood.

***Caution:*** In high dosages, it slows the respiratory system and heart. Only take under medical supervision.

### *Basil (Ocimum basilicum)*

Also known as ***St. Joseph Wort*** and ***sweet*** or ***common basil,*** and ***luole*** in Chinese healing system. Aromatic herb often used in Italian cooking.

*Source:* Herb.

*Principal body systems it benefits:* Digestive system, hepatic (blood) system.

*Principal health related actions:* Antispasmodic, carminative, galactoagogue, stomachic.

*Suggested uses:* Improves blood circulation. Aids and supports digestive system and related organs, eases stomach cramps, nausea, constipation, enteritis, gas, intestinal catarrh, gastric catarrh. Helps alleviate whooping cough symptoms. Externally applied to relieve itching from hives and soothe blood shot eyes. Subdues headaches and stimulates mental cognitive processes.

*Dosage:* Put 2 teaspoons (10 ml) of dried herbs in a tea strainer and add to 1 cup (8 ounces, 237 ml) of hot water; drink 1 to 3 cups a day. Add 1 tsp (5 ml) of honey if you want to boost its cough relieving benefits.

### *Bayberry Bark (Myrica cerifera)*

*Source:* Root bark and rhizome.

*Principal body parts it benefits:* Gallbladder, liver.

*Principal health related actions:* Astringent, alterative, anti-inflammatory, cholagogue, tonic.

*Suggested uses:* Cankers, hay fever, hemorrhage, clears mucous membranes, sinus congestion, wounds. Stops bleeding from uterus, lungs and colon. Improves circulation. For sores, it may be used externally as a poultice. The powder relieves nasal congestion and sinus problems when sniffed. Use in tea as a gargle for sore throats.

*Dosage:* Drink in a tea using 1 teaspoon of the dried herb. For liquid extracts, blend 10 to 20 drops, or as per label, in water or juice. You can massage the liquid extract onto varicose veins and hemorrhoids as needed. Look for 'standardized extract' on the capsules' label and follow directions.

***Caution:*** Large doses can cause vomiting and nausea.

## *Bilberry (Vaccinium myrtillus)*

Was used by Royal Air Force pilots during World War II to improve sight and prevent night blindness. Its active ingredients are anthocyanosides, the antioxidant protectors of small blood vessels and rebuilders of the light-adapting retinal pigments in the eyes. The prescription eye enhancing and protecting drug, Myrtocyan R, is derived from bilberry.

*Source:* Fruit.

*Principal health related actions:* Antiseptic, astringent, improves myopia (nearsightedness). It does this by speeding up the regeneration of visual purple (retinol purple) in the eyes. Protects and helps the vascular system. May have anticancer properties.

*Suggested uses:* Aids in preservation of eyesight and night vision. Prevents eye damage. Regulates bowels. Stimulates appetite. Helps improve circulation.

*Dosage:* For liquid extracts, blend 10 to 20 drops in juice or water, and drink it, up to three times a day. For capsules, look for 'standardized extract' on the label and take one 500 mg capsule up to three times a day. More effective when taken with an equal amount of vitamin C each time.

***Caution:*** Only use commercially prepared extracts or capsules from a reputable supplier which uses the fruit of this plant. Do not exceed the recommended dosages. The leaves of this plant can be poisonous when used over long time periods.

## *Bistort (Polygonum bistorta)*

*Source:* Root, leaf.

*Principal body part it benefits:* Blood.

*Suggested uses:* It is an astringent. Beneficial as a gargle and mouthwash for mouth inflammations, sore gums, and sore throats. Stops bleeding and hemorrhaging. Helps expel worms.

## *Black Cohosh (Cimicifuga racemosa)*

*Source:* Root.

*Principal body systems and parts it benefits:* Circulation, large intestines, liver, nervous system, female hormones.

*Principal health related actions:* Alterative, antispasmodic, diaphoretic, diuretic, emmenagogue, expectorant, sedative.

*Suggested uses:* Natural supplier of estrogen. Beneficial for almost all female problems such as hot flashes, and general discomfort from menopause and menstruation. Eases labor and birthing. Helps reduce pain due to neuralgia. Alleviates the soreness and swelling resulting from rheumatism. Relieves and reduces muscle spasms. Reduces the urge to cough by relaxing bronchial tubes. Helpful for treating asthma.

*Dosage:* For tinctures, take 10 to 30 drops in water or juice, once a day. For capsules, take one standardized extract up to three times a day.

***Caution:*** Never use during pregnancy. During labor, black cohosh should only be used under your doctor's supervision. Discontinue use if headaches occur. The headaches probably indicate your body has sufficient amounts of estrogen. Excessive doses may cause poisoning. You may use sarsaparilla and/or ginseng instead, for their progesterone. If a woman cannot tolerate black cohosh for female problems, she can substitute with blessed thistle.

## *Black Walnut (Julgans nigra)*

*Source:* Leaves, hulls.

*Principal body parts it benefits:* Skin, blood, bowels.

*Principal health related actions:* Antiseptic. Antifungal. Promotes bowel regularity. Antiparasitic. Unripe green hulled black walnut can rid the body of infestations by parasites, ringworm and worms. It kills parasites by oxygenating the blood.

*Suggested uses:* Use as a tincture, extract or powder. May be used topically as a poultice for skin problems, or taken internally for ringworm, worms, and other parasites, as well as poison oak and poison ivy. Helps relieve constipation. In powdered form it aids restoration of tooth enamel when used to brush teeth. May help eliminate warts, athlete's foot, and jock itch. Rub the extract onto the skin and it may help with herpes, psoriasis, eczema and skin parasites.

*Dosage:* For tinctures, blend 10 to 30 drops in juice or water, as per label and drink it daily. You can massage the extract directly onto the skin, twice a day.

***Caution:*** To avoid toxicity use only commercially prepared black walnut extracts.

### *Blessed thistle (Cnicus benedictus)*

Also known as ***holy thistle***.

*Source:* Aerial portions of the herb.

*Principal body parts it benefits:* Female problems involving hormones, lactation, menstrual cramps. Liver, spleen, stomach.

*Principal health related actions:* Alterative, antiseptic, astringent, bitter, hemostatic, vulnerary.

*Suggested uses:* To enrich and increase production of a nursing mother's milk. Beneficial for liver, pulmonary and urinary problems. Stimulates bile production in the liver. Improves circulation and memory. If a woman cannot tolerate black cohosh for female problems, she can use blessed thistle instead. Stimulates appetite. Reduces fevers. An ancient remedy given to girls before the onset of puberty, since it supposedly alleviates and prevents potential cramping problems. Until further studies are done, we do not recommend this use, as it may interfere with the natural hormonal changes that are occurring.

*Dosage:* For extracts, blend 10 to 20 drops in water or juice and take daily. For capsules, follow instructions of standardized extracts.

***Caution:*** Do not use during pregnancy.

### *Blue Cohosh (Caulophyllum thalictroides)*

Used to be known as ***Lydia Pinkhams***.

*Source:* Root.

*Principal body part it benefits:* Liver.

*Principal health related actions:* Anthelmintic, antispasmodic, diaphoretic, diuretic, emmenagogue.

*Suggested uses:* To ease the affects of dysmenorrhea and amenorrhea (menstrual irregularities), cramps, as well as childbirth pain. Expel intestinal worms.

**Caution:** Mildly toxic. Large doses may cause headaches, convulsions or thirst. Use activated charcoal to counteract negative side effects. Activated charcoal is a safe product used for intestinal disorders such as gas, diarrhea and food poisoning. It is available in pharmacies and health food stores.

### Boneset (Eupatorium perfoliatum)

*Source:* Leaves.

*Principal health related actions:* Diaphoretic, expectorant, febrifuge, laxative.

*Principal body parts it benefits:* Bowels, liver, lungs, stomach, uterus.

*Suggested uses:* Relieves constipation. Alleviates cold and flu symptoms of upper respiratory congestion and coughs. Loosens phlegm, opens nasal passages, reduces fever.

*Dosage:* For extracts, take 10 to 35 drops in juice or water, each day.

### Brigham tea (Ephedra nevadensis)

*Source:* Herb.

*Principal body parts it benefits:* Blood, sinuses.

*Suggested uses:* Excellent tonic best taken in spring. Blood purifier, clears sinus congestion.

**Caution:** May cause nervousness and restlessness as it contains ephedrine (adrenaline), a sympathetic nervous system stimulant. Do not use during pregnancy.

### Buchu (Barosma crenata or Barosma betulina)

*Source:* Leaves.

*Principal body part it benefits:* Bladder.

*Suggested uses:* Beneficial for urinary disorders, such as infections, urine retention, irritation, weakness and mucus. When buchu is taken with uva ursi it is more effective.

**Caution:** Do not use during pregnancy.

### Buckthorn (Rhamnus frangula)

*Source:* Bark.

*Principal body parts it benefits:* Bowels, skin.

*Suggested uses:* It is primarily used as a laxative that is not habit forming. It is also useful for treating constipation, gallstones, hemorrhoids, perspiration, skin problems, warts, worms.

**Caution:** If nausea occurs, discontinue use since this indicates that the body has had enough. Do not use during pregnancy.

### *Bupleurum (Bupleurum Chinese)*

Also known as ***Ch'ai hu***, it is recognized as the premium Chinese herb for detoxifying the liver.

*Source:* Root

*Principal body parts it benefits:* Gallbladder, liver, pericardium, uterus.

*Principal health related actions:* Alterative, analgesic for head or chest pains, antinauseant, antipyretic (reduces fever).

*Suggested uses:* Counteracts anxiety and dizziness. Detoxifies the liver. Relieves pain. Strengthens eyes and limbs. Excellent for toning leg muscles and premenstrual syndrome.

*Dosage:* 2 to 5 grams per day.

### *Burdock (Arctium lappa)*

*Source:* Root. Burrs and leaves also have specific uses.

*Principal body parts it benefits:* Blood, skin.

*Suggested uses:* Excellent blood purifier that does not cause irritation or nausea. Anti-inflammatory properties help reduce arthritic swelling and deposits on the joints. Treatment for genital and urinary tract infections. External or internal use benefits skin problems. The burrs from burdock are diuretic. Externally, the leaves are used for wounds, burns and other skin problems.

*Dosage:* Take as a capsule, drink in a tea or apply externally as a poultice. One tsp burdock root to three cups of water. Boil 30 minutes. Drink three cups a day.

**Caution:** Do not use during pregnancy or with children under two years old.

### *Butcher's broom (Ruscus aculeatus)*

*Principal health related actions:* Treatment for varicose veins, restoring circulation to vein. It is a diuretic helping to remove excess water from the body. The flowers help regulate and support the heart beat, preventing heart rhythm fluctuations.

***Camomile*** – see Chamomile.

***Capsicum*** – see Cayenne.

### *Cascara Sagrada (Rhamnus purshiana)*

Also known as ***Doans Pills***.

*Source:* Dried bark.

*Principal body parts it benefits:* Colon, gallbladder, liver.

*Principal health related actions:* Laxative, tonic.

*Suggested uses:* Acts on large intestines (stimulates peristalsis the dilations and contractions of the alimentary canal that move the contents onward). Useful for digestive problems such as constipation and dyspepsia. When taken internally it stimulates secretions in the pancreas, liver and stomach. For chronic constipation, you can stimulate the peristaltic action of the colon by slowly decreasing the dose taken. Tones the bowels. Best taken before bed, it soothes and relaxes the body's elimination system. Liver tonic. Most beneficial when taken on an empty stomach.

***Caution:*** Not for use by lactating or pregnant women. Do not use if suffering from diarrhea, abdominal pain or taking medication. Excessive use of laxatives can cause the bowels to become lazy.

### *Cat's Claw (Uncaria tomentosa)*

*Source:* Bark.

*Principal health related actions:* Antiviral, antioxidant, anti-tumor.

*Suggested uses:* Anti-inflammatory. Immune system booster. Stimulates pancreatic secretions and gastric juices. Beneficial in treatment of irritable bowel syndrome, Crohn's disease and other problems of the body's waste disposal system.

### *Catnip (Nepeta cataria)*

*Source:* Herb.

*Principal body part it benefits:* Stomach.

*Suggested uses:* An old remedy for helping alleviate colic, catnip was brewed in a tea and given to infants. Use it in a tea to stop vomiting. For toothaches, chew on fresh catnip leaves. It raises your mood and leaves you with a sense of well-being. It is also useful in treating childhood diseases, colic, flu, insomnia, morning sickness, nervous disorders.

***Natural Insecticide Tip:*** An active ingredient in catnip repels many types of insects.

## *Cayenne (Capsicum annum, Capsicum frutescens)*

*Source:* Fruit.

*Principal health related actions:* Digestive, stimulant.

*Suggested uses:* Aids digestion and stimulates appetite. Relieves bowel pains, gas and cramps. Increases production of gastric juices. Under medical supervision it may be tried as an aid for regulating the heart and blood pressure; it cleanses the circulatory system, while strengthening the heart rate. When used with garlic, it helps to lower blood pressure.

***Caution:*** Irritates hemorrhoids. Not to be used if you have gastrointestinal problems.

## *Chamomile (Matricaria chamomilla)*

Also spelled Camomile

*Source:* Flower.

*Principal health related actions:* anti-inflammatory, antispasmodic, anti-infective, calmative, mild sedative.

*Suggested uses:* Eases anxiety. Good antibacterial action. Reduces inflammation of the mucous membrane. Aids in parasite and worm elimination. Beneficial for prevention of migraines. Good cleanser for those who have used prescription or illicit drugs for a long-term. Excellent hair rinse, adding luster to hair. Calms nerves and upset stomach. Soothes ulcers. When externally used as a poultice, it has a cooling effect.

***Caution:*** Rare cases of allergic reaction have been noted in those with a severe hypersensitivity to ragweed pollen. In large doses, it acts as an emetic that does not depress the digestive system.

## *Chaparral (Larrea divaricata, Larrea mexicana)*

*Source:* Herb.

*Principal body parts it benefits:* Blood, skin.

*Suggested uses:* Used externally on acne, sores and wounds, as an astringent. Works synergistically with red clover to purify the blood and help rid the body of tumors and growths. Also useful in treating arthritis.

***Chasteberry*** – see Vitex.

***Chaste Tree*** – see Vitex.

### *Chickweed (Stellaria media)*

*Source:* Herb.

*Principal body parts it benefits:* Skin.

*Suggested uses:* Beneficial when scrubbed on acne. Helps stop bleeding and/or inflammations in the bowels, lungs and stomach. As a poultice it helps heal boils, sores and rashes. Aids respiratory system in expelling mucus. Beneficial for weight loss since it dissolves body fat.

***Note:*** Chickweed is high in vitamin C.

### *Chrysanthemum (Chrysanthemum morrifolium)*

Also known as 'chu hua' or 'ye ju' by Chinese health practitioners, the dried chrysanthemum flowers are a Chinese symbol of longevity. If you are a guest of a Chinese family and treated to a cup of tea with chrysanthemum petals floating in it, they are wishing you a long life. In the Chinese healing system, it clears heat and is a cooling herb.

*Source:* Flowers.

*Principal body system and parts it benefits:* Blood, digestion, liver and nerves.

*Principal health related actions:* Alterative, antipyretic, carminative.

*Suggested uses:* Chrysanthemum tea is beneficial for treating skin diseases and conjunctivitis. May lower blood pressure. Used to treat dizziness, fever and headaches. Reduces inflammation, abscesses and boils. Fights pneumonia.

*Dosage:* 3 to 10 grams, steeped for making a tea.

### *Citrus Peel (Citrus reticulata)*

Also known as ***chen pi*** in the Chinese healing system, it is used as a warming herb.

*Source:* Orange or tangerine peel.

*Principal body parts it benefits:* Lungs, spleen, pancreas, stomach.

*Principal health related actions:* Antiemetic, antitussal, digestant, expectorant, stimulant, stomachic.

*Suggested uses:* Prevents mucus formation. Alleviates cold symptoms. Helps neutralize abdominal swelling, indigestion and diarrhea. Improves digestion. Counteracts vomiting and muscle fatigue. Used as an energy promoting stimulant.

*Dosage:* Chew thoroughly, then swallow 4 to 6 grams at mealtime. May also steep peel in boiling water to make a tea.

### ***Cnidium (Ligusticum chuanxiong)***

Also known as ***Chinese Lovage*** and ***chuanxiong*** in the Chinese healing system, it is used as a warming herb.

*Source:* Root.

*Principal body parts it benefits:* Bladder, gallbladder, liver, reproductive organs.

*Principal health related actions:* Antispasmodic, emmenagogue, stimulant.

*Suggested uses:* Aids in regulating menstrual cycles. Beneficial for regulating the bowels and alleviating abdominal pains. Treats skin conditions such as itching, boils and carbuncles. Used as a substitute for, and also with dong quai.

*Dosage:* 4 to 5 grams, steeped in boiling water to make a tea.

### ***Coltsfoot (Tussilago farfara)***

*Source:* Leaves.

*Principal health related actions:* Anticatarrhal, antispasmodic, demulcent, expectorant.

*Suggested uses:* Pulmonary (lung) coughs and colds. Used for asthma, bronchitis and emphysema.

**Caution:** Do not ingest. Though not established, controversy exists concerning coltsfoot's possible toxicity upon the liver.

### *Comfrey (Symphytum officinale)*

*Source:* Root.

*Principal health related actions:* Astringent, antiphlogistic, expectorant, hemostatic, regenerative, sedative.

*Suggested uses:* Bruises, muscular and nervous inflammations; pain from fractures, phlebitis, rheumatism and painful joints, sprains, strains, varicose veins, varicose ulcers.

***Caution:*** For external use only. The German Commission E endorses topical application of comfrey for its anti-inflammatory benefits on bruises, sprains and dislocations. First apply an ice pack to the affected area, then wrap in a comfrey soaked bandage. Comfrey contains a toxic nervine, consolidin, and should never be used internally. Do not use on injuries with fractured bones. Though not established, controversy exists concerning comfrey's possible toxicity upon the liver. Not for use by pregnant or lactating women.

### *Cordyceps (Cordyceps sinensis)*

Also known as ***Chinese caterpillar fungus*** and since ancient times it has been used as a tonic to promote vitality and fight fatigue. Nourishes both yin and yang, cool and warm, states. Access to cordyceps used to be very rare until the Chinese created a method of mass production, using fermentation to produce the active ingredient in cordyceps.

Principal health related actions: One of Chinese medicine's antidotes for old age, restoring energy and vigor. It helps the body naturally raise antioxidant levels, which fight free radical damage, thought to be a major cause of heart diseases, arthritis and a host of other age-related diseases. Chinese athletes use it to increase performance and Chinese doctors prescribe it to weakened heart patients to restore energy levels. It is believed to enhance oxygen absorption and utilization in the lungs. Oxygen helps increase energy and endurance. Clears phlegm. Stops bleeding. Tones kidneys.

*Dosage:* Take up to 1000 mg (one gram) a day, at meal time.

### *Cranberry (Vaccinium macrocarpon)*

Harvard Medical School studies indicate that drinking one 8 ounce glass of cranberry juice a day has positive health benefits.

*Source:* Twigs and fruits.

*Principal body part it benefits:* Urinary tract.

*Principal health related actions:* Bacteriostatic effect, antioxidant. Its antioxidant properties are due to the cranberry's proanthocyanidins, anthocyanidins, ellagic acid, mineral and vitamin content.

*Suggested uses:* Helps clear and heal urinary tract infections. Cleanses the urinary tract. Additional research is needed to uncover the full potential of its antioxidant and cancer tumor fighting properties.

*Dosage:* Drink one 8-ounce glass of cranberry juice a day or the equivalent amount in caplets.

***Caution:*** Many grocery store and commercially prepared cranberry juices are not appropriate for healing. They may have too much sugar, or lack pure cranberry juice and its active ingredients. If you want the maximum healing benefits from cranberry juice, make sure you get pure, cold-pressed juice or capsules with pure ingredients. If a week of treatment does not clear the urinary problem, then consult with your doctor, naturopath or nutritionally orientated healer. Sexually active adults may keep reinfecting each other, unless both are treated.

### *Damiana (Tunera aphrodisiaca)*

*Source:* Leaves and flowers.

*Principal health related actions:* Antidepressant, aphrodisiac, nervine, tonic.

*Suggested uses:* Laxative, general tonic. Relieves anxiety and enhances sexual enjoyment and performance.

### *Dandelion (Taraxacum officinale)*

*Source:* Leaves and roots.

*Principal body part it benefits:* Blood, joints, kidneys, liver.

*Principal health related actions:* Antirheumatic, diuretic, tonic.

*Suggested uses:* Aids healing of kidney and liver disorders, natural diuretic, digestive aid, reduces blood pressure. Appears to help prevent iron deficiency, anemia, chronic rheumatism, gout and stiff joints.

*Dosage:* Try dandelions in salads.

### *Devil's Claw (Harpagophytum procumbens)*

*Source:* Root.

*Principal body part it benefits:* Joints.

*Principal health related actions:* Analgesic, anti-inflammatory, anti-rheumatic, sedative.

*Suggested uses:* Arthritis, rheumatism, helps reduce swelling, relieves pain and improves joint mobility.

***Caution:*** Should be avoided during pregnancy.

### *Dong Quai (Angelica sinensis)*

Also known as ***tang kuei*** and ***female ginseng***. Believed to be beneficial for men and women. In the Chinese healing system it is used as a warming herb.

*Source:* Root.

*Principal body system and part it benefits:* Female reproduction system, blood.

*Principal health related actions:* Antispasmodic, immunostimulant, tonic.

*Suggested uses:* Treats all symptoms of menopause as an alternative to estrogen treatment therapy (ERT). Helps regulate hormonal system. General tonic for female reproductive system. Reduces affects of premenstrual syndrome (PMS) and reduces high blood pressure. Beneficial antispasmodic for cramps, hypertension and insomnia. It is an excellent blood purifier and treatment for anemia.

***Caution:*** Do not use during pregnancy or if you have excessive menstrual flow. Ask your nutritionally orientated healer if angelica (angelica archangelica) is an appropriate substitute in these situations.

*Dosage:* 4 to 6 grams in a tea daily or in capsule form as per directions.

### *Don sen (Codonopsis pilosula)*

Also known as ***Tang shen***. In the Chinese healing system it is used as a warming herb to improve one's vital (chi) energy. Its tonic actions are milder than ginseng.

*Source:* Root.

*Principal body parts it benefits:* Increases energy in the heart, pancreas, spleen and stomach.

*Principal health related actions:* Tonic for spleen and stomach.

*Suggested uses:* Restores energy. Used to treat diabetes. Builds disease resistance. Conditions and improves spleen and pancreas' functions, alleviating problems such as diarrhea, vomiting, lack of appetite and tired limbs. Treats inflammations and infections. Strengthens stomach by improving weak digestion and reducing levels of acidity.

*Dosage:* 6 to 14 grams can be taken daily by men or women, at any time of the year because its tonic actions are milder than ginseng. Increase Don sen's energy producing and disease-fighting benefits by taking it with astragalus.

### ***Echinacea (Echinacea angustifolia/purpurea)***

*Source:* Root.

*Principal health related actions:* Antibiotic, antifungal, immunostimulant.

*Suggested uses:* Boosts levels of properdin, a chemical in the body that aids the immune system in fighting bacteria and viruses. Boosts and stimulates immune function generally. Targets the cold symptoms of fatigue and general malaise. Cortisone-like activity aids wound healing.

*Dosage:* Take 10 to 20 drops of tincture or extract, in a little water or juice, two to four times a day or as per labels directions. Do not take longer than 10 days.

***Caution:*** Contraindicated in autoimmune diseases, such as Multiple Sclerosis (MS) and Acquired Immune Deficiency Syndrome (AIDS). Not recommended for those with allergies to plants in the sunflower family.

### ***Elderberry extract (Sambucus nigra, one of the many species of elder)***

Is loaded with natural healing elements, such as essential oils, glycosides and organic acids that detoxify the body and clean the blood. Very good source of vitamin C, calcium and phosphorus. Contains a higher concentration of B vitamins than other fruit. The high levels of potassium promote diuresis (kidney activity) and the flushing out of toxins and waste.

*Source:* Flowers and berries.

*Principal body system it benefits:* Immune system.

*Principal health related actions:* Alterative, diaphoretic, expectorant, stimulant.

*Suggested uses:* Improves and strengthens immune system function. Help detoxify the body. Reduces cold and flu symptoms. In vitro (test tube) studies show it inhibits the AIDS virus. Excellent flu fighter. Purifies the blood and kidneys. Enhances energy and vitality. Expectorant that helps the respiratory passages clear themselves of phlegm and mucus. Diaphoretic (promotes perspiration) which aids the body in eliminating toxins.

*Dosage:* At the first sign of flu or cold, take 1000 mg of caplets or 2 tablespoons (30 ml) of elderberry concentrate in 1 cup (8 ounces, 250 ml) of water. Reduce to 500 mg of caplets or 1 tablespoon of elderberry extract every four hours, until all symptoms disappear or for a maximum of four days.

***Note:*** A three-day elderberry mini-cleanse program is an excellent aid when starting a weight reduction program.

### *Eleuthero (Eleutherococcus senticosus)*

A relative of Siberian ginseng, eleuthero is used in the Chinese healing system as a warming herb. Its calming properties make it the top Chinese remedy for insomnia.

*Source:* Roots, leaf.

*Principal body system and parts it benefits:* Circulation, heart, lungs, nerves.

*Principal health related actions:* Antispasmodic, cardiac tonic.

*Suggested uses:* Excellent for insomnia. Used as a treatment for arthritis. Beneficial for chronic lung problems and bronchitis. Used to lower cholesterol levels and reduce blood pressure, making it a heart and cardiovascular system tonic. Aids low blood oxygen levels. Used to treat stress and impotence due to stress.

*Dosage:* A mild herb that requires large amounts to be effective, depending on the severity of the ailment. Take up to 30 grams daily. When the leaves are used, much less is needed, since they are far stronger. Use between 3 to 8 grams daily.

### *Ephedra (Ephedra sinica)*

Also known as ***Ma huang***. In the Chinese healing system, it is used as a warming herb. American ephedra is much milder, and is used the same way.

*Source:* Stems, branches.

*Principal health related actions:* Astringent, diaphoretic, expectorant, stimulant.

*Principal body parts it benefits:* Adrenals, heart, lungs.

*Suggested uses:* Beneficial in treating asthma, bronchitis, coughs and other mucous-causing conditions. Beneficial for flus, colds and fevers without sweat. Long-acting stimulant. Used in cold remedies and allergy medications.

*Dosage:* Use American ephedra, also known as ***desert tea,*** since it is milder. Take 2 to 10 grams.

**Caution:** Do not use if you have high blood pressure, hyperactive thyroid, tachycardia (rapid heart rate), headaches. Not recommended for those who are exhausted or low in energy due to weakened adrenal glands. Use with caution.

### *Evening Primrose Oil (Oenothera biennis)*

Evening primrose oil is an essential fatty acid (EFA). For a better and more complete understanding of EFAs, see Chapter 5, "Fats and Oils – The Good, the Bad & the Ugly!"

*Source:* Plant.

*Principal health related action:* Anti-spasmodic.

*Suggested uses:* Helpful in treating PMS and MS. Prevents heart disease, stroke and maintains healthy skin. Excellent source of gamma-linolenic acid (GLA) and mixed tocopherols.

**Caution:** Overconsumption can result in oily skin.

### *Eyebright (Euphrasia officinalis)*

*Source:* Herb.

*Principle body part it benefits:* Eyes.

*Principal health related actions:* Astringent, tonic.

*Suggested uses:* Strengthens eyes. Aids the body in dissolving cataracts, soothing conjunctivitis (inflammation of the mucous membrane that covers the front of the eye and lines the inside of the eyelid), and healing lesions.

***Fang-feng (Ledebouriella divaricata)*** – see Sileris.

### *Fennel Seeds (Foeniculum vulgare)*

*Source:* Seeds.

*Principal body system it benefits:* Digestive system.

*Principal health related actions:* Soothes digestive tract and aids digestion. Relieves flatulence. Use as an expectorant for colds and coughs to clear the lungs. Stimulates appetite.

*Dosage:* Thoroughly chew, then swallow a teaspoon of the seeds with a cup of water. For stomach aches and pains, when using tinctures and extracts, blend 10 to 15 drops with a little water, swish in mouth with saliva, then swallow. For colds and coughs, drink a teaspoon of honey mixed with 10 to 20 drops of fennel seed oil and 1/2 a cup of warm water each day.

### *Fenugreek (Trigonella foenum-graecum)*

*Source:* Seeds.

*Principal health related actions:* Demulcent, expectorant, restorative.

*Suggested uses:* Beneficial for stomach and intestinal problems. Expectorant for colds and coughs. Strengthens those recovering from illness or suffering tuberculosis. Increases milk flow. Induces breast enlargement. Defatted fenugreek seed powder for non-insulin-dependent diabetics resulted in better glucose tolerance test results according to a 1988 study in the *European Journal of Clinical Nutrition.*

*Dosage:* Use as a gargle for sore throats. Non-insulin-dependent diabetics take 50 gm of defatted fenugreek seed powder, twice daily, with your physician's or naturopath's assistance.

### *Feverfew (Tanacetum parthenium)*

*Source:* Leaves.

*Principal health related actions:* Anti-inflammatory, emmenagogue.

*Suggested uses:* Migraine headache prevention. Beneficial against arthritis and swelling. Improves liver function. Stimulates digestion.

*Dosage:* Take standardized extract caplets or tablets, as per label. It may take weeks or longer for enough active ingredient to accumulate in your system, to be effective.

***Caution:*** Not for use by lactating or pregnant women.

## *Fo-Ti (Polygonum multiflorum)*

Also known as ***Ho Shou Wu***, ***He Shou Wu***, or ***Ho Shou***, and in America commercially known as ***Shen Min***®. In the Chinese healing system fo-ti is a warm herb, promoting longevity.

*Source:* Root.

*Principal parts it benefits:* Blood, kidneys, liver, pancreas, spleen.

*Principal health related actions:* Alterative, diuretic, hepatic (blood system) tonic.

*Suggested uses:* Anti-aging tonic properties that promote vigor, vitality and energy. The Chinese medical system considers it a longevity herb, since it strengthens the bones, muscles, ligaments and tendons. Treats any deficiency disease. Used to lower blood pressure, prevent blood clots, strengthen the heart and promote fertility in men and women. Believed to prevent gray hair and balding or thinning hair, by nourishing the body from within. In Western terms, gray hair may signal nutrient deficiencies or imbalances that this Chinese herb helps restore or rebalance. Has anti-tumor properties. Used to treat diabetes and hypoglycemia.

*Dosage:* Available in extracts or capsules. If using the root steep 5 to 15 grams daily in a tea, as per package directions or as a Doctor of Chinese medicine directs. Take one 500 mg capsule three times daily, on an empty stomach, an hour before or two hours after a meal. Depending on the dosage and potency, it takes from six months to a year to help return gray hair to its original color.

***Caution:*** A high dosage can cause mild diarrhea, a skin rash or numbness in legs and arms. Decrease dosage to amount prescribed by physician or naturally oriented health provider.

***Note:*** Yellow dock has tonic properties similar to fo-ti.

## *Fu ling (Poria cocos)*

In the Chinese healing system, fu ling is a neutral herb. It comes in two colors, white and red. Red fu ling, also known as ***muk sheng,*** is better used for restless and nervous states, while white fu ling is used primarily as a diuretic.

*Source:* Whole fungus.

*Principal body part it benefits:* Kidneys, spleen.

*Principal health related actions:* Diuretic, expectorant, nervine.

*Suggested uses:* White fu ling is considered one of the best diuretics. Beneficial treatment for congested lungs, insomnia and weak kidneys. Helps body eliminate excess water and mucus. Beneficial for rebalancing the negative emotional states of apprehension, instability and fear. Tones and nourishes the pancreas, spleen, stomach and nerves. Treats childhood hyperactivity.

Red fu ling is the preferred choice for restless and nervous conditions.

***Fu tzu*** – see Aconite.

## *Garlic (Allium sativum)*

Known as 'hu suan' in Chinese medicine.

*Source:* Bulb.

*Principal health related actions:* Antibiotic, antifungal, anti-inflammatory, antiparasitic, antitoxic, antiviral.

*Suggested uses:* Reduces high blood pressure, blood cholesterol and blood sugar levels. Thins blood. Benefits conversion of sugar in the blood, into carbohydrates in the liver. Supports immunity of the respiratory system. The French cure for a hangover is a soup made of garlic and onions. Anticancer and digestive tonic. Protects against poisons. Chinese also use garlic oil for its anti-inflammatory properties to treat middle ear infections. Taken orally and in suppository form, it is effective against yeast infections. Garlic is an inexpensive and excellent treatment for amoebic dysentery (ulcerative inflammation of the colon causing severe diarrhea, often with blood and mucus); according to studies it is as effective as the drug metronidazole. Helps rid body of pinworms, thread worms and parasite infestations. Topically used to treat insect and snake bites.

*Dosage:* Available as suppositories, capsules, pills, dried powder, garlic juice, garlic oil capsules, raw garlic, aged garlic. Look for organically grown and aged garlic in the form that is best suited to dealing with your condition. In capsules, try odorless aged garlic, 1 capsule up to 3 times a day. Cook with raw or crushed cloves.

***Caution:*** Should not be used by lactating women, since it can pass through the breast milk and cause colic in babies. Excessive consumption of raw garlic, 10 or more raw cloves a day, for a prolonged period of time may be toxic and cause an allergic reaction.

### *Ginger (Zingiber officinale)*

Also see HMP-33

HMP-33 is the standardized extract Europeans use to successfully treat osteoarthritis and rheumatoid arthritis. Recently, Americans have discovered this powerful healing substance, which has been used for hundreds of years in the Indian Ayurvedic medical system.

*Source:* Root.

*Principal health related actions:* Carminative, cholagogue, diaphoretic, stimulant.

*Suggested uses:* Targets the cold symptoms of fever and muscle aches. Fights the most common cold-causing culprit – rhinoviruses. Relieves abdominal cramping and indigestion. Promotes bile flow. Helps prevent and/or relieve motion sickness, colds, dizziness and nausea. Lowers blood clotting. See HMP-33 for additional benefits.

*Dosage:* For tea, grate 3 to 8 gm of ginger root, steep in hot water. Use in salads, soups and cooking. Take two 500 mg capsules a day.

***Caution:*** People with gallstones should consult their doctor prior to using ginger. Not recommended for pregnant or lactating women.

### *Ginkgo Biloba (Ginkgo biloba)*

*Source:* Leaves

*Principal health related actions:* Antiasthmatic, bronchodilator, platelet activating factor (PAF) inhibitor.

*Suggested uses:* Improves memory in patients with Alzheimer's disease and memory loss, cerebral vascular insufficiency. Inhibits blood clotting. Neutralizes free radicals. Beneficial for asthma, Raynaud's symptoms, stress, tinnitus and vertigo.

*Dosage:* Use standardized extracts with 24 percent flavoglycosides. Take one to two capsules a day.

***Caution:*** Take with food. Rare cases of headaches or stomach upset have been reported. Possible drug interaction with Aspirin, Warfarin or anticoagulants. Not recommended for pregnant or lactating women.

### *Ginseng*

- ***American Panax Ginseng (Panax quinquefolium)***
- ***Siberian Ginseng (Eleutherococcus senticosus)***
- ***Chinese/Korean Ginseng (Panax ginseng or Panax schin-seng)***
  Also known as ***jen sheng***.

There are over 100 varieties of ginseng, depending on the plant's root. The Chinese consider red ginseng, from shiu chu root, the best. In the Chinese healing system, ginseng is a warming herb. It is regarded the best herbal tonic and longevity herb.

*Source:* Root.

*Principal health related actions:* Alterative, cardiac tonic, demulcent, hepatic tonic, stimulant, stomachic, general body tonic.

*Principal body system and part it benefits:* Heart, circulation, entire body.

*Suggested uses:* Antifatigue – overcomes deficiencies, insomnia, poor appetite, nervousness, weaknesses. Enhances the immune system. Aids adrenal gland function. Antistress. Stimulates both mental and physical activity. Normalizes blood pressure. Prevents atherosclerosis. Reduces blood cholesterol levels. Nourishes blood. Treats anemia. Beneficial in treating diabetes, since it reduces blood sugar levels.

***Caution:*** Those with high blood pressure or who are pregnant should consult with their health care provider or doctor before taking ginseng. Do not use it to treat diseases exhibiting the following Yang conditions and symptoms; burning sensations, constipation, high fever, inflammation, irritability, overweight, cloudy urine.

*Dosages:* There are many grades and varieties of ginseng available. Choosing the most beneficial one for you may require a little more research on your part. Your mind, body and spirit will thank you.

### *Goldenseal (Hydrastis canadensis)*

*Source:* Root

*Principal health related actions:* Anti-inflammatory, alterative, astringent, hemostatic, mild laxative, tonic.

*Suggested uses:* Acts as an anti-inflammatory. Alleviates constipation. Boosts the immune system which lessens cold and flu symptoms. Treatment for liver diseases such as cirrhosis and hepatitis. Cleanses and dries the mucous membranes. Beneficial for stomach and digestive system disorders, such as acid indigestion, gastritis, colitis, duodenal ulcers, menorrhagia. A tonic for the female reproductive system, vaginitis (inflammation of the vagina), used in douches to relieve candida-caused fungal infections. Helpful for eczema, ringworm and other skin disorders and inflammations. Mouthwash for gingivitis and to prevent gum disease.

*Dosage:* Available in capsule, powders, tinctures and extracts. Used in herbal formulae combination usually having one or more of these alteratives – garlic, echinacea, chaparral and myrrh. For stomach ulcers, it is best when combined with myrrh. For vaginal douches, dissolve 1 tablespoon (15 ml) in warm boiled water, douche once cooled. Repeat every three days up to a maximum of five douches.

***Caution:*** Do not use during pregnancy. Not recommended for individuals who are prone to or have high blood pressure or deficient conditions. Eating fresh goldenseal may inflame mucous tissue. Never use for longer than two weeks at a time.

## *Gotu Kola (Centella Asiatica)*

*Source:* Nut.

*Principal body systems it benefits:* Circulatory system, respiratory system.

*Principal health related actions:* Expectorant, decongestant, analgesic, nerve and circulatory system tonic.

*Suggested uses:* For centuries it has been used as an aphrodisiac in Africa. Alleviates cold and upper respiratory infection symptoms, such as fever and congestion. Nerve tonic. Promotes relaxation. Enhances memory and brain function. Used to treat physically rooted emotional disorders, which can be the case with depression. Mild diuretic. Treats skin inflammation. By strengthening capillaries and veins, it improves blood flow. Treatment for inflammation of the veins, phlebitis and leg problems, such as cramps, heaviness, tingling and swelling. Aids delivery, obstetric manipulations and healing of episiotomy tears.

*Dosage:* Look for standardized extract preparations to ensure a minimum amount of the active ingredient. If using liquid extracts, blend 5 to 10 drops in juice or water and take up to three times a day. If using capsules, take up to three a day.

***Caution:*** Do not use if pregnant. If you have an overactive thyroid, check with your doctor before using.

***Griffonia simplicifolia*** – see 5-HTP.

### *Gugulipid (Commiphora mukul)*

Also on page 302.

*Source:* Stem.

*Principal health related action:* Anticholesterenic.

*Suggested uses:* Studies indicate it lowers blood cholesterol by 14 to 27 percent and triglycerides by 22 to 30 percent. Prevents and reduces buildup of atherosclerotic plagues. Increases liver metabolism of LDL cholesterol. Benefits heart metabolism.

**Caution:** Not for use during pregnancy.

### *Hawthorn Berries (Crataegus oxyacantha)*

*Source:* Berries.

*Principal health related actions:* Antiscelrotic, cardiac tonic, diuretic, hypotensive, vasodilator.

*Suggested uses:* To lower blood pressure and reduce the effects of hypertension. Strengthens heart muscle by oxygenating and increasing blood flow to the heart. Improves circulation and cardiovascular health. Alleviates the severity of angina attacks. It is a sedative, antispasmodic and diuretic.

*Dosage:* see Caution.

**Caution:** In lower dosages, it is generally safe to use according to the manufacturer's instructions. Highly concentrated forms of hawthorn berry should only be used in consultation and under supervision of your health care provider.

***He Shou Wu*** – see Fo-ti

### *Honeysuckle (Lonicera japonica)*

Also known as ***Yin hua***. It is used in the Japanese healing system. The Chinese healing system uses it as a cooling herb, in all of the detoxifying formulas.

*Source:* Flowers.

*Principal body parts it benefits:* Blood, liver.

*Principal health related actions:* Antipyretic, alterative.

*Suggested uses:* Excellent detoxifier. Beneficial in treating acute inflammations and infections, especially skin problems such as poison oak and other rashes. For acute flus and fevers it is used with chrysanthemum.

*Dosage:* Can apply externally on affected skin or take as an infusion.

***Caution:*** Not for long term use. Do not use for chronic conditions.

### Hops (Humulus lupulus)

*Source:* Fruit.

*Principal body systems it benefits:* Nervous system, gastrointestinal system.

*Principal health related actions:* Anodyne, diuretic, febrifuge, hypnotic, sedative, tonic.

*Suggested uses:* Calms the body. Stimulates appetite. Relieves cramps, muscle spasms and gas. Alleviates indigestion. Helps alleviate water retention. Treats insomnia, nervous diarrhea, and restlessness.

*Dosage:* To aid digestion, take 1 cup of cold hop tea an hour before meals or as an excellent after dinner tea, mix 1-2 teaspoons in 1 cup of warm water; drink once a day. Available in capsules; follow label directions. Make a hop pillow to promote sleep; sprinkle grain alcohol (vodka) over hops, then fill a pillowcase or small cloth bag with it.

***Caution:*** Avoid prolonged use or excessive dosages.

### Horse Chestnut (Aeculus hippocastum)

*Source:* Bark, leaves, fruit.

*Principal body parts it benefits:* Veins, lungs.

*Principal health related actions:* Astringent, expectorant, vagotonic (tones and strengthens veins).

*Suggested uses:* Soothing treatment for varicose veins, hemorrhoids, leg ulcers, recurrent neuralgia, and sunburn. Bark for diarrhea. Tones and strengthens veins. Promotes sweating. The fruit is helpful in reducing cold symptoms, fever, respiratory catarrh (inflammation of the mucous membranes of the nose and air passages with increased flow of mucus), and bronchitis.

*Dosage:* Use a commercially prepared mixture for external applications or make one yourself. Mix 1 teaspoon (5 ml) of chestnut powder in 32 ounces (4 cups) of water. Gently apply it to varicose veins, leg ulcers, sunburns or hemorrhoids. For a tea, steep 1 teaspoon (5 ml) of bark in warm water. For capsules follow directions.

***Caution:*** Consuming excessive amounts of the green walnut shells, leaves and seeds may cause poisoning. Roasting the seeds appears to destroy their poison.

### *Horseradish (Armoracia lapathifolia)*

*Source:* Root.

*Principal body systems it benefits:* Respiratory and digestive systems.

*Principal health related actions:* Diuretic, expectorant, rubefacient, stomachic.

*Suggested uses:* Beneficial diuretic for bladder infections, rheumatic and gout problems. Use externally to relieve rheumatism; horseradish increases blood flow to the joints which may account for its ability to alleviate rheumatic discomfort. Aids clearing of putrefaction due to colitis and intestinal problems. Combined with warm water and honey, it soothes and clears respiratory problems such as asthma, coughs and catarrhal lungs. When infused in wine, it stimulates the nervous system and promotes perspiration.

*Dosage:* Only undried horseradish root is effective. It stores well for months in the refrigerator. You can use the undried root in a vinegar based preparation, poultice or syrup. To make a poultice add fresh horseradish to cornstarch. Apply it to the affected area and cover with a gauze bandage.

***Caution:*** Do not consume large amounts of horseradish at one time. If night sweats or diarrhea occur, stop taking it immediately.

### *Horsetail (Equisetum arvense)*

Also known as ***Silica***.

*Source:* Herb.

*Principal body parts it benefits:* Bones, connective tissue, hair, nails, skin.

*Principal health related actions:* Astringent, diuretic. Aids calcium absorption by the body.

*Suggested uses:* Used for arteriosclerosis. To nourish and repair broken nails, hair loss, skin. Helpful for genitourinary complaints. Eliminates white spots in nails. Mild diuretic. Increases amount of white blood cells. Used to treat inflamed or enlarged prostrate. Rids skin of excess oil. Used in herbal beauty products.

*Dosage:* Follow product label directions.

***Caution:*** Large quantities can cause toxic reactions.

***Ho Shou Wu*** – see Fo-Ti
in America known commercially as ***Shen Min®***

***Huang Chi*** – see Astragalus.

***Jie Geng*** – see Platycodon.

### *Juniper (Juniperus communis)*

*Source:* Berries.

*Principal body parts it benefits:* Kidneys, stomach.

*Principal health related actions:* Antiseptic, carminative, diuretic, stimulant.

*Suggested uses:* Alleviates urinary tract problems, such as gallstones and urine retention. Treatment for gout, a painful inflammation of joints due to an accumulation of uric acid deposits in the joints. Improves digestion. Helps eliminate stomach cramps and gas.

*Dosage:* In tea up to 3 cups a day. Available in tincture and extracts, take between 10 to 25 drops three times a day.

***Caution:*** Not for use during pregnancy. Avoid if suffering from a kidney ailment. Cease taking juniper if excessive urination occurs.

### *Jujube date (Ziziphus jujuba)*

Also known as ***Da T'sao***. In the Chinese healing system it is used for its neutral energy balance. Its primary use is for calming the body.

*Source:* Whole date.

*Principal body parts it benefits:* Nerves, pancreas, spleen, stomach.

*Principal health related actions:* Digestive, nervine, nutritive, tonic.

*Suggested uses:* In the Orient, it is used in cooking to boost the flavor and health benefits of stews and soups. Source of energy for the body. Beneficial in treating apprehension, clamminess, exhaustion due to nervousness, dizziness, forgetfulness, insomnia.

*Dosage:* Used in many herbal combinations and alone.

### *Kava Kava (Piper methysticum)*

*Source:* Root and stem.

*Principal body parts it benefits:* Kidneys, liver, nerves.

*Principal health related actions:* Analgesic, anti-anxiety, antiseptic, antispasmodic, diuretic, aids sleeping, stimulant, tonic.

*Suggested uses:* Since 1990, Germany has approved Kava Kava for anxiety disorders. Non-addictive natural relaxant. Helpful for dealing with insomnia and getting a deep restful night's sleep. Reduces water retention and pain.

*Dosage:* Take powder or capsules as per labels directions. Use capsules standardized to 30 percent Kavalactones. Take two 150 mg capsules a day, or if 250 mg capsules, take one to three a day, or as per health care providers directions. With tinctures, blend 10 to 30 drops with water or juice. To alleviate pain, apply a poultice of Kava Kava directly onto the painful wound.

***Caution:*** Not recommended for pregnant women or lactating women, those suffering from Parkinson's disease or depression. Do not take large dosages for prolonged periods, as toxins could accumulate in the liver.

***Ko Ken*** or ***Kuzu root*** – see Pueraria

### *Kudzu*

An herb, used by ancient Chinese healers for treatment of alcoholism and hangover prevention, plus a host of other benefits. Refer to page 306.

### *Licorice (Glycyrrhiza glabra)*

Also known as ***Gan T'sao*** or ***Gan Cao***. In the Chinese healing system, it is used as a neutral herb. Licorice is regarded as a very important herb and is added to many detoxifying and tonic herbal remedies since it generally does not interfere with the beneficial properties of other herbs. It contains chemicals similar to adrenal cortical hormones, as well as DGL (derived from licorice root stripped of glycyrrhizin acid), and flavonoids. It has successfully been used to treat chronic fatigue syndrome patients with abnormally low blood pressure.

*Source:* Root.

*Principal body parts it benefits:* Intestines, liver and spleen, lungs, stomach and the entire body.

*Principal health related actions:* Alterative, blood pressure elevator, demulcent, diuretic, expectorant, laxative.

*Suggested uses:* Adrenal insufficiency, anti-inflammatory, antioxidant, antiviral, gastric ulcers, hypoglycemia, reduces fever. Beneficial for bronchial complaints, colds, coughs, sore throats, flus. Stimulates liver's bile production and relieves ulcers and stomach aches. Detoxifies blood. Helps lower cholesterol. Used to treat chronic fatigue syndrome, those with low blood pressure. Studied for its potential as a cancer treatment. Israeli researchers have discovered it may prevent atherosclerosis, hardening of the arteries. May be an effective treatment for Lupus, according to Japanese researchers at Tokyo's Oriental Medical Research Center. It may also have anti-depressant possibilities, but St. John's Wort is a better choice for depressive states at this time. Its stimulating properties offer stress relief.

*Dosage:* Look for it in Chinese herbal formulas for the above conditions. One to three 500 mg capsules per day. In tea, use 2 to 10 grams. Chronic fatigue syndrome patients, refer to Caution section below.

***Caution:*** Do not use if you have high blood pressure, hypokalemia (deficiency of potassium in the blood), edema, cirrhosis of the liver, cholestatic liver disorders, diabetes, take digoxin-based drugs, retain water, or are pregnant. Chronic fatigue patients should consult with their primary health care provider before trying licorice root, the dosage varies considerably depending on weight, age, and other factors. The 'tilt table test' is used to identify the CFS low blood pressure abnormality; passing out very quickly, after being held in an upright position on the table, indicates that you have this condition. If high blood pressure is a problem, consider trying DGL which is derived from licorice root, but is stripped of the glycyrrhetinic acid present in licorice, which can raise blood pressure.

### ***Lilly of the Valley (Convallaria majalis)***

A heart stimulant that supports a weak heart, edema, gout, rheumatic pain, and dysmenorrhea (painful menstruation).

## *Longan berries (Euphoria longana)*

Also known as ***Long yen rou*** and ***Dragon's Eye's***. In the Chinese healing system, it is used as a neutral herb.

*Source:* Berries.

*Principal body parts it benefits:* Heart, pancreas, spleen.

*Principal health related action:* Nourishing tonic

*Suggested uses:* Longan berries are used in many foods and medicines. It counteracts anemia, strengthens female reproductive organs and is beneficial for rebalancing mental conditions such as forgetfulness and hyperactive thought processes.

***Special note:*** Excellent remedy for dealing with hypoglycemia and sweet cravings. Cook this combination: millet, aduki beans and longan berries. Eat with sweet squash.

*Dosage:* Use 5 to 15 grams in a tea, daily.

***Caution:*** Stop using if suffering abdominal distension or diarrhea.

***Lu Hui*** – see Aloe Vera

***Luole*** – see Basil

### *Lycii (Lycium Chinensis)*

Also known as ***Gay Gee***. In the Chinese healing system, it is used as a cooling herb; lycii strengthens and nourishes the kidneys and liver. It increases longevity and promotes a sunny disposition.

*Source:* Berries.

*Principal body parts it benefits:* Blood, kidneys, liver, lungs.

*Principal health related actions:* Alterative, antipyretic, nourishing tonic.

*Suggested uses:* Beneficial for treating bronchial inflammations. Helps clear the eyes of cloudy vision. Reduces thirst. Helps cool fevers. Beneficial for treating high blood pressure and some types of cancer. Used to treat diabetes. Detoxifies blood by nourishing and supporting the liver and nourishing the kidneys.

*Dosage:* In a tea, use 5 to 10 grams, daily.

***Caution:*** Never use for acute (short term) colds or acute fevers. Best used for chronic colds with low grade fevers due to nutrient deficiencies, and where perspiration is present.

### *Marshmallow (Althaea officinalis)*

*Source:* Root, leaves.

*Principal body system and parts it benefits:* Throat, chest, gastrointestinal system.

*Principal health related actions:* Anti-inflammatory, antiseptic, emollient, demulcent, mucilaginous.

*Suggested uses:* Calms the body. It contains mucilage, a water soluble fiber, which is antiseptic and anti-inflammatory, and soothes the swollen mucous membranes in the throat. Alleviates the sore throat and irritated chests from bronchitis and bad coughs. Excellent expectorant, helping coughs get rid of phlegm. Beneficial for gastrointestinal problems such as colitis, enteritis and ulcers.

*Dosage:* Put 1 tablespoon (15 ml) of the dried herb in a tea strainer and steep in 1 cup (8 ounces, 237 ml) of hot water. Remove strainer. Drink up to 3 cups a day of this tea. In capsules, look for standardized extracts and follow label directions.

***Ma huang*** – see Ephedra.

***Mi Die Xiang*** – see Rosemary.
Used by Chinese doctors principally for its calming properties on the nervous system and as a treatment for stomach aches and headaches.

### *Milk Thistle (Silyburn marianum or Cardus marianus)*

*Source:* Seeds, leaves.

*Principal body parts it benefits:* Liver, spleen.

*Principal health related actions:* Antidepressant, hepatoprotective, cholagogue, demulcent, detoxifier, tonic.

*Suggested uses:* Enhances liver function and liver cell reproduction. Promotes flow of bile, critical for breakdown of fats. Detoxifies poisons, such as alcohol, nicotine, carbon monoxide and others that get into the bloodstream. Tonic for liver, kidneys, gallbladder, spleen and stomach. Beneficial for sufferers of liver diseases such as cirrhosis, jaundice and hepatitis. The liver is the main storage site for vitamins A, D, E and K.

*Dosage:* When using 250 mg capsules, standardized to 80 percent Silymarin, take one to two capsules, with meals, three times a day. In tinctures or extracts, 10 to 15 drops in a little water, three times a day or as per instructions.

***Note:*** If you are constantly exposed to smoke, pollutants or other chemical stressors, it would be wise to cleanse your liver at least twice a year using milk thistle, or even better, a synergistic herbal combination with milk thistle in it. It contains powerful flavonoids and Silymarin.

### *Mistletoe (Phoradendron flavescens)*

The variety known as American Mistletoe.

*Source:* Leaves.

*Principal health related actions:* Emetic, nervine.

***Caution:*** Only use under medical supervision. The berries from this plant are poisonous. Do not use if pregnant as it can induce an abortion. May increase blood pressure and and uterine contractions.

### *Mistletoe (Viscum album)*

The variety known as European Mistletoe.

*Source:* Plant, berries.

*Principal body system it benefits:* Circulatory system.

*Principal health related actions:* Cardiac, diuretic, stimulant, vasodilator.

***Caution:*** Use with great care and under medical supervision, preferably with a naturally orientated health care practitioner.

### *Oats (Avena sativa)*

Also known as ***Oat Fiber***.

*Source:* Stems, seeds.

*Principal health related actions:* Antidepressant, cardiac tonic, nervine.

*Suggested uses:* Debility, depression, menopausal symptoms and stress. Beneficial for skin conditions. Take a sitz bath (sitting in water up to the hips) to ease hemorrhoids. Alleviates indigestion. Tonic for impotence. Excellent natural relaxant, the extract calms the body. To reduce cholesterol by 10 to 15 percent, eat 2 to 4 ounces of oat fiber each day. This provides a good preventative measure against heart disease.

*Dosage:* For external preparations the straw is used. Excellent source of B vitamins. It is great in regular, foot and sitz baths. Oat fiber is available in foods. Try an extract to alleviate the symptoms of indigestion; take 5 to 20 drops, up to three times a day.

**Caution:** Take your time. Gradually increase the amount of fiber you eat. Give your body the time it needs to adjust to this powerful health promoting change. Too much at once can çause temporary bloating, cramps and gas.

## *Olive (Olea europaea)*

*Source:* Bark, fruit, leaf.

*Principal health related actions:* The oil has cholagogue, demulcent, emollient and laxative properties. The leaves have antiseptic, astringent and tranquilizing properties.

*Suggested uses:* A tea made from the leaves reduces nervous tension. Olive oil taken internally acts as a laxative by promoting muscle contractions in the bowels, it also increases the secretion of bile. In combination with lemon juice, it softens, dissolves and enables gallstones to pass. Thought to dissolve cholesterol. Beneficial for the heart and mucous membranes. Used as a massage oil, it soothes burns, bruises, insect bites, itching, and sprains. In combination with essential oil of rosemary and tea tree oil, it is an excellent dandruff treatment and hair/scalp tonic.

*Dosage:* For a tea, steep 1 to 3 teaspoons of the leaf in a cup of hot water for 8 to 10 minutes. For massage, use as needed. As a laxative, drink 1 to 2 ounces. To alleviate and clear the gallbladder of gallstones: Get 1 quart of cold-pressed extra virgin olive oil plus 4 to 5 lemons. Before going to sleep, start taking a quarter cup of the olive oil, followed by 1 tablespoon (15 ml) of freshly squeezed lemon juice, every 15 minutes until you have completely drunk the quart of olive oil. Then lie in bed on your left side and go to sleep. Periodically you will wake up through the night to relieve yourself. During those times, you will be passing the gallstones in your feces. This method for clearing your body of gallstones can be repeated as needed. We recommend waiting a few days between treatments. If this treatment does not help, surgery may be required.

## *Onion (Allium cepa)*

*Source:* Bulb.

*Principal health related actions:* Anthelmintic, antiseptic, antispasmodic, carminative, diuretic, expectorant, stomachic, tonic.

*Suggested uses:* Onion juice is often used as an expectorant and diuretic. It may help lower blood pressure and strengthen the heart. In the stomach it stops the fermentation and putrefactive processes. When onion juice is taken with honey, it alleviates hoarseness, coughs and allergies. It helps disinfect wounds. Restores sexual vigor which has been affected by mental stress or illness.

*Dosage:* Take 1 teaspoon (5 ml) of onion juice, three to five times daily. For hoarseness and coughs take it with a teaspoon of honey as needed. For minor cuts and wounds apply onion juice directly to affected area. For earaches, roast an onion in the oven until the outside is brown, cut in half, let cool until warm, and hold over the ear for ten minutes. A half-a-cup of raw or cooked onions, taken at the beginning of a meal, will prevent blood platelet accumulation.

## *Pai shu (Atractylodes macrocephala koidz)*

In the Chinese healing system, it is used as a warming herb, primarily for its diuretic properties. Often combined with and used to enhance the effectiveness of other Chinese tonic herbs.

*Source:* Root.

*Principal body parts it benefits:* Kidneys, pancreas, spleen, stomach.

*Principal health related actions:* Diuretic.

*Suggested uses:* First, it eliminates excess sodium, then other electrolytes; this process creates the diuretic properties for which this herb is known. Fortunately during this process, it does not stress the filtration process of the kidneys, and is therefore gentler than other diuretics. Restorative tonic for pancreas and spleen. Beneficial for treating abdominal distension, diarrhea, edema, indigestion, vomiting.

*Dosage:* Use 4 to 10 grams per cup of hot water. Drink one or two cups a day.

***Caution:*** Very low toxicity.

## *Papaya (Carica papaya)*

*Source:* Fruit.

*Principal body part it benefits:* Stomach.

*Principal health related actions:* Digestive aid: contains papain, which is similar to the enzyme pepsin that aids in the digestion of protein.

*Suggested uses:* Try papaya to alleviate indigestion. Excessive use of antacids can cause problems, which you can avoid with papaya tablets or juice. Helps metabolize protein in the body.

*Dosage:* Drink 1 teaspoon (5 ml) to 1 tablespoon (15 ml) of papaya juice as needed. Eat dried papaya slices, a sweet after-dinner treat. Commercially prepared chewable tablets are available, take one tablet up to three times a day, with meals, to relieve symptoms.

**Caution:** Not recommended for people with ulcers. For more information on enzymes refer to Chapter 4.

### *Parsley (Petroselinum sativum)*

*Source:* Leaves, fruit, root, seeds.

*Principal health related actions:* Antispasmodic, antiseptic, antirheumatic, aperient, carminative, diuretic. The seeds carry the properties of an emmenagogue, expectorant, sedative.

*Suggested uses:* Parsley is rich in B-vitamins, vitamin C and chlorophyll, a natural breath freshener and body detoxifier. A natural diuretic. Alleviates gas. Calms the stomach after eating. Good for bronchial and lung congestion problems, such as asthma and coughs. Eases difficult menstruation, and can be used to induce menstruation. Aids healing of urinary tract infections. Dissolves and rids the body of gravel and stones.

*Dosage:* You can eat parsley raw or make a tea by steeping stems and chopped leaves in hot water for a few minutes. Have one to three times a day. Use parsley in salads, sandwich spreads, soups, et cetera. As a tincture, use 10 to 30 drops as per label.

**Caution:** Parsley oil and juice should not be used by pregnant women.

### *Passionflower (Passiflora incarnata)*

*Source:* Leaves, fruit.

*Principal health related actions:* Antispasmodic, anodyne, hypnotic, hypotensive, gentle sedative.

*Suggested uses:* Alleviates insomnia and promotes a restful night's sleep. Beneficial for nervous disorders and headaches. Helpful for neurological or emotionally upsetting problems such as Parkinson's, epilepsy, neuralgia, hysteria, anxiety and shingles. Calms muscle spasms.

*Dosage:* The fruit is edible and delicious in fruit juice blends, balancing their sweetness with a tartness. As a tea, cut leaves and steep for a few minutes in hot water. As a tincture, use 10 to 50 drops or as per label instructions as needed each day. Calming benefits are enhanced when combined equally with valerian, wood betony and skullcap.

***Caution:*** Not to be taken during pregnancy. With some people, it can cause sleepiness. Do not use when operating machinery or driving.

### *Pau d'arco (Tabebuia impetiginosa or Tabebuia avellandedae)*

*Source:* Inner bark of Lapacho tree.

*Principal body parts it benefits:* Blood, lungs, liver.

*Principal health related actions:* Alterative (blood purifiers), antibacterial, antifungal, anti-diabetic, antiparasitic, antitumor, bitter tonic, digestive, hypotensive.

*Suggested uses:* Helpful for fighting fungal infections (athlete's foot, candida, et cetera), and parasitic infestations, aids digestion and can lower blood sugar levels. Good ulcer healer and for skin diseases. Helpful for respiratory conditions. In South America, it is used to treat leukemia and cancers. Human studies demonstrate that pau d'arco's lapachol derivatives have cancer fighting abilities: the growth of cancers and tumors were inhibited and slowed by pau d'arco.

*Dosage:* Available in capsules, extracts and teas. Follow package directions. For 500 mg capsules take one capsule three times a day. If using to treat life threatening problems, consult with a nutritionally orientated health practitioner and/or doctor.

***Caution:*** No known toxicities. Not recommended for pregnant or lactating women.

### *Pennyroyal (Hedeoma pulegioides is used in America, Mentha pulegium in Europe)*

*Source:* Leaves.

*Principal body parts it benefits:* Female reproductive organs, liver, lungs.

*Principal health related actions:* Antispasmodic, carminative, diaphoretic, emmenagogue, mild sedative.

*Suggested uses:* As an herbal remedy used for colds, flus, fevers. Promotes chest-clearing coughs. Promotes the start of menstruation. Relieves and alleviates premenstrual syndrome and menstrual cramping. Helps induce sweating. Beneficial for relief of gas and nausea. As an oil it is used as a mosquito and bug repellent for humans and pets. Put a few drops on pets.

*Dosage:* As a dried herb, take 1 tablespoon (15 ml) with 1 cup (8 ounces, 237 ml) of warm water, once a day, or as per health practitioner's instructions. As an extract, use as per the manufacturers guidelines, usually 15 to 60 drops in water or juice each day to alleviate symptoms. To help induce sweating, take at night before sleep; this can be beneficial when fighting colds and flus, and can aid in breaking a fever. Apply a few drops of oil as a bug repellent for humans and pets.

***Caution:*** Should not be used by pregnant women, as it can induce abortions and result in serious complications, such as hemorrhaging. Should be used only with the guidance of your nutritionally orientated health care practitioners and/or herbalists to facilitate labor and delivery. Never exceed recommended dosage or take for longer than a week.

### *Peony (Paeonia lactiflora)*

Also known as ***Shao-yao***. In the Chinese healing system it is used as a cooling herb.

*Source:* Root.

*Principal body parts it benefits:* Blood, liver, skin, uterus.

*Principal health related actions:* Antispasmodic, alterative, hepatic (blood system) tonic, sedative.

*Suggested uses:* Beneficial for treating menstrual pains and menstrual cycle irregularities. Used to treat liver imbalance diseases and restore optimal function. Peony is usually combined with licorice root. Peony nourishes and purifies the blood and is a good treatment for anemia. Beneficial for treating infections and skin eruptions.

***Caution:*** Use only under medical supervision. The plant and its flowers are poisonous and can be fatal.

## *Periwinkle (Vinca major, vinca minor)*

*Source:* Herb.

*Principal health related actions:* Astringent, sedative.

*Principal body systems and parts it benefits:* Blood system, female reproductive system, skin.

*Suggested uses:* Excellent remedy for diarrhea. Helpful for excessive menstruation or hemorrhages. Stops bleeding in the nose and mouth. Drink periwinkle tea for hysteria, fits and other nervous conditions. Chew on it for toothaches.

## *Peppermint (Mentha piperita)*

*Source:* Leaves.

*Principal body parts it benefits:* Head, stomach.

*Principal health related actions:* Antispasmodic, carminative, diaphoretic.

*Suggested uses:* Aids digestion and lessens flatulence. Alleviates colds and influenza. Soothes coughs and is effective for breaking up mucous. Relaxes stomach muscles. Soothes tired aching feet. Promotes burping. Beneficial for reducing symptoms of migraines and tension headaches. It is calming on the body. Known to help with insomnia, since it promotes a restful sleep. Endorsed by the German Commission E and British medical community for its ability to alleviate spastic colon, and reduce or eliminate the symptoms of irritable bowel syndrome.

*Dosage:* Use a commercially prepared tea and drink one or two cups each day or put one drop of the essential oil on a sugar cube and suck on it. It is a great substitute for regular teas or coffees. With headaches drink a strong cup of peppermint tea, then lie down for 20 to 30 minutes. Check with your doctor before giving it to infants for colic and children for upset stomach.

For spastic colon and irritable bowel syndrome, take one or two standardized enteric-coated peppermint oil capsules containing 2 milliliters of peppermint oil, between meals. Enteric-coated capsules pass through the stomach into the intestines, before dissolving.

For tension headaches, put a drop or two of the essential oil on your finger and draw it across you forehead from temple to temple, on your eyebrows and along your hairline. If the back of your neck aches, rub oil on this area as well. Repeat as needed.

**Caution:** Do not inhale the essential oil or other inhalants of the oil for long periods of time. Never use inhalants for babies. Have your health care provider confirm that tension headaches are the cause of your headaches before using peppermint oil. If peppermint oil gets in your eyes, immediately wash them with water.

### Plantain (Plantago major and Plantago lanceolata)

*Source:* The plant, leaves and seeds.

*Principal body system and parts it benefits:* Bladder, gallbladder, kidneys, respiratory system, small intestine.

*Principal health related actions:* Alterative, anti-allergenic, anti-inflammatory, aperient, demulcent, diuretic, expectorant, hemostatic.

*Suggested uses:* The aucubin in plantain makes it a beneficial herb for treatment of urinary tract infections, since it aids uric acid secretion from the kidneys. Helpful for hepatitis and other internal inflammations. Beneficial for respiratory problems resulting in mucous congestion. An antidote for venomous insect stings and bites as well as animal bites. Aid for stopping bleeding. Plantain supports healing injuries and wounds. Smoking cessation aid. CigNo®, an all-natural herbal supplement containing plantain, helps reduce nicotine cravings and supports the respiratory system. CigNo® is available in an herbal capsule and an homeopathic mouth spray.

*Dosage:* Make a tea, using 3 to 9 grams. Drink one to three times a day. In ointments, apply onto skin and hemorrhoid problem areas. Apply leaves to stings and bites. For nicotine cravings follow manufacturers directions.

### Platycodon (Platycodon grandiflorum)

Also known as ***Jie Geng***. In the Chinese healing system it is used as a warming herb.

*Source:* Root.

*Principal body part it benefits:* Lungs.

*Principal health related actions:* Expectorant, lung tonic.

*Suggested uses:* Treats respiratory problems, such as asthma, bronchitis, coughs, pneumonia and other lung ailments. It clears the lungs of infected mucus. Use for a sore throat.

*Dosage:* Available in Chinese herbal shops. Use as directed or 4 to 8 grams in a tea, taken as needed, daily.

### *Pleurisy root (Asclepias tuberosa)*

*Source:* Root.

*Principal body parts it benefits:* Colon, lungs, and upper respiratory tract (bronchioles).

*Principal health related actions:* Carminative, cardiac tonic, diaphoretic, diuretic, expectorant.

*Suggested uses:* Beneficial for treating pleurisy, colds, the flu and a range of respiratory problems since it promotes sweating and clears mucus from the chest. Aids digestion.

*Dosage:* When using an extract, take 5 to 35 drops in water or juice, every three hours to relieve symptoms. May take 1 tablespoon (15 ml) of the herb in 1 cup (8 ounces, 237 ml) of warm water or a warm juice, once a day. Follow package directions.

***Caution:*** The fresh root may cause vomiting and nausea. Only use commercial preparations of pleurisy root.

### *Poke Weed (Phytolacca americana)*

*Source:* Root, berries.

*Principal body systems and parts it benefits:* Kidney, lungs, spleen. Glandular and lymphatic systems.

*Principal health related actions:* Alterative, antibacterial, anti-inflammatory, antirheumatic, antiviral, cathartic, emetic.

*Suggested uses:* Beneficial for inflamed or swollen glands. Reduces arthritic and rheumatic inflammations. Good for lymphatic and blood cleansing and purification. The berries offer a homeopathic weight-loss remedy.

*Dosage:* Start with a small amount to see if you have a sensitivity to this herb. Available loose, in tinctures, capsules and as a tea. Follow package directions.

***Caution:*** Symptoms of sensitivity or toxicity to this herb include gastrointestinal problems. Although rare, taking poke weed can be fatal for those extremely sensitive to it.

### *Psyllium (Plantago psyllium, P. ovata, P. indica, P. arenaria)*

*Source:* Husks of seeds and the seeds. Its main ingredient is fiber.

*Principal health related action:* Bulk-lubricating laxative.

*Principal body systems and parts it benefits:* Digestive system. Bowels and the elimination system. Colon, stomach, spleen.

*Suggested uses:* Natural powerful laxative. Relieves irritation due to hemorrhoids. Beneficial for gastrointestinal problems and irritations. Aids in cardiovascular disease prevention.

*Dosage:* Mix 1 teaspoon of ground seeds or powder in 1 cup (8 ounces, 237 ml) of liquid. Drink it two to three times a day. Metamucil is a commercially prepared laxative, whose main ingredient is psyllium. Follow package directions.

**Caution:** If you have colitis or an ulcer, check with your doctor before using psyllium. Sensitive people may have an allergic reaction to psyllium. Check with your allergist before use. Since psyllium is a fiber, if you are just starting to add fiber to your diet, do so gradually, giving your body time to adjust. Fiber is the toothbrush for you digestive system. It helps remove toxins and materials the body does not need or want. Allow yourself two to four weeks for your body to make this adjustment. It is important to drink liquids when taking psyllium. Liquids, preferably water, will increase psyllium's benefits. Drink 8 or more glasses a day, as your bodily needs dictate. A lack of liquids can cause stomach discomfort, gas or bloating.

### *Pueraria (Pueraria lobata)*

Also known as ***Ko Ken*** or ***Kuzu root***. In Chinese medicine it is used as a cooling herb.

*Source:* Root.

*Principal body parts it benefits:* Lungs, stomach.

*Principal health related actions:* Antipyretic, diaphoretic, demulcent, refrigerant, spasmolytic.

*Suggested uses:* Beneficial for treating colds, flus, fever, gastrointestinal problems, hypertension, dizziness, tinnitus. Relieves minor aches and pains, particularly in the upper back and neck, by neutralizing body acidity.

*Dosage:* In a tea ball use 3 to 10 grams with 1 cup of hot water. Drink once or twice a day.

### *Pumpkin (Cucurbita pepo)*

*Source:* Seeds.

*Principal health related actions:* Anthelmintic, demulcent, diuretic, taeniacide.

*Suggested uses:* The linoleic acid and zinc components in pumpkin seeds reduce the size and symptoms of an enlarged prostrate. Zinc inhibits the enzyme that converts testosterone to dihydrotestosterone (DHT), the hormone that causes the over production of prostate cells. Aids in expelling tapeworms.

*Dosage:* Take one 1 gram (1000 mg) capsule of cold-pressed pumpkin seed oil a day.

***Puncture Vine*** – see Puncturevine page 316.

### *Pygeum (Pygeum africanum)*

*Source:* Bark

*Principal body systems it benefits:* Male genitourinary and reproductive systems.

*Principal health related actions:* Anti-inflammatory, antiedema, diuretic. Decreases symptoms of benign prostate hypertrophy (BPH). Men suffering from prostate enlargement have found this herb to be helpful, especially when combined with saw palmetto, stinging nettle, lycopene, and pumpkin seeds. A side benefit appears to be its ability to increase male sex drive and improve the ability to have an erection.

*Suggested uses:* Beneficial for treating BPH, cancer of the prostrate, dysuria, painful urination, prostatitis, incontinence, urinary tract disorders. May improve sex life.

*Dosage:* In capsules, take up to 1500 mg each day, with 1 cup of water. Inform your health care provider that you are using it.

***Caution:*** For prostate cancer and life-threatening problems, seek medical advice and a partnership with a doctor interested in following your wishes.

### *Raspberry leaves (Rubus idaeus)*

*Source:* Fruit, leaves.

*Principal body parts it benefits:* Kidneys, liver, reproductive organs, spleen.

*Principal health related actions:* Astringent, mild alterative, cardiac, hemostatic, parturient, tonic.

*Suggested uses:* Beneficial for fever blisters and sore throats. Used prenatally to tone the uterus. In this way, it helps to shorten delivery time by preparing the uterus to facilitate childbirth. Prevents miscarriage. Good for controlling excessive or frequent menstrual bleeding and irregularities. Eases menstrual cramps. A tonic that nourishes and strengthens the blood. Fresh, it acts as a mild laxative.

*Dosage:* Take as a tea during last two months of pregnancy, after childbirth, before and after menstruation, and to soothe sore throats and reduce fevers. Available in liquid extract and as a dried herb.

**Caution:** If pregnant, use it only under a medical practitioner's supervision and not until the last two months.

### *Red Clover (Trifolium pratens)*

*Source:* Blossoms.

*Principal body parts it benefits:* Blood, heart, liver, lungs.

*Principal health related actions:* Alterative, anti-tumor, antispasmodic, expectorant.

*Suggested uses:* Fights cancerous growths. Clears phlegm. Soothes and calms coughs. Beneficial treatment for skin inflammations, eczema and wrinkles. Calms the body, relaxes the muscles. A tonic that improves overall health.

**Caution:** When treating cancers or tumors, seek professional help before use to create and monitor a plan most suitable for your physical and emotional needs. Do not use during pregnancy.

### *Rehmannia (Rehmannia glutinosa)*

Also known as ***Sok Day-Sang Day***. It is an important cooling herb in the Chinese healing system.

*Source:* Root.

*Principal body parts it benefits:* Blood, bones and tendons, kidneys, liver.

*Principal health related actions:* Alterative, cardiac tonic, diuretic, hemostatic, uterine tonic.

*Suggested uses:* Sang day is the unprocessed root best used for treating the kidneys and helping the body eliminate excess acid. Sok day is the processed form, better for nourishing blood. Good for heart weakness and treatment of anemia. Aids recovery from illness and alleviates fatigue. Used for treating infertility in women and menstrual irregularities. During pregnancy, it is used as a tonic by the Chinese. After delivery, it helps stop postpartum hemorrhaging.

Many Chinese herbal formulations use it because it nourishes and cleanses the blood, strengthens the kidneys and promotes healing of bones and tendons.

*Dosage:* Make a tea using 4 to 8 grams of either sang day or sok day (as per your needs) and 1 cup of hot water. Drink 1 to 3 cups a day. In combination formulas, follow directions on the label.

### ***Rosehips (Rosa species)***

*Source:* Fruit.

*Principal body parts it benefits:* Blood, nerves.

*Principal health related actions:* Astringent, diuretic, tonic.

*Suggested uses:* Great source of vitamin C and B-complex vitamins for stressful and nervous situations. Blood purifier. Helps prevent infections.

### ***Rosemary (Rosmarinus officinalis)***

Also known as ***Mi Die Xiang***.

*Source:* Flowering tops, leaves.

*Principal body parts it benefits:* Liver, pancreas, spleen, stomach.

*Principal health related actions:* Anti-inflammatory, anticarcinogenic, antipyretic, antiseptic, astringent, diaphoretic, nervine, stomachic.

*Suggested uses:* Rosemary calms upset stomach and aids digestion. Improves circulation, but can result in high blood pressure. The acetylcholinesterase inhibitors in rosemary prevent the neurotransmitter, acetylcholine, from breaking down. This is beneficial. Acetylcholine is vital for memory and mental functioning. Low levels of acetylcholine have been associated with Alzheimer's disease.

Rosemary strengthens hair and cleanses scalp. Offers pain relief for headaches and other inflammatory joint conditions, such as arthritis. Reduces severity of common cold symptoms. Promotes liver function. Increases bile secretion, which is important for proper digestion.

Penn State University researched rosemary's cancer fighting potential, particularly with tumor formation in its early stages. Encouraging results indicated it has anticancer properties. If you or your family has a history of cancer, you may want to start cooking with rosemary daily.

*Dosage:* Available as a commercially prepared tea or you can make a tea with 3 to 10 grams of the leaves, and drink one to three times a day. Available as a tincture; follow manufacturer's directions. In capsules, take up to 1000 mg a day.

***Caution:*** If constantly consumed in excessively high amounts, it can be toxic. This is not the case when used moderately and frequently in cooking or in tea. If suffering from or prone to high blood pressure, monitor your intake of rosemary.

### *St. John's Wort (Hypericum perforatum)*

*Source:* Herb.

*Principal health related actions:* Anti-inflammatory, antidepressant, anti-anxiety, astringent, sedative. New research indicates its antidepressant benefits are due to its 'serotonin reuptake inhibitor' properties, meaning it keeps the serotonin levels more constant, which is what Prozac does. It used to be thought that hypericin was the active ingredient, but it now appears that a synergy between numerous chemicals of the herb's complex chemical mixture account for its beneficial properties.

*Suggested uses:* Excellent antidepressant. Reduces stress, anxiety and irritability. Ointment alleviates rheumatism and back pain. Promotes a restful night's sleep. Supports immune system as an antiviral. May benefit AIDS patients by supporting their immune systems. Excellent anti-inflammatory and beneficial on dry skin. It is a muscle relaxer, and is used to treat menstrual cramps. Aids treatment of gastric ulcers and other gastrointestinal disorders. The oil is used for burns and skin irritations since it has antiseptic and painkilling properties.

Researchers at New York University have found it has retrovirus inhibiting properties. In other words, if interferes with the human immunodeficiency virus (HIV) development into AIDS. The inhibiting properties were also noted in animals.

*Dosage:* For external applications on the skin, use St. John's Wort oil. It soothes minor skin irritations and is beneficial on rough dry skin. For mild to moderate depression we suggest a 300 milligram (mg) capsule or tablet containing a standardized extract of 0.3 percent hypericin, three times a day. This gives you 1 mg of this herb's main active ingredient daily. New research indicates that severe depression in patients not suffering delusional or psychotic symptoms, has effectively been treated with double the dosage. In America, the formula used in the German studies is sold under the brand name Kira.

***Caution:*** Although safe for humans, hypericin can make the skin photosensitive. Avoid excessive exposure to sunlight. Mild reversible side effects have occurred in some users, ranging from gastrointestinal complaints to allergic reactions. Compared to prescription antidepressants, the number and severity of side effects are negligible. Commission E, Germany's herb regulatory body endorses St. John's Wort for depression. When using this herb for long term relief of depression, as a substitute for another anti-depressant or to treat any serious emotional state, we recommend you seek professional medical help and supervision. If you are severely depressed or suicidal, see a health care professional immediately. Do not stop taking any antidepressants without first discussing this with your doctor or health care professional.

## *Salvia (Salvia miltiorrhiza)*

Also known as ***Dang Shen, Danshen Wan*** and ***Red Sage Root***. The Chinese healing system use it as a cooling herb. It is a species of sage.

*Source:* Root.

*Principal body parts it benefits:* Heart, liver.

*Principal health related actions:* Alterative, blood stimulant, emmenagogue, reduces cholesterol and lipids.

*Suggested uses:* Vital herb for relieving blood stagnation and promoting regular menstruation. It is a complete blood tonic, due to it having alterative properties. For women, it is very helpful when dealing with obstructed or excessive menstruation. Beneficial for boils, abdominal distension, erysipelas, itch, spasmodic rheumatism.

*Dosage:* Used in teas (4 to 10 grams with 1 cup of hot water) and as a liquid extract for injection into affected areas by a trained Chinese medicine practitioner who knows which acupuncture points to use.

***Sang Day*** – see Rehmannia

### *Sarsaparilla (Smilax officinalis, S. medica, S. ornata)*

*Source:* Rhizome or roots.

*Principal body parts it benefits:* Kidneys, liver, stomach.

*Principal health related actions:* Alterative, anti-inflammatory, antipruritic, diaphoretic, helps reduce heat, tonic.

*Suggested uses:* Believed to be an aphrodisiac. Beneficial alterative for skin problems such as psoriasis and eczema. Bodybuilders use it as a non-steroidal way of building muscle mass. It is used to treat venereal diseases, such as gonorrhea and syphilis, but professional medical help should always be consulted for any sexually transmitted disease. Tonic for the liver and liver-related problems, such as hepatitis, gout and jaundice.

*Dosage:* In tinctures or extracts, take 10 to 30 drops in liquid and follow label directions.

**Caution:** Always consult with your health care provider when dealing with sexually transmitted diseases and liver problems. Do not use if taking blood thinners.

### *Saw Palmetto (Serenoa serrulata)*

*Source:* Berries.

*Principal body system and part it benefits:* Prostate gland, reproductive system.

*Principal health related actions:* Diuretic, endocrine agent, expectorant, sedative, tonic.

*Suggested uses:* Treatment for enlarged prostrate or benign prostatic hypertrophy (BPH). Studies indicate saw palmetto is about 90 percent effective in treating BPH, benefits happened faster (4 to 6 weeks) and without the side effects or toxicity associated with the much more expensive drug Proscar. Anti-allergic. Anti-inflammatory. Treatment for congested chests due to colds and coughs. Beneficial for urinary tract disorders, impotence in men and infertility in women. Saw palmetto blocks the enzyme that converts testosterone to dihydrotestosterone (DHT), the hormone that causes the over production of prostate cells. DHT can also be a cause of male-patterned baldness. Saw palmetto is even more effective when used in synergistic blends with other herbs or antioxidants, such as lycopene, pumpkin seed extract, pygeum and stinging nettle.

*Dosage:* Use as an extract for chest congestion. Take 20 to 45 drops in water or juice each day, or as per label. For BPH, two products in the United States have received a lot of positive study results and/or consumer satisfaction feedback, Pros-Forte™ (Vitaline Corporation) and ProstAvan® (Melaleuca Corporation). For minor prostate discomfort or enlargement, follow package directions. If results are not forthcoming within 6 weeks, try larger dosages under the supervision of your health care provider, until you find an amount that works effectively. No negative long term or serious side effects have been reported by users of saw palmetto.

### *Schizandra*
### *(Schisandra Fructus, Schisandra Chinensis, Wu Wei Tsu)*

A Chinese herb believed to increase stamina and energy. Highly prized herb for its *Ooh! La! La!* properties, see below. In the Chinese healing system, it is considered a warming herb.

*Source:* Seeds.

*Principal body system and parts it benefits:* Reproductive system, liver, kidneys.

*Principal health related actions:* Adaptogen (energizes RNA and DNA molecules to rebuild), antidepressant, aphrodisiac, sedative, tonic.

*Suggested uses:* Chinese women highly prize its youth tonic and sexual enhancing properties. It is believed to keep one beautiful and youthful. For men it supposedly increases sexual stamina. Reputed to have antidepressant properties. Seeds have over a dozen liver-protecting properties and are used by Chinese doctors to treat viral hepatitis and other liver problems. According to natural products pharmacists, schisandra chinensis, in particular has powerful liver protecting properties. Alleviates insomnia. Aids eyesight.

*Dosage:* Available in capsules and extracts. Use as label directs. In China, after the hepatitis subsides, patients take 1 to 8 teaspoons each day, for a month.

***Scutellaria*** – see Skullcap.

***Shao-yao*** – see Peony.

### *Sileris (Ledebouriella divaricata)*

Also known as ***Fang-feng***. In the Chinese healing system, it is used as a warming herb.

*Source:* Root.

*Principal body parts it benefits:* Liver.

*Principal health related action:* Antispasmodic.

*Suggested uses:* Helps relieve chills, flus, dull headaches, joint pain, muscle spasms, rheumatoid numbness, tetanus. Used in the oft-prescribed immune system building formula, Jade Screen Powder, for colds and flu. The formula combines astragalus, atractylis and sileris which can be used long-term, on a daily basis for enhanced immune system functioning.

***Silica*** – see Horsetail.

### *Skullcap (Scutellaria lateriflora)*

Also known as ***Scutellaria*** or ***Huang Chi***. There are many varieties of this plant in the world. The Chinese use a different variety, scutellaria baicalensis, and consider it a cooling herb.

*Source:* Root.

*Principal body parts it benefits:* Heart, gallbladder, large intestines, liver, lungs.

*Principal health related actions:* Antipyretic, antispasmodic, astringent, diuretic, hemostatic, laxative.

*Suggested uses:* Very beneficial plant for nerves due to its calming properties. Used to treat alcoholics and alleviate withdrawal symptoms. In Chinese medicine, its cooling properties sedate by ridding the body of the excess heat coming from the heart, liver and lungs. Relieves stress-induced menstrual cramps and muscle pains. Used to treat stagnant blood conditions, such as carbuncles, infections, jaundice, pneumonia, sores. Used to treat rabies. Long ago it was claimed to calm and reduce excessive sexual desires.

*Dosage:* Drink 1 cup of skullcap tea daily. Steep 1 tablespoon (15 ml) of dried herb in 1 cup (8 ounces, 237 ml) of hot water. Look for capsules with a standardized extract and follow package directions. For liquid extracts blend 3 to 10 drops in water, have daily or as per package directions.

### *Slippery Elm (Ulmus fulva)*

*Source:* Inner bark.

*Principal body parts it benefits:* Esophagus, throat.

*Principal health related actions:* Astringent, demulcent, emollient, mucilage.

*Suggested uses:* Duodenal or gastric ulcers. Inflammation of stomach, coughs, colitis, sore throat. Soothes skin disorders.

*Dosage:* Suck on lozenges up to 5 times a day.

***Sok Day*** – see Rehmannia.

### *Stevia*

Also known as ***sweet grass***. Coke a-Cola® used it as the sweetener for Diet Coke in Japan. When the company decided to standardize Diet Coke's formulation around the world, Stevia was dropped in favor of an artificial sweetener. There is a lot of controversy about artificial sweeteners' possible link to brain tumors and/or other problems. Another controversy surrounds the use of artificially sweetened soft drinks before meals. Studies document that those who have an artificially sweetened drink before meals eat about 11 percent more, in terms of calories, than those who do not consume artificially sweetened drinks. While artificial sweeteners are not recommended for cooking, Stevia is. It is an approved noncaloric sweetener in Japan, which can be used instead of sugar for cooking and baking.

*Source:* Grass.

*Principal health related actions:* Gentler on the body than sugar or artificial sweeteners. Does not provoke insulin problems as sugar does. Approximately 200 times sweeter than sugar.

*Suggested uses:* For people wanting to reduce their sugar intake. Extremely sweet, only a pinch is needed. In cooking and baking.

*Dosage:* Available in health food stores. Just a pinch will do.

### *Suma (Pfaffia paniculata)*

Also known as ***Brazilian ginseng***.

*Source:* Root.

*Principal body parts it benefits:* Lung, spleen, pancreas.

*Principal health related actions:* Adaptogen, demulcent, energy tonic, nutrient.

*Suggested uses:* For people with low energy, poor stamina or chronic fatigue. If you are recovering from the flu, use suma to perk yourself up. Considered equal to Siberian or Panax ginseng for its adaptogenic energy tonic properties. It strengthens the immune system. Speeds wound and fracture healing. Dr. Brazzach, Sao Paulo University's Head of the Pharmaceutical Department is a leading authority on suma. His interest was aroused when his wife cured herself of breast cancer by eating large amounts of the suma root. Since then he has successfully used it on many serious diseases, with incredible results – leukemia, various types of cancer, chronic fatigue syndrome, Epstein-Barr disease, Hodgkin's disease, and diabetes. Relieves and alleviates menopausal symptoms.

*Dosage:* Orally, take 1 or 2 tablets or capsules, up to three times a day or as per package directions. For a tonic, start by taking 3 grams in warm water, four times a day, then slowly increasing your dosage to 6 grams in warm water, four times a day.

### *Tienchi (Panax notoginseng)*

In the Chinese healing system, it is used as a warming herb.

*Source:* Root.

*Principal body parts it benefits:* Heart, blood, liver.

*Principal health related actions:* Cardiac tonic, hemostatic.

*Suggested uses:* Used internally to stop nosebleeds and externally applied directly onto wounds. Prevents fatigue. Considered a good heart tonic since it helps normalize blood pressure, circulation, heart rate and cholesterol. Beneficial for weight maintenance. Helpful for stress. 'Yunan Baiyao' is a patented Chinese medicinal using Tienchi as its principal ingredient. It is thought to be the best formula for dealing with bleeding, cuts, gunshot wounds, wounds in general, and chronic stomach aches.

*Dosage:* Drink a tea made with 4 to 10 grams of tienchi, as needed.

### *Thyme (Thymus vulgaris)*

Also known as ***garden thyme*** or ***common thyme.***

*Source:* Leaves, flowers.

*Principal body parts it benefits:* Liver, lungs, stomach.

*Principal health related actions:* Anthelmintic, antiseptic, antispasmodic, antitussal, carminative, diaphoretic, expectorant, sedative.

*Suggested uses:* Beneficial for short and long term respiratory infections and/or conditions, including bronchitis, colds, coughs, laryngitis and whooping cough. Aid for gastrointestinal conditions such as diarrhea, gas, and indigestion. Use as a tea, to promote a more restful sleep, if you suffer from nightmares. Treat shingles and other skin conditions such as bruises, sprains and swelling. Used in toothpastes and mouthwashes for its powerful antiseptic properties.

*Dosage:* Use when cooking. For a tea, steep 2 teaspoons (10 ml) of dried herb, or 1 teaspoon (5 ml) of fresh herb, in 1 cup (8 ounces, 237 ml) of hot water. Drink a mouthful of tea at a time, up to 1 1/2 cups a day. In extracts or tinctures generally, 10 to 20 drops, three times a day, or as per label directions. As an essential oil, 1 to 2 drops on a sugar cube or mixed into a tablespoonful (15 ml) of honey, taken two or three times a day. For additional ways of using thyme in bath water, orally, and externally, refer to Chapter 15, Aromatherapy.

**Caution:** Excessive use can lead to overstimulation of the thyroid gland and symptoms of poisoning.

### *Turmeric (Circuma longa)*

This herb is one of the many spices in curry along with cayenne, coriander, cumin, garlic and onion, seasonings whose healing properties can help prevent blood clots and reduce cholesterol. This results in reduced incidence of heart disease and stroke for frequent curry eaters. Curried foods are a wonderful way to get the benefits of turmeric.

*Source:* Rhizome.

*Principal body parts it benefits:* Gastrointestinal tract, heart, liver, lungs.

*Principal health related actions:* Alterative, analgesic, antibacterial, antiseptic, aromatic, astringent, cholagogue, emmenagogue, stimulant.

*Suggested uses:* Beneficial for reducing the swelling and pain of arthritis. Turmeric is a thousands-of-years-old Indian healer's treatment for obesity. As a liver tonic, it helps improve liver function. Stimulates the liver's bile flow and ability to break down fats in foods. This result may also regulate menses and reduce the effects of PMS, since it gently balances and regulates hormonal function through its actions upon the liver. Beneficial in treating stomach problems, blood clots, gallbladder diseases, menstrual disorders, liver ailments and hepatitis. Used to prevent and dissolve gallstones. Improves blood circulation. Helps impede blood clots by preventing blood cells from sticking together; this aids in wound healing for bruises and injuries. Aids prevention of gallbladder problems.

*Dosage:* Take 1 capsule, up to three times a day. Use in oils and liniments externally to treat bruises and injuries. Eat a lot of curried food. When combined with chickpeas, you are also getting a complete protein, which is very healthy for you.

**Caution:** Large doses of turmeric are not recommended in cases of painful gallstones, obstructive jaundice, acute bilious colic and extremely toxic liver disorders.

### *Uva Ursi (Arctostaphylos uva-ursi)*

Also known as ***Bearberry***.

*Source:* Leaves.

*Principal body parts it benefits:* Bladder, kidneys, urinary tract system.

*Principal health related actions:* Astringent, diuretic, urinary antiseptic.

*Suggested uses:* Modern research shows it is beneficial for kidney and bladder problems. Treat urinary tract infections, help alleviate pain from nephritis, cystitis, urethritis and pyelitis. Excellent diuretic. When Uva ursi is taken with Buchu, it is more effective for healing bladder weakness.

*Dosage:* Take one tablet or capsule up to three times a day for relief of symptoms. For a tea, steep 3 to 9 grams or 1 tablespoon (15 ml) of the dried herb in 1 cup (8 ounces, 237 ml) of warm water. Drink 1 cup a day.

**Caution:** Stop using if nausea or vomiting occur. Do not take during pregnancy, if suffering from liver or kidney problems or during acute cystitis.

### *Valerian (Valeriana officinalis)*

*Source:* Root.

*Principal body system and parts it benefits:* Heart, liver, nervous system.

*Principal health related actions:* Antispasmodic, anodyne, carminative, hypnotic, nervine, hypotensive, sedative, stimulant.

*Suggested uses:* Beneficial for insomnia, nervousness, anxiety, panic attacks and extreme emotional stress. Balancing agent for exhaustion and hyperexcitability. Alleviates gas, pains, spasms and other conditions due to stress, such as muscle cramps due to PMS and menstrual cramps.

*Dosage:* Take one tablet or capsule up to three times a day. For liquid extracts or tinctures, mix 5 to 15 drops in water or juice daily, or as per label directions.

***Caution:*** Avoid high dosages over long periods of time. Not recommended during pregnancy, if taking muscle relaxants, antihistamines, psychotropic drugs, narcotics or having impaired kidney or liver function.

### *Vitex (species Verbenaceae)*

Also known as ***Chaste tree, Chasteberry*** and ***vitex agnus castus***.

*Source:* Fruit.

*Principal body system and part it benefits:* Female reproductive and hormonal systems.

*Principal health related actions:* Hormone rebalancer, tonic.

*Suggested uses:* Europeans use it as an alternative to estrogen replacement therapy. It helps alleviate negative side effects of menopause. Herbalists treat fibroid tumors with vitex. Treatment for PMS and other female reproductive system complaints such as amenorrhea (abnormal absence of menstruation). Reputed to promote lactation (milk production) after birth, as well as reduce breast tenderness.

*Dosage:* For tinctures or extracts, blend between 10 to 30 drops in water or juice and take up to three times a day. Follow label directions to maximize benefits. In tablet or capsule form, take 1 up to three times a day.

### *White Willow (Salix alba)*

The synthetic drug, aspirin, also known as acetylsalicylic acid, is derived from an active ingredient in white willow. The manufactured drug can result in stomach problems and life-threatening internal bleeding, which 9000 people a year die from in the United States. White willow on the other hand, has many components that buffer the affect of salicum and it contains tannins, beneficial to your digestive system. White willow is a good substitute for aspirin, with fewer side effects.

*Source:* Bark

*Principal body parts it benefits:* Heart, kidneys, liver.

*Principal health related actions:* Analgesic, alterative, anti-inflammatory, astringent, antiperiodic, febrifuge, tonic, vermifuge.

*Suggested uses:* Reduces fevers. Symptomatic relief of headaches and sciatic aches and pains. Beneficial for certain stomach ailments and heartburn. It is a mild analgesic and reduces inflammation of rheumatic and arthritic conditions. Pain killing properties beneficial for neuralgia.

*Dosage:* Take 1 or 2 capsules every two to three hours as required.

**Caution:** If you are allergic to aspirin, do not use white willow until you have consulted with your allergist or health care practitioner.

***Wild Ginger (Asarum heterotropoides)***

Also known as ***Xi Xin***. In the Chinese healing system, it is used as a warming herb. Refer to HMP-33.

*Source:* Root.

*Principal body parts it benefits:* Heart, kidney, liver, lungs.

*Principal health related actions:* Antiparasitic, antispasmodic, diaphoretic, emmenagogue, stimulant.

*Suggested uses:* Unblocks obstructed menstrual flow. Alleviates lung, head and nose congestion. Helps keep the digestive system free of parasites.

*Dosage:* For tea, grate 3 to 8 gm of ginger root, steep in hot water. Use in salads, soups and cooking. Take two 500 mg capsules a day. Follow package directions.

**Caution:** The American variety is milder and slower acting than the Chinese type. The Chinese variety is so powerful that doses larger than 3 grams can be mildly toxic and should only be used in smaller amounts. People with gallstones should consult with their doctor prior to use. Not recommended for pregnant or lactating women.

***Wild Yam (Dioscorea villosa or Dioscorea paniculata)***

*Source:* Root.

*Principal body parts it benefits:* Gallbladder, kidneys, liver, spleen, pancreas.

*Principal health related actions:* Anti-inflammatory, antispasmodic, cholagogue, mild diaphoretic, expectorant.

*Suggested uses:* Aid for dealing with menopause, menstrual cramps and ovarian pain. Wild yam is used in the natural remedy preparation that Dr. Pettle recommends for menopausal symptoms in Chapter 10. It is helpful for biliary colic, gallstone pain, intestinal and abdominal cramps. Beneficial for certain types of rheumatism and intestinal colic. Helpful for chronic conditions due to gas and/or flatulence.

*Dosage:* In a tea, use 3 to 8 grams in a cup of hot water and drink 1 to 2 cups a day. With tinctures and extracts, use 10 to 30 drops, or as per label instructions.

### Witch hazel (Hamamelis virginiana)

*Source:* Principally, the bark, and secondarily, the twigs and leaves.

*Principal body system and parts it benefits:* Heart circulation, intestines, skin, stomach.

*Principal health related actions:* Astringent, anti-inflammatory, hemostatic.

*Suggested uses:* Helps heal cuts and abrasions. Good unscented aftershave for men and women. Known as a skin tonic, since it revitalizes skin by eliminating excess oil. Relieves discomfort from varicose veins and hemorrhoids. Naturally orientated healers and herbalists use it for vaginal and penile discharges, diarrhea, dysentery, hemorrhages, prolapsed uterus or intestines, and menorrhagia. It can be used in vaginal douches. It is a general tonic used to restore the womb to its normal size after a miscarriage or abortion.

*Dosage:* Can be used internally in a suppository for hemorrhoids. Apply externally by hand or with a soft cloth or cotton ball onto irritated areas as needed. T use as a skin tonic, splash on and gently wipe off.

***Caution:*** For penile and vaginal discharges, consult with your health care provider, to ensure proper diagnosis and treatment of the condition.

### Wormwood (Artemisia absinthium)

*Source:* Aerial parts.

*Principal body parts it benefits:* Gallbladder, liver, stomach.

*Principal health related actions:* Anthelmintic, anti-inflammatory, antiparasitic, cholagogue, stomachic.

*Suggested uses:* Used to cleanses the body of parasites. Alleviates aches and pains. Gastritis, hot stomach aches and inflammation of the gastrointestinal tract. Beneficial for treating jaundice and hepatitis. May be a treatment for drug-resistant forms of malaria.

When combined with goldenseal, garlic, black walnut hulls, licorice root and ginger, it creates a powerful intestinal worm and parasite cleanser.

**Caution:** Take as per package directions. Do not use for longer than 30 days, unless otherwise directed by your health care provider.

***Xi Xin*** – see Wild Ginger.

### *Yarrow (Achillea millefolium)*

Also known as ***Soldier's woundwort, Nosebleed,*** and ***Milfoil.***

*Source:* Herb.

*Body systems most affected:* Lung, liver.

*Principal health related actions:* anti-inflammatory, antipyretic, antispasmodic, astringent, carminative, diaphoretic, hemostatic, stomachic.

*Suggested uses:* Beneficial for colds, fevers, flu, hemorrhoids, painful menstruation, as well as hypertension. For external application for hemorrhoids combine yarrow with witch hazel.

**Caution:** Not recommended during pregnancy.

### *Yellow Dock (Rumex crispus)*

*Source:* Root.

*Body systems most affected:* Colon, liver.

*Principal health related actions:* Alterative, blood tonic, cholagogue, mild laxative.

*Suggested uses:* Anemia (iron deficiency), excellent blood purifier, gastrointestinal diseases, certain inflammatory liver and gallbladder problems, liver congestion, mild laxative, skin conditions such as acne, eczema, herpes, psoriasis and skin eruptions. As a tonic for the body.

***Caution:*** Stop using yellow dock if it causes excessive urination, nausea or diarrhea.

***Note:*** The Chinese herb fo-ti also called he shou wu, has similar tonic properties as yellow dock.

## *Yerba santa (Eriodictyon californicum)*

Also known as ***Mountain balm*** and ***Holy herb***

*Source:* Leaves.

*Body systems most affected:* Lungs, spleen.

*Principal health related actions:* Alterative, carminative, expectorant, sialagogue.

*Suggested uses:* Treats upper-respiratory congestion by reducing coughing, clearing phlegm from the chest, alleviating bronchial congestion resulting from allergies, asthma and hay fever. Promotes salivation, thereby aiding digestion, dryness and thirst.

*Dosage:* Make a tea using 1 tablespoon (15 ml) in 1 cup (8 ounces, 237 ml) of warm water and drink 1 cup a day. For extracts and tinctures, blend 10 to 15 drops in water or juice each day, or as per label directions.

## *Yohimbe (Pausinystalia johimbe)*

*Source:* Bark of a tree from West Africa.

*Biochemical components:* An FDA-approved yohimbe extract, yohimbine hydrochloride, is used to treat impotence. It works by dilating the blood vessels. Unfortunately yohimbine hydrochloride can cause a sudden and potentially dangerous drop in blood pressure. It is not recommended for people with heart problems, low blood pressure or those on antidepressants. This powerful drug can cause anxiety attacks. The following information deals with the weaker Yohimbe herbal medicines you can purchase over-the-counter.

*Possible principal health related actions:* aphrodisiac, builds muscles, increases male potency, remedy for impotence.

*Suggested uses:* Usually combined with other natural substances, to enhance male sexual function, such as zinc, L-arginine and Ginkgo biloba.

***Caution:*** Consult with your doctor or naturally orientated healer before trying yohimbe products to determine the your best dosage range. Stop using yohimbe if sweating, nausea or vomiting occur. Avoid if you have a history of high blood pressure, psychosis, use tranquilizers, or antidepressants.

***Yucca (Yucca liliaceae)***

Also known as ***Spanish bayonet***.

*Source:* Root.

*Body systems most affected:* Liver, stomach.

*Principal health related actions:* Alterative, anti-inflammatory, antirheumatic, laxative, purgative.

*Suggested uses:* Alleviates arthritic and rheumatic joint pain, lessens inflammation.

*Dosage:* For extracts or tinctures, blend 10 to 30 drops in water or juice and take it up to three times a day, following the label directions. For tablets or capsules, take 1 up to three times a day to reduce symptoms.

***Caution:*** Sometimes yucca causes intestinal cramping. Combine with anti-rheumatic herbs such as prickly ash bark or ginger to counteract Yucca's potential intestinal cramping effect. Excessive long-term use can result in reduced absorption of vitamins A, D, E, and K. Consult your naturopath or nutritionally orientated doctor to design a supplementation program for the fat-soluble vitamins, if long term use of Yucca is required.

# chapter 15

# Aromatherapy

## — The Top 40 Essential Oils

## When, how and what to use them for

A Marriott Hotel in Florida greets its guests with an aromatherapeutic, stress-relieving blend of orange blossom, jasmine, lavender, lemon and peppermint. The Japanese use essential oils to increase productivity – lemon to start the day with a boost, rose at lunch time to sooth staff and tree-trunk in the late afternoon to reenergize them. Virgin Atlantic Airways uses it to alleviate jet lag in passengers. Bakeries use it to increase sales. What is it? Aromatherapy.

Basically there are four ways to use the aromatherapeutic essential oils from plants – orally, externally, nasally (inhalation) and in cooking. Aromatherapy uses the essential oils that are distilled from a whole plant or a specific part of the plant. These are powerful substances that can affect your health and well-being.

An essential oil can contain as many as 200 organic chemicals, the combination determining the essential oil's properties. Different essential oils affect different aspects of the body. For example, essential oil of grapefruit is thought to help suppress appetite and stimulate the immune system.

The essential oils are very delicate and volatile. Improper storage or exposure to sun, heat or air can deplete their beneficial properties. With proper storage, a small bottle will last years.

When using essential oils to create aromatherapy massage oils, it is preferable to use 100 percent pure botanical essential oils. Synthetic oils may not have the same therapeutic properties. It's the chemistry of the oil that counts. Read the label to see if it is diluted in a carrier base or 100 percent natural. The purer the oil, the greater the likelihood it will have therapeutic properties. Smell does not indicate whether or not it is a 100 percent pure botanical oil. Buyer beware. Ask.

Synergy means that the benefit derived from a combination of materials is greater than that provided by the individual components alone. Here's a partial list of recommended oils for different emotional states: For anxiety, use basil, bay, lemon balm, orange, sandalwood, ylang-ylang. For depression, use basil; and for hormonal depression, such as PMS, try clary sage. For tension, use Canadian pine, lemon balm, rosewood, ylang-ylang. And for insomnia, use tangerine or orange. When you go to sleep, put a drop of orange on your pillow and below your nose, then savor the aroma.

Orange irritates the skin if it is not diluted, so be careful. Orange drops leave stains, which usually wash out. For massage, very little is needed for total coverage. The oils also nourish the skin and body.

One stress relieving mixture includes the essential oils of Roman chamomile (3 drops), lavender (4 drops), and orange (3 drops) mixed into a base of 1/4 cup (60 ml) safflower and 1/4 cup (60 ml) almond cold-pressed oils. For different emotional states, you can use different oils in various combinations, with up to 12 drops of essential per half cup of base oils. Experiment with combinations of one or more of the oils to create the synergistic blend that works best for you.

Essential oils are prone to rapid deterioration if stored improperly. This is due to oxidation when exposed to air. In addition, exposure to sunlight or extremes of heat or cold can decrease the beneficial properties of an essential oil.

For example, when tea tree oil is exposed to air, the active microbial agent in it, terpinen-4-ol, begins to decrease. Technically, the Gamma-terpinene content decreases and the para-cymene content increases. Generally, tea tree oil is hardy and does not easily suffer a significant loss of potency when exposed to air, heat or light.

When stored properly, it and other essential oils have a shelf life of approximately three years, and have been known to stay potent even longer.

Ten points to remember when storing and using undiluted pure essential oils:

- Store in an airtight, dark glass container. (In certain instances, such as a diluted mixture, or when small amounts of oil are thoroughly mixed into a base, a clear plastic container is suitable.)
- Store away from extreme heat or cold.
- Store away from light.
- Store in a dry, cool place.

- Keep out of reach of children and pets.
- Clearly label the bottle.
- Only use in minute quantities (1-3 drops), unless otherwise prescribed.
- Some essential oils can be toxic to small pets, such as dogs and cats. Consult with your veterinarian before using them on pets.
- Do not use an essential oil from a family of plants you are allergic to.
- Consult a professional before using essential oils for therapeutic purposes, especially if you are using medications.

### *Four Key Ways to Use an Essential Oil*

*Orally* 2 to 3 drops in a teaspoonful of non-pasteurized honey or on a sugar cube, two to three times a day.

*Inhalation* Put a few drops in an essential oil diffuser. Use the diffuser according to the manufacturer's directions. Add a few drops to a bowl of hot water, then inhale. Add a few drops to the water in a facial steamer. Put a couple of drops on a cotton ball or handkerchief, then inhale. Sniff the oil directly from the bottle.

*Cooking* Blend a few drops with extra-virgin (cold-pressed) olive oil. Then add a few drops of this mixture to your recipe.

***Quick tip:*** 3 drops of an essential oil = one teaspoon (5 ml) of a dried herb.

*Externally* For massage, mix 5 to 9 drops into 3 oz (6 tablespoons, 90 ml) of cold-pressed safflower oil.

For a bath, put 7-9 drops in 3 oz (6 tablespoons, 90 ml) of cold-pressed sweet almond oil.

For a non-oily lotion, dilute 5 drops of essential oil with 1/2 cup (4 oz, 118 ml) of aloe vera nectar.

Massage involves touching the skin by rubbing or kneading a part of the body. It stimulates circulation, aids the lymphatic system and increases the production and release of oxytocin, a powerful natural healing hormone in the body. Combine that with the beneficial properties of an essential oil and you have a dynamic therapeutic combination.

When using an essential oil for massage, mix it with a light vegetable oil as a carrier. A carrier oil is what you put an essential oil into.

Different carrier oils have different properties. Cold-pressed, unadulterated oils are preferred. They do not contain the harsh chemicals used in the processing of many oils, nor are they processed at high temperatures that may weaken or destroy some or all of their beneficial properties.

Try the following cold-pressed carrier oils: jojoba, sweet almond, corn or grapeseed. Soya, sunflower, apricot kernel, avocado, hazelnut, peanut and olive oil can also be used in creating your own carrier oil blend.

While jojoba oil is a liquid wax that does not go rancid, the other oils can. To prolong their shelf life, add a little wheat germ oil, which has vitamin E and antioxidant properties.

For massage purposes, a little essential oil diluted in a carrier oil, will provide a lot of coverage. Before each application, gently roll the container of essential oil and carrier oil between your palms. Apply to the affected area two to four times daily at the beginning, then reduce to twice daily.

### *Carrier Oils*

The highly concentrated essential oils are often diluted in a carrier oil for external applications, such as an aromatherapy massage or an aromatherapy bath. If you choose to use only one carrier oil, use one from the 100 percent list and add the essential oil to this carrier.

To create a blended carrier oil, determine which oils best match your skin condition. Choose one from the 100 percent carrier oil list and one from the 10 percent carrier oil list. For example, if your skin is dry and dehydrated, you may decide to use apricot kernel oil from the 100 percent list and boost the beneficial properties of the carrier oil by adding avocado pear oil from the 10 percent carrier oil list.

To make your carrier oil blend with 10 percent of its volume being avocado pear oil, you blend one teaspoon of avocado pear oil with 9 teaspoons of apricot kernel oil. This is called a 10 percent carrier oil dilution by volume.

Carrier oils that match various conditions are indicated below. For example, sweet almond oil is good for inflammation, so that could be a base carrier oil to blend with essential oils for conditions such as bursitis, carpal tunnel syndrome or repetitive strain syndrome.

***Note:*** If you or a child are allergic to peanuts, properly processed oils such as sweet almond, hazelnut or even peanut do not contain the protein that causes these allergic reactions and should not pose a problem. To be on the safe side, speak to your doctor, allergist or health care provider if in doubt.

### *100 Percent Carrier Oils*

| | |
|---|---|
| Apricot Kernel Oil | good for prematurely aged, dry, inflamed, and sensitive skin. |
| Corn Oil | soothes all skin types. |
| Grapeseed Oil | good for general use. |
| Hazelnut Oil | provides mildly astringent action. |
| Peanut Oil (Arachis Nut) | good for general use. |
| Safflower Oil | good for general use. |
| Soya Oil | good for general use. |
| Sunflower Oil | good for general use. |
| Sweet Almond Oil | relieves itching, dryness, soreness and inflammation. |

### *10 Percent Carrier Oils*

Maximum of 10 percent of the total volume of the carrier oil

| | |
|---|---|
| Avocado Pear Oil | good for dehydrated skin, eczema. |
| Borage Seed Oil | good for heart disease, multiple sclerosis, menopausal problems, PMS, psoriasis and eczema, prematurely aged skin. Stimulates and regenerates skin. |
| Carrot Oil | good for itching, premature aging, psoriasis and eczema. Rejuvenating and reduces scarring. |
| Evening Primrose Oil | good for heart disease, multiple sclerosis, menopausal problems, PMS, psoriasis and eczema, prematurely aged skin. Helps prevent premature aging of skin. |
| Jojoba Oil | good for acne, hair care, inflamed skin, psoriasis and eczema. It is highly penetrative. This is the oil used by Native Americans for smooth, soft and healthy skin. |
| Olive Oil (Extra virgin) | good for cosmetics, hair care, rheumatic conditions. Soothing. |
| Sesame Oil | good for arthritis, eczema, psoriasis, rheumatism. |
| Wheatgerm Oil | good for eczema, psoriasis, prematurely aged skin. |

### *Check out these top 11 essential oils every home should have:*

| | | | |
|---|---|---|---|
| Lavender | Tea Tree | Lemon | Rosemary |
| Peppermint | Thyme | Chamomile | Clove |
| Eucalyptus | Geranium | Clary sage | |

### *Synergistic Combinations*

Essential oils blend very well together. The benefits to an individual can be significantly increased if the right oils are used in the best proportion for the condition being dealt with. We recommend you purchase a couple of good books on aromatherapy if you want to maximize the benefits to you and your family. You will save time, energy and money once you become acquainted with the powers of aromatherapy. One book we recommend is *The Tea Tree Oil Bible* (AGES Publications, 1999). Ordering information is at the back of this book.

### *Sample Uses*

| | |
|---|---|
| Anxiety | Basil, chamomile, jasmine, eucalyptus, marjoram, Neroli, ylang-ylang, thyme. |
| Depression | Chamomile, lavender, jasmine, nutmeg, thyme. |
| Dizziness and fainting | Cinnamon, peppermint, nutmeg, rosemary, wintergreen. |
| Headaches | Peppermint, chamomile, cardamom, lemon, lavender, rosemary, wintergreen. |
| Hysteria | Chamomile, lavender, jasmine, neroli, nutmeg, rose, peppermint, rosemary. |
| Irritability | Chamomile, cypress, lavender, jasmine, marjoram, nutmeg, vanilla, melissa, rose. |
| Menstrual cramps | Clary sage, chamomile, cypress, eucalyptus, marjoram, juniper, peppermint, rose, rosemary, ylang-ylang. |
| Impotence | Cinnamon, cypress, clove, frankincense, ginger, juniper, patchouli, peppermint, thyme, vanilla, sandalwood, ylang-ylang. |

## *The Top 40 Essential Oils*

### *Basil (Ocimum basilicum)*

*Part of plant used:* Whole plant.

*Principle geographic sources:* United States, Europe, Madagascar, Seychelles Islands.

*Main symptom indications and uses:* Anxiety, depression, migraines, nervous spasms, bronchitis, colds, fatigue, gout, loss of concentration, aches and pains.

*Primary system targeted:* Nervous.

*Methods of use:* Orally, externally, cooking. See page 249.

### *Bay (Laurus nobilis)*

*Part of plant used:* Leaves.

*Principal geographic sources:* South America, West Indies.

*Main symptom indications and uses:* Allergies, anxiety, asthma, colds, congestion, flu, infections, insomnia, psychosis, rheumatism, spasms.

*Primary systems targeted:* Dermal (skin), neurological, respiratory.

*Methods of use:* Orally, externally, inhalation. See page 249.

### *Bergamot (Citrus bergamia)*

*Part of plant used:* Peel of fruit.

*Principal geographic sources:* Guinea, Italy, Morocco.

*Main symptom indications and uses:* Acne, coughs, cuts, bruises, perfume, tension, scrapes, skin ulcers. It is also used as an antidepressant to counteract stress.

*Primary system targeted:* Dermal.

*Method of use:* Externally. See page 249.

***Caution:*** A very toxic essential oil. Avoid if you are sensitive to sunlight. Only for external use.

### *Canadian pine (Abies balsamea)*

*Parts of plant used:* Leaves and bark.

*Principal geographic sources:* United States, Canada.

*Main symptom indications and uses:* Arthritis and rheumatism, convalescence and fatigue, spasms, tension.

*Primary systems targeted:* Blood, musculoskeletal.

*Methods of use:* Orally, externally, inhalation. See page 249.

**Caution:** Excessive amounts may cause indigestion.

### *Carrot seed (Daucus carota)*

*Parts of plant used:* Root, seeds.

*Principal geographic sources:* England, France.

*Main symptom indications and uses:* Eczema, psoriasis, flatulence, gout, ulcers; used as a diuretic.

*Methods of use:* As a carrier (base) oil. See page 249.

### *Cedar (Juniperus virginiana)*

*Parts of plant used:* Tree, wood.

*Principal geographic sources:* United States, Canada.

*Main symptom indications and uses:* Only for household applications and/or as an insecticide. Do not use for therapeutic purposes.

*Methods of use:* For a disinfectant, add 30 to 90 drops to a gallon of soapy water. It leaves a clean, fresh scent.

**Caution:** It is a very toxic essential oil. Only use for household cleaning and/or as an insecticide.

### *Cinnamon (Cinnamomum zeylanicum)*

*Parts of plant used:* Twigs, leaves.

*Principal geographic sources:* India, Madagascar, Sri Lanka.

*Main symptom indications and uses:* Chills, colds, constipation, coughs, fatigue, flatulence, flu, lose of appetite, viral infections, rheumatism, sexual stimulant, warts.

*Primary systems targeted:* Gastrointestinal, neurological.

*Methods of use:* Orally, inhalation, cooking. See page 249.

**Caution:** Cinnamon is dermacaustic – avoid contact with skin and avoid excessive use, as excessive doses may be highly stimulating. Not recommended for diabetics.

### *Citronella (Cymbopogon nardus)*

*Parts of plant used:* All parts.

*Principal geographic sources:* South America and Madagascar.

*Main symptom indications and uses:* Insecticide, deodorant, stimulant, tonic, for skin irritation and wrinkles.

*Primary system targeted in body:* Skin.

*Method of use:* Externally. See page 249.

### *Clary sage (Salvia sclarea)*

*Parts of plant used:* Flowering tops.

*Principal geographic sources:* France, Russia, Spain.

*Main symptom indications and uses:* PMS and menstrual pains, general aches and pain, menopausal problems, hormone depression, bad circulation, nervousness, acts as a sedative.

*Primary system targeted:* Female urogenital

*Methods of use:* Orally, externally, cooking. See page 249.

**Caution:** Never use during pregnancy.

### *Clove (Eugenia caryophyllata)*

*Part of plant used:* Flower bud.

*Principal geographic sources:* East and West Indies, Molucca Islands, Philippines.

*Main symptom indications and uses:* antiseptic and analgesic; use for arthritis, bronchitis, chills, diarrhea, parasites, flatulence, infections, nausea, rheumatism, toothaches, viruses.

*Primary systems targeted:* Digestive system. Immune system.

*Methods of use:* Orally, cooking. See page 249.

**Caution:** Never use during pregnancy. Dermacaustic – avoid contact with skin.

### *Cypress (Cupressus sempervirens)*

*Parts of plant used:* Leaves, twigs.

*Principal geographic source:* Mediterranean.

*Main symptom indications and uses:* Hemorrhoids, congested prostate, circulatory conditions, excessive sweating, menopausal problems, nervous tension, rhinitis (inflammation of the nose or its mucous membrane), sinusitis, varicose veins, whooping cough, as an astringent on wounds.

*Primary systems targeted:* Male urogenital, female urogenital, circulatory.

*Methods of use:* Orally, externally, inhalation. See page 249.

### *Eucalyptus (Eucalyptus globulus)*

*Parts of plant used:* Leaves, twigs.

*Principal geographic sources:* California, Australia, Brazil, China, Tasmania, Spain.

*Main symptom indications and uses:* As an antiseptic and anti-inflammatory; for arthritic and rheumatic pain, coughs, bronchitis, inflammation, muscular pain, neuralgia, sinusitis, skin infections, sores, sore throats, ulcers.

*Primary systems targeted:* Musculoskeletal.

*Methods of use:* Externally, inhalation. See page 249.

### *Frankincense (Buswellia thurifera)*

*Part of plant used:* Bark.

*Principal geographic sources:* China, Ethiopia, Somalia, Southern Arabia.

*Main symptom indications and uses:* For bronchitis, coughs, colds, fevers, inflammation, laryngitis, nervous conditions, sores, skin eruption, stress, tension, wound healing; as perfume, calmative.

*Primary system targeted:* Neurological.

*Methods of use:* Externally, inhalation. See page 249.

**Cautions:** A very toxic essential oil. Never take Frankincense orally. Only for external use.

### *Geranium (Pelargonium graveolens)*

*Part of plant used:* flowers, leaves, stalks.

*Principal geographic sources:* Algeria, China, Egypt, France, Madagascar, Morocco, Russia.

*Main symptom indications and uses:* For depression, diabetes, diarrhea, inflammation, circulatory problems, kidney stones, menstrual problems, neuralgia, oily skin, skin irritation, eczema, sores, sore throats: as a perfume.

*Primary system targeted:* Skin.

*Methods of use:* Orally, externally, inhalation. See page 249.

### ***Ginger (Zingiber officinalis)***

*Part of plant used:* Roots.

*Principal geographic sources:* China, India, Japan, West Africa.

*Main symptom indications and uses:* Chills, cold, fever, loss of appetite, as an immune system stimulant.

*Primary systems targeted:* Digestive, immune.

*Methods of use:* Orally, cooking. See page 249.

### ***Grapefruit (Citrus paradisi)***

*Part of plant used:* Rind of fruit.

*Principal geographic sources:* United States, Israel.

*Main symptom indications and uses:* Aid for drug withdrawal, a tonic, anticarcinogenic and immune system stimulant; for cholesterol, depression. infections, liver and kidney problems, migraines, obesity; used as a perfume, cholesterol, depression, infections.

*Primary systems targeted:* Blood (hepatic), immune.

*Methods of use:* Orally, cooking. See page 249.

### ***Jasmine (Jasminum officinalis)***

*Part of plant used:* Flower.

*Principal geographic sources:* Algeria, China, Egypt, France, Morocco.

*Main symptom indications and uses:* Anxiety, aphrodisiac, depression, lethargy, menstrual problems, nervous tension; a relaxant.

*Primary systems targeted:* Brain, nervous.

*Methods of use:* Inhalation. See page 249.

### ***Juniper (Juniperus communis)***

*Part of plant used:* Berry.

*Principal geographic sources:* United States, Canada, Europe, North Asia, North Africa.

*Main symptom indications and uses:* Acne, rashes, liver problems, coughs, obesity, respiratory distress, rheumatic pain, fever, skin inflammation – ulcers; as a diuretic for urinary infections (e.g. cystitis).

*Primary systems targeted:* Skin, respiratory.

*Methods of use:* Orally, externally, inhalation. See page 249.

### *Lavender (Lavendula spica)*

*Part of plant used:* Flower.

*Principal geographic sources:* France, England, Yugoslavia, Tasmania.

*Main symptom indications and uses:* Burns, acne, arthritis, asthma, bacterial problems, boils, congestion, cough, cuts, earache, eczema, fainting, headaches, infections, inflammation, influenza, insomnia, migraines, muscular pains, neuralgia, rheumatic pains, sore throat, sinusitis, toothache, nervous tension, ulcers, wounds.

*Primary systems targeted:* Skin, respiratory.

*Methods of use:* Orally, externally, inhalation. See page 249.

### *Lemon (Citrus limonum)*

*Part of plant used:* Rind.

*Principal geographic sources:* United States, Argentina, Brazil, Israel.

*Main symptom indications and uses:* Used as an astringent, antiseptic, mood enhancer and tonic for anxiety, blood pressure, concentration, digestive problems, fever, gallstones, oily skin, skin infection and irritation, sore throat; also used as a perfume.

*Primary system targeted:* Skin.

*Methods of use:* Inhalation, externally, cooking. See page 249.

### *Lemon balm (Melissa officinalis)*

*Parts of plant used:* Flower, leaf.

*Principal geographic sources:* North America, Europe. North Asia.

*Main symptom indications and uses:* Anxiety, skin eruptions, tension, wounds.

*Primary systems targeted:* Nerves, skin.

*Methods of use:* Orally, externally, inhalation. See page 249.

### *Lemongrass (Cymbopogon citratus)*

*Part of plant used:* Whole plant.

*Principal geographic sources:* Brazil, Central Africa, Sri Lanka.

*Main symptom indications and uses:* Used as an insect repellent, antiseptic and tonic; used for respiratory problems, sore throats, fevers, headaches, infections.

*Primary systems targeted:* Respiratory, skin.

*Methods of use:* Externally, inhalation. See page 249.

### *Lime (Citrus aurantifolia)*

*Part of plant used:* Rind.

*Principal geographic sources:* Mexico, Brazil, Italy, West Indies.

*Main symptom indications and uses:* Used as a tonic and astringent. For alcoholism, anorexia, anxiety, depression, headaches, fevers, sore throats, rheumatism.

*Primary systems targeted:* Respiratory, brain.

*Methods of use:* Orally, externally, inhalation. See page 249.

### *Mandarin (Citrus Noblis)*

*Part of plant used:* Rind.

*Principal geographic sources:* Argentina, Brazil, China, Italy, Spain.

*Main symptom indications and uses:* Used as a tranquilizer and tonic. Anxiety, weak digestive system, insomnia, liver problems, nervousness.

*Primary systems targeted:* Digestive, nervous.

*Methods of use:* Orally, externally, inhalation, cooking. See page 249.

### *Marjoram (Origanum marjorana)*

*Parts of plant used:* Flower, leaf.

*Principal geographic sources:* France, Egypt, Germany, Portugal, Hungary, Spain.

*Main symptom indications and uses:* Anxiety, asthma, loss of appetite, arthritic and rheumatic inflammation, bloating, bronchitis, circulatory problems, diarrhea, headaches (e.g. stress induced, migraines), insomnia, intestinal cramps, menstrual problems, muscular problems; used as an immune system stimulant and a perfume.

*Primary systems targeted:* Circulatory, digestive, neurological.

*Methods of use:* Orally, externally, inhalation, cooking. See page 249.

### *Neroli (Citrus bigaradia, the orange blossoms)*

*Part of plant used:* Flower.

*Principal geographic sources:* France, Morocco, Italy, Egypt, Tunisia.

*Main symptom indications and uses:* Anxiety, dermatitis, depression, diarrhea, hysteria, insomnia, menopausal problems, nervous tension; its positive mood altering affect makes it beneficial as a cardiac tonic.

*Primary systems targeted:* Neurological, skin.

*Methods of use:* Inhalation, externally. See page 249.

### *Orange (Citrus aurantium)*

*Part of plant used:* Rind.

*Principal geographic sources:* United States, Brazil, Spain, France.

*Main symptom indications and uses:* Sedative, anticarcinogenic, antiseptic, perfume, and tonic; used for anxiety, cholesterol, constipation, depression, infections, insomnia, muscular spasms, nervous conditions, wrinkles.

*Primary systems targeted:* Immune, skin.

*Methods of use:* Orally, externally, inhalation, cooking. See page 249.

### *Oregano oil (Origanum vulgare)*

*Parts of plant used:* Flowering tops, leaves. Recently, oregano oil has become fashionable, so we decided to give you additional information about it. In Greece and Crete, it is known for its ability to slow food spoilage through its antibacterial, antifungal, antiparasitic and antioxidant activity. In North American supermarkets, the related herbs marjoram and thyme are often incorrectly labeled as oregano and do not have wild oregano's powerful healing properties.

*Principal geographic sources:* Europe, North Africa, Egypt and Asia.

*How it works:* The oil is extracted from the leaves which contain phenols. Isomeric phenols, mainly carvacrol, in dilutions as low as 1 part per 50,000 destroys Aspergillus mold, Candida albicans, E. coli, Staphylococcus and other bacteria. Another phenol constituent, Thymol, boosts the immune system. Their compounds also shield against toxins by acting as free radical scavengers, thereby preventing additional tissue damage while encouraging healing.

*Principal health related actions:* Antibacterial, antifungal, antioxidant, anti-parasitic, antiviral.

*Main symptom indications and uses:* Acne, allergies, arthritis, asthma, athlete's foot, bronchitis, candidiasis, canker sores, colds/flus, cold sores, colitis, congestion, croup, dandruff, diarrhea, digestive problems, earache, eczema, fatigue, gastritis, gum disease, muscle pain, neuritis, prostatitis, psoriasis, respiratory problems, rheumatism, ringworm, rosacae, seborrhea, sinusitis, varicose veins, viral infections, warts, and wounds.

*Methods of use:* Orally, externally, inhalation, cooking. See page 249. Blend 3 to 5 drops of oregano oil with one teaspoon (5 ml) of extra virgin olive oil to improve palatability. Put 2 to 3 drops of the blend under the tongue, several times daily.

### *Oregon grape root (Mahonia aguifolium and Mahonia repens)*

*Parts of plant used:* Root and rhizome. (Its main biochemical component is berberine alkaloid.)

*Principal parts it benefits:* Gallbladder, liver.

*Main symptom indications and uses:* Astringent, alterative, anti-inflammatory, cholagogue, tonic. Used for cankers, hay fever, hemorrhage, mucous membranes, sinus congestion, wounds. Stops bleeding from uterus, lungs and colon. Improves circulation. Beneficial for liver problems, and menstrual irregularities. For sores, it may be used externally as a poultice. The powder relieves nasal congestion and sinus problems when sniffed. In tea, use as a gargle for sore throats.

*Dosage:* As a tincture, take 10 to 20 drops, three times a day or as per manufacturers directions.

*Caution:* Large doses can cause nausea and vomiting. Not to be taken over long periods for sufferers of hypothyroidism or anemia.

### *Parsley (Petroselinum sativum)*

*Part of plant used:* Seed.

*Principal geographic sources:* Europe, United States, Canada.

*Main symptom indications and uses:* Used as a diuretic and sedative. Used for acne, anemia, foul breath, digestive disturbance, intoxication, kidney problems, menstrual problems, menopausal problems, nervous conditions, rheumatism.

*Primary systems targeted:* Digestive, blood.

*Methods of use:* Orally, cooking. See page 249.

**Caution:** Never use during pregnancy.

### *Patchouli (Pogostemon cabin)*

*Part of plant used:* Leaf.

*Principal geographic sources:* Japan, China, Madagascar, Indonesia.

*Main symptom indications and uses:* Used as an antiseptic, insecticide and diuretic for acne, eczema, fungal infections, skin inflammations; also used as a perfume, aphrodisiac, tonic, and for dandruff (seborrhea).

*Primary system targeted:* Skin.

*Methods of use:* Orally, externally, inhalation. See page 249.

### *Peppermint (Mentha piperata)*

*Part of plant used:* Leaf.

*Principal geographic sources:* United States, Canada, Europe, China.

*Main symptom indications and uses:* Used as a stimulant. Used for arthritis, digestive spasms, sluggish digestion, fatigue, fevers, flatulence, indigestion, intoxication, inflammation, nausea, sluggish liver, tired aching feet, tension headaches.

*Primary systems targeted:* Digestive, neurological.

*Methods of use:* Orally, externally, cooking. See page 249. Excellent for tension headaches. Put a drop or two on your finger or a cotton ball and draw it across you forehead from temple to temple, on your eyebrows and along your hairline. Do the same for the back of your neck. Repeat as needed.

**Caution:** In high dosages, it may be toxic. The essential oil is not recommended for use in hypertension cases. Have your health care provider confirm that tension headaches are the cause of your headaches, before using peppermint oil. If peppermint oil gets into your eyes, immediately wash them out with water.

### *Pine (Pinus sylvestris)*

*Parts of plant used:* Needles, twigs.

*Principal geographic sources:* United States, Canada, Europe, Russia, North Asia.

*Main symptom indications and uses:* Used as a diuretic. For fatigue, catarrh, chest infections, circulation problems, colds, kidney and bladder problems, muscle aches and pains, rheumatism, respiratory problems, sore throats.

*Primary systems targeted:* Blood, respiratory.

*Methods of use:* Orally, externally, inhalation. See page 249.

***Caution:*** Excessive amounts may cause indigestion.

### *Roman chamomile (Chamaemelum nobile)*

*Parts of plant used:* Flower, leaf.

*Principal geographic sources:* Bulgaria, England, France, Hungary, Yugoslavia.

*Main symptom indications and uses:* Acne, poor circulation, dermatitis, headache, insomnia, menstrual pains, migraines, nervousness, neuralgia, spasms.

*Primary systems targeted:* Urogenital in females, circulatory in males and females.

*Methods of use:* Orally, externally, inhalation. See page 249.

### *Rose Bulgar (Rosa damascena)*

*Parts of plant used:* Flower, petals.

*Principal geographic source:* Bulgaria.

*Main symptom indications and uses:* Anxiety, antiseptic, aphrodisiac, depression, poor circulation, menopausal problems, tonic.

*Primary systems targeted:* Circulatory, brain, respiratory.

*Methods of use:* Externally, inhalation. See page 249.

### *Rose Morac (Rosa damascena)*

*Parts of plant used:* Flower, petals.

*Principal geographic source:* Morrocco.

*Main symptom indications and uses:* Aphrodisiac, depression, poor circulation, menopausal problems, stress, sedative, tonic.

*Primary systems targeted:* Circulatory, brain, respiratory.

*Methods of use:* Externally, inhalation. See page 249.

### *Rosemary (Rosmarinus officinalis)*

*Parts of plant used:* Flower, leaf.

*Principal geographic sources:* France, Japan, Spain, Yugoslavia.

*Main symptom indications and uses:* Analgesic, liver decongestant, heart tonic, decongestant, nerve stimulant. For arthritis, gout, hair, rheumatism, obesity, poor circulation, congestion, immune stimulant, muscular pains and aches, skin, sprains, spinal injuries.

*Primary systems targeted:* Circulatory, immune, respiratory.

*Methods of use:* Orally, externally, inhalation, cooking. See page 249.

### *Rosewood (Aniba rosaeodora)*

*Parts of plant used:* Wood, bark.

*Main symptom indications and uses:* Healing, inflammation, skin eruption, tension. Used as a perfume.

*Primary systems targeted:* Skin.

*Methods of use:* Externally, inhalation. See page 249.

### *Sandalwood (Santalum album)*

*Part of plant used:* Wood.

*Principal geographic sources:* India, Indonesia.

*Main symptom indications and uses:* Used as a sedative, mood enhancer, sexual stimulant, perfume. For anxiety, depression, acne, bacterial infections, cystitis, fungal infections, inflammation, menstrual problems, skin infections.

*Primary systems targeted:* Neurological, skin.

*Methods of use:* Externally, inhalation. See page 249.

***Cautions:*** A very toxic essential oil. Only for external use.

### *Tea tree (Melaleuca alternifolia)*

*Part of plant used:* Leaf.

*Principal geographic source:* Australia.

*Main symptom indications and uses:* Antibacterial, antifungal, antiviral, disinfectant, general stimulant, immune stimulant, penetrating. For acne, burns, flus, fungal, gangrene, warts, yeast to zona. There are over 100 conditions and hundreds of ways to use and benefit from tea tree oil for health, home, beauty, plant and pet care. We refer you to *The Tea Tree Oil Bible* (AGES Publications, ordering information in the back of this book).

*Primary systems targeted:* Blood, skin, neurological.

*Methods of use:* Orally, externally, inhalation. See page 249.

***Caution:*** Avoid excessive use, as high doses may be highly stimulating. If you or a child swallow 1 teaspoon (5 mg) or more, call your local poison control center. Generally, it is not toxic.

### *Thyme (Thymus vulgaris)*

*Part of plant used:* Herb.

*Principal geographic sources:* Mediterranean, Egypt.

*Main symptom indications and uses:* Used as a tonic, stimulant and immune system booster. For bacterial infections, sore throat, lethargy, roundworm, sores, urinary infections, wounds.

*Primary systems targeted:* Ear, nose, throat.

*Methods of use:* Orally, externally, inhalation, cooking. See page 249.

***Cautions:*** Excessive amounts may cause indigestion.

### *Ylang-ylang (Cananga odorata)*

*Part of plant used:* Flower.

*Principal geographic sources:* Comoro Islands, Indonesia, Philippines.

*Main symptom indications and uses:* Used as a general tonic, mood enhancer, perfume, skin tonic, sedative, aphrodisiac. For anxiety, depression, high blood pressure, tension.

*Primary systems targeted in body:* Neurological, skin.

*Methods of use:* Externally, inhalation. See page 249.

***Caution:*** Avoid excessive use, as high doses may be extremely stimulating.

# chapter 16

# Homeopathy

## What, how and when to use Homeopathic Remedies with everyday health problems

### *What is homeopathy and who uses it?*

The Royal Family uses it. Europeans use it. It is estimated that over 500 million people worldwide use this seemingly magical tool to deal with illness and disease. In Great Britain, an experiment with sick cows given homeopathic remedies, cleared their diseases. Many veterinarians use homeopathic remedies in their practices.

German physician Samuel Hahnemann, founded homeopathy in the early 1800s, based on the principle of "like cures like". There are two different approaches used to create and apply homeopathic remedies. The classical method uses only one single-component remedy at a time. The physician prescribes it in a potency, meaning the number of times the substance is diluted and shaken, specifically adjusted to the patient, at that moment in time. Then the physician waits to see what happens before prescribing anything else. Complex homeopathy involves multiple substances, given at the same time, usually in low potencies.

A homeopathic nosode is a super-diluted remedy, that takes the energy imprint from a disease such as tuberculosis, bacterial infection, influenza, measles and about 200 others. No physical traces of the disease are in the nosode. It stimulates the body to rid itself of all 'taints' or residues it holds of a disease, whether contracted or inherited. Only qualified homeopaths administer a nosode.

A homeopathic miasm is the taint or energy residue of previous, even inherited, illness. Inherited predispositions for chronic diseases are much more subtle than genetic ones. These broad focused remedies benefit families and people predisposed to specific illnesses such as cancer, sexually transmitted diseases, psoriasis and tuberculosis. The remedies are usually available from health food stores, pharmacies and homeopathic practitioners. How do they work? Primarily by stimulating your body's natural wisdom to heal itself and utilize its self-balancing mechanisms.

The example and remedies listed here are based on personality traits, environmental and other stress inducing situations. The key is to find the remedy best suited for you and your particular situation. The better the fit, the greater the chance of success. Relief can occur within minutes, hours or days. Use one remedy at a time, observe its effects before trying another. Your body takes time to correct the imbalances and problems. Be patient. Potency technically refers to the dilution of the substance. The greater the dilution, the more powerful or potent the homeopathic remedy is. In essence, there may not even be one molecule of the actual substance used to energize the water in the solution. Why it works remains the subject of much theorizing.

### *When and how to take a homeopathic remedy*

The remedies are usually in pellet or liquid form. They should be placed directly under the tongue, and held there for one to three minutes, until they dissolve and are absorbed by the mucous membrane. The best time to take them is on an empty stomach, between meals and an hour or so after or before brushing the teeth.

### *What if the wrong remedy is used, will I get sick?*

No. That is one of the wonderful aspects of homeopathy. One cannot overdose with it and if a remedy doesn't work for you, there will be no side effects. Since exactly how and why the mechanism works are not fully understood, a trained practitioner is especially important when administering to the unique symptoms of a sick person. The powerful targeted single remedies are only available through consultation with a naturopathic doctor, homeopath or suitably trained health care professional.

One exception to the rule is the homeopathic remedy, thuya. In high doses thuya may cause the cancer to spread. It should only be administered by a trained homeopath or naturopath.

### *What homeopathic remedies would you use for stress?*

Homeopathy has thousands of formulas. Depending on the nature and traits of the individual and condition, a classical homeopathic practitioner will recommend a course of treatment starting with one remedy at a time. Their remedies are significantly more powerful than those you would buy over-the-counter.

The following is a sampling of remedies for stress-related problems. First is the name of the remedy, followed by a dosage range or amount in parentheses. The key to successfully using these off-the-shelf preparations is to choose the one best suited for you and your situation. The closer personality traits and specific situations match the weak spots or underlying tendencies, the greater the chances of the remedy working for you. Read them and, if need be, refer to a book on homeopathy. If you are still unsure, see an homeopathic practitioner or naturopath trained in using these remedies.

| ***Remedy*** | ***Dilution*** | ***Condition*** |
|---|---|---|
| Colubrina | (12c-30c) | Usually for stress caused by sleep deprivation or prolonged office work, mental work or studying. |
| Nat. Mur. | (6c-12c) | Relieves symptoms that appear after anger, fright or grief. |
| Sepia | (6c-12c) | For chronic stress or overwork, such as motherhood or pregnancy. |
| Pulsatilla | (12c) | Stress characterized by rapid mood swings, symptoms which wander from place to place or constantly changing physical symptoms. |
| Sulfur | (12c) | For a variety of states, this is a deep and broad acting remedy. |
| Staphysagria | (12c-30c) | For grief that has been 'swept under the rug', anger or indignation. |

## *Some conditions and appropriate homeopathic remedies*

### *Burns*

| | |
|---|---|
| Arnica | First remedy of choice. |
| Cantharis | Second choice for burns. |
| Calendula | Use for minor burns. Soothes pain, prevents infection and speeds healing. |
| Causticum | Use when pain occurs with blister formation and restlessness. |
| Aloe Vera | Promotes healing and relieves pain. |

### *Coughs*

| | |
|---|---|
| Drosera | Used for barking coughs to the point of choking, ticklish throat, dry cough, shortness of breath. |
| Spongia | Used when one exhibits symptoms of croupy cough, wheezing and shortness of breath. After drinking warm drinks, you cough more effectively. |
| Phosphorus | Sensation of cough being in your lungs. Symptoms include a dry cough, tightness in the chest, tickling behind the breastbone. |
| Causticum | Severe cough accompanied by a painful raw throat. |
| Bryonia | Very painful dry cough, that causes one to hold their ribs while coughing. The cough worsens with movement. It is better with heat, a compress bandage wrapped around the ribs, and rest. |

### *Dental Problems and Surgery*

| | |
|---|---|
| Aconite | Helps deal with underlying emotions (anxiety, fear, nervousness) one may have during dental problems and surgery. |
| Arnica | Trauma after tooth extraction. Sore gums. |
| Hypericum | Used for nerve pain caused by drilling, tooth extraction and/or root canals. Also see *Injury and Trauma.* |
| Phosphorus | Used for relief from the after effects of anesthetics and excessive bleeding. |
| Staphysagria | Good remedy for dental work, nerve pain and sharp wounds. Use when symptoms are due to stitching, and when the area is sore and tender and worsens when touched slightly, but feels better under strong pressure. |

### *Digestive System conditions*

| | |
|---|---|
| Carbo Vegetabilis | Use when symptoms of nausea are combined with a sour acid taste in the mouth, flatulence and digestive distress after eating. |
| Chamomilla Vulgaris | Infants with diarrhea. Emotional hypersensitivity affecting the digestive system. |
| Colubrina | Constipation, indigestion and hemorrhoids. |
| Ipeca | Vomiting and nausea, distended abdomen and constantly swallowing saliva. Symptoms are worsened by bending over. Ipeca is used by pregnant women. |

| | |
|---|---|
| Lycopodium | For migraine headaches of digestive origin. Other symptoms include noisy flatulence, nausea and liver congestion. |
| Magnesium Phosphoricum | Colic in infants and abdominal cramping. |

### *Emotional Trauma*

Also refer to ***Flower Remedies*** in the next chapter.

| | |
|---|---|
| Gelsemium Sempervirens | For use in stage fright, anticipatory anxiety of situations. In cases where fear has a tendency to cause trembling weakness, diarrhea and lapses in memory. |
| Iamara | This is the remedy of choice for grief, depression, stress and hypersensitivity to emotion. |
| Rescue Remedy® | Combines five flower remedies – Cherry Plum, Clematis, Impatiens, Rock Rose and Star of Bethlehem – for a variety of stressful situations. Many health care professionals, veterinarians and consumers have indicated it produces calming and stabilizing results. It comforts and calms individuals who experience severe upset, get serious news and experience traumatic events, which may lead to a dazed and/or numb state of mind. It also appears to be helpful in less severe circumstances, such as examinations, arguments, and visits to the dentist. Rescue Remedy® is a must for your self-health care medicine cabinet. |

***Note:*** Rescue Remedy® – It is not a traditional single dose homeopathic remedy, and would not normally be included with these remedies. Rescue Remedy® uses a very gentle homeopathic approach, which is covered in the next chapter on Flower Remedies.

### *Fever*

| | |
|---|---|
| Belladonna | The initial remedy of choice for the sudden onset of a fever, acute feverish states, high temperatures accompanied with hot perspiration. Also for general or local spasms, bright redness, congestion, throbbing pain. |
| Ferrum Phosphoricum | For gradual onset of a low grade fever. |
| Aconite | For sudden onset of fever, restlessness, fear and anxiety, and burning sensation. The symptoms worsen in |

| | |
|---|---|
| | the evening. Fever, chills and throbbing pulse are not accompanied by perspiration. |
| Natrum Muriaticum | For the early stages of fever when liquids do not alleviate an excessive thirst and the skin is dry. |

### *Headaches*

| | |
|---|---|
| Aconite | Headaches with a violent start, tingling and numbness, burning pain, extreme restlessness and anxiety. The pain moves to the nose and forehead. At night the symptoms get worse. You feel better when lying down in the open air. |
| Belladonna | For a sudden intense onset of pain and throbbing temples. Your face becomes hot and red and the pupils your eyes dilate. The headache worsens with eye movement, light and noise. It eases when bending your head back or lying down. |
| Gelsemium Sempervirens | Use when the following symptoms occur: eyelids and head feel heavy, vision blurs or you feel lethargy, trembling, weakness. |
| Nux Vomica | For tension and stress headaches, with digestive upset. For example, a dull headache in front of the head, like a hangover. The pain intensifies in cold weather or noisy surroundings, in the morning, when there is light. |
| Sanguinaria | Use when you feel a thrusting or bursting pain in the right side of the head going from the back of the head to the eye. It is accompanied with burning flashes of heat in the head. Symptoms worsen in the presence of strong odors and motion. Symptoms lessen if one vomits, sleeps or applies pressure to the head. |

### *Infant Illness*

| | |
|---|---|
| Metallum Album | This is the first choice for food poisoning, nausea and vomiting in infants. |
| Belladonna | For teething, sore throat and ear infections in children. |
| Calcarea carbonica | For infants who get colic from intolerance to milk. When teething is delayed. |

### *Injury and Trauma*

| | |
|---|---|
| Arnica | This is the first remedy of choice for all trauma and |

| | |
|---|---|
| | tissue injury. For example, bruises, physical fatigue, a fall or shock. It is also effective after childbirth. |
| Hypericum | Good for injuries due to crushed or damaged nerves or nerve tissue. For post-operative pain that feels like a cutting knife combined with shooting sensations. Lacerations and puncture wounds. Also see *Dental Problems and Surgery.* |
| Apis | Helpful when an injury has a bright red smooth swelling, sting and burning pain. An animal or insect sting may also cause the condition. Exhibited symptoms are made worse from sudden jarring movements and heat. |
| Ledum | Beneficial for insect bites, animal scratches and bites, black eyes and puncture wounds, for example from rusty nails. Symptoms are alleviated by applications of cold, such as an ice pack. |
| Symphytum | Fractured bones. |
| Rhus Toxicodendron | Strained ligaments, muscles or tendons. |
| Ruta | Tendinitis. |
| Bellis Perennis | Use for traumas in top of deep tissue areas – abdomen, pelvis, legs. Beneficial for bruises, swelling and soreness. Very helpful for tendinitis and other repetitive strain injuries. |
| Bryonia | Good for falls, sprains and dislocation of joints. Promotes the healing of bone and tendon, particularly beneficial for rib fractures. If the slightest movement causes a worsening of symptoms, like fractured ribs, then definitely use Bryonia. |
| Calendula | Helps heal cuts, scraps, bleeding and other external wounds. Its antiseptic and disinfectant aspects prevent infection, sooth pain and speed healing. |
| Natrum Sulphuratum | Use for brain and head injuries or traumas, such as concussion, confusion, epilepsy, irritability, memory loss. Also good for spine and lower back injuries. |
| Staphysagria | Good remedy for dental work, nerve pain and sharp wounds. Use when symptoms are due to stitching or when the area is sore and tender and worsens when touched slightly, but under strong pressure feels better. |

# chapter 17

# Flower Remedies

## — Homeopathy of a Different Sort

## The Top 38

### *History and purpose of flower remedies*

In the 1930s, the noted British physician, homeopath, bacteriologist and researcher, Dr. Edward Bach, realized that his patients' illnesses were intimately related to their negative states of mind. He concluded that negative moods caused health threatening imbalances. Emotionally stressful states, such as hopelessness, jealousy, fear, lack of self-confidence and worry, diminished internal ability to resist disease.

According to Bach, a negative state of mind had to be replaced with the opposite virtue to regain the inner harmony needed to heal. Using plants and trees, he created a revolutionary therapeutic system that is safe, natural and gentle. Through observation, he classified negative states of mind common to most people. He discovered the corresponding flower from plants or trees, for each state of mind, which helped to alleviate the specific negative mood. There are hundreds of other homeopathic flower remedies, in addition to the core ones listed here.

### *How to choose the appropriate flower remedy*

These remedies use the homeopathic model of healing from within. They offer simple and safe ways to deal with emotionally distressing states. They can be taken by anyone without danger of side effects or overdose. To familiarize yourself with each remedy, read the descriptions which follow, taking particular note of the personality traits within yourself, your responses are to the problematic situations and what you would like to change. Choose up to six situations or traits that cause you the most distress or unhappiness. If only vague or general impressions such as fear, worry or tension are initially evident, it is important to ask yourself why those moods exist or reflect on the specific nature of those moods. Awareness and thoughtful reflection should guide you to the appropriate selection of the correct remedy or remedies. Keep in mind that each remedy represents a negative state of mind.

### *When to use flower remedies*

Use as soon as stressful situations occur or for short periods of time to rebalance your inner self.

Pets and farm animals, often have specific personality traits and attitudes too. By observing their condition you can determine their emotional state, such as fear, possessiveness, jealousy, anguish, trauma, et cetera, and choose the remedy best suited for them.

### *How to use flower remedies*

Follow the directions on the bottle. Generally, you may take 2 to 3 drops of an undiluted flower remedy under the tongue, or in 1/4 of a glass of spring water or juice, sipping frequently until the glass is empty.

After you have chosen up to six different flower remedies that best match your emotional state, take them one at a time for three to seven days, to see if the one you are taking is the most effective for you. If you are in distress, start with Rescue Remedy® to stabilize yourself.

For pets and small farm animals, combine 4 drops of Rescue Remedy® with 2 drops of the most appropriate other remedy in their drinking water. You may sprinkle this dilution over their food. For larger animals, put 4 drops on a sugar cube or add 10 drops per gallon of drinking water.

### *How to store your remedy*

When stored away from direct sunlight and at room temperature, genuine concentrated flower remedies can last indefinitely. Government regulations, created for other products in the health care field, may require producers to put expiry dates on them, even though this may not necessarily be appropriate for that product.

## *The Top 38 Flower Remedies*

| | |
|---|---|
| Agrimony | For people who are so greatly distressed by disagreements that they would not reveal their problems or opinions just to keep the peace. They hide their cares and concerns behind a cheerful facade. |
| Aspen | For apprehension or vague fears about something terrible happening due to unknown origins. Good for children with nightmares. |
| Beech | For people who are hypercritical and judgmental of others. Encourages tolerance, understanding and acceptance of difference. |
| Centaury | For weak-willed, timid and quiet people who often disregard their purpose for being. Their over-anxiousness to help makes them act more as servants than helpers. |
| Cerato | For people lacking the self-confidence and judgement to make decisions, without frequently seeking advice from others who misled them. |
| Cherry Plum | For people who fear losing control over their mind or body; who impulsively do things which they know to be wrong. |
| Chestnut Bud | For people who fail to learn from observing others or from their own experiences. Mistakes are repeated before the lesson is learned. |
| Chicory | For people excessively concerned for the needs of people close to them. They enjoy constantly correcting what they consider wrong. They may be overprotective and possessive. |
| Clematis | For people who are spacey, dreamy, and drowsy. They live more in the future than the present, hoping for happiness. |
| Crab Apple | For people with poor self-image or who somehow feel unclean or contaminated. |
| Elm | For people feeling inadequate, depressed or overwhelmed by their obligations and responsibilities. |
| Gentian | For children in school and adults who are easily discouraged when they have small delays or hindrances in daily life. |

| | |
|---|---|
| Gorse | For feelings of extreme hopelessness, when it seems like no relief or solution will come. Heals inner will. |
| Heather | For people who are disturbed by feelings of envy, hate, jealousy, suspicion and revenge. People who make mountains out of molehills. When one is in a state of antipathy to love. |
| Honeysuckle | For people who reflect upon the past as a happier time. The good-old-days preoccupy them with feelings of nostalgia and homesickness, which prevents them from living in the present. |
| Hornbeam | For those 'Monday morning' blues when your body or mind seems to need strengthening before you can get going and do your daily work. |
| Impatiens | For people who cannot tolerate the inability of others to keep up. Those quick in action and thought who desire no delays, leading them to want to work alone. |
| Larch | For people lacking confidence and who feel inferior in their abilities. They make little or no attempt to succeed, as they anticipate failure. |
| Mimulus | For people who fear things they have experienced such as: poverty, being alone, accidents, the dark, other people. |
| Mustard | For people suddenly experiencing gloom, depression, melancholy or deep sadness for unknown reasons. It is as if a dark cloud suddenly blocked out all the sunshine – joy and light – in their lives. |
| Oak | For people who ceaselessly struggle on, despite hardships and great odds, never giving up even when overworked or ill. Overly focused on achieving goals. |
| Olive | For total physical and/or mental exhaustion, when you have no more strength to persist. |
| Pine | For people who blame themselves, who are never content with their efforts or results – even when they succeed they feel they could have done better. They may take responsibility for the mistakes of others. |

| | |
|---|---|
| Red Chestnut | For individuals who are overanxious about the safety and well-being of others, often overlooking and neglecting their own needs. |
| Rock Rose | For emotional states of extreme fear such as terror, hysteria, alarm and panic that are caused by illness, accident, nightmares, et cetera. |
| Rock Water | For people who are rigid in their ways of living. They stick to ideals and beliefs, often without joy in their life. They are very hard on themselves, often trying to be examples for others. |
| Scleranthus | For those who are ambivalent, having difficulty in deciding between two things, switching from one choice to the other. For those torn between two lovers. It may show itself more generally in the form of mood swings. |
| Star of Bethlehem | For individuals suffering from great stress brought about by trauma. For the emotional and mental effects manifested from accidents, loss of someone close, serious news, et cetera. |
| Sweet Chestnut | For individuals suffering from unbearable anguish. When your body or mind appears to have reached its limit. At those times when all that seems to remain is annihilation or destruction. |
| Vervain | For individuals who wish to convert those around them to their fixed ideals and principles. They always philosophize and teach, possibly in overbearing and over-enthusiastic ways. They may be overactive and high-strung. |
| Vine | For individuals who can be tyrannical and dictatorial. When their actions are not to the extreme, they may make good leaders. |
| Walnut | For people needing constancy and protection against external influences during major periods of transition. Examples include changing job, moving, ending old or forming new relationships, et cetera. |
| Water Violet | For individuals who are aloof and self-reliant, preferring to be alone even during times of illness and trouble. |

| | |
|---|---|
| White Chestnut | For individuals who cannot stop ideas, thoughts or arguments, which they do not want, from entering their minds. For those who have unwanted thoughts and chatter. It is as if they are circling round and round disturbing their concentration and peace of mind. Beneficial for people with ADD or ADHD. |
| Wild Oats | For individuals who have ambition to do something distinguishing or of prominence in life, yet have a problem deciding on which occupation or career to follow. This can cause delay and dissatisfaction. |
| Wild Rose | For individuals who are resigned and indifferent to all that happens. They surrender without complaint, making no effort to improve their situation, and find no joy in life. |
| Willow | For individuals who are bitter or resentful over negative events or adversities. They have feelings of not deserving life's injustices. |

***Note:*** Rescue Remedy® is a combination of five flower remedies – Cherry Plum, Clematis, Impatiens, Rock Rose and Star of Bethlehem – used for a variety of stressful situations. Many health care professionals, veterinarians and consumers have indicated it produces calming and stabilizing results. It creates comfort and calm in those severely upset, receiving serious news or experiencing traumatic events, which may lead to a dazed and/or numb state of mind. It also appears to be helpful in less severe circumstances such as examinations, arguments, visits to the dentist and stage-fright. Rescue Remedy® is a must for your self-health care medicine cabinet.

# chapter 18

# Leading Edge Remedies

## What, how and when to use them.

## Nutraceuticals, Phytochemicals, Oldies and Goodies, Plus More

Nutraceuticals are substances from natural sources that can positively affect one's health. These unusual healing products are not herbs, minerals or vitamins. In the proper dosage and concentration, they may stimulate and support the body's healing process. It is their wide range of effectiveness and safety which offers benefits for a variety of health conditions. Properly used, they can eliminate the need for prescribed drugs and, most importantly, the potential side effects prescription drugs can cause.

Nutraceuticals are usually prepared in standardized concentrations and taken in capsules and tablets.

We recommend you use nutraceuticals that are natural source products, clearly labeled as standardized extracts and cite the amount of active ingredient(s) you are getting. Specific information on this is in Chapter 9, "Price versus Value", which examines bio-availability, and shows you how to get the most out of your supplements.

Phytochemicals refer to the medicinal qualities of plant life, such as the vitamins, minerals, and thousands of healing substances in the herbs and foods we eat. Some of these remedies have been passed down through the ages, others are recent discoveries.

Use this section, in combination with the index, to discover a broader range of healing substances and options for what interests you.

## 5-HTP

A natural antidepressant, appetite suppressant and sleeping aid. The active ingredient comes from the griffonia simplicifolia, a small bean or seed harvested in Western Africa.

*Biochemical components:* 5-HTP (5-hydroxytryptophan) is an amino acid, that easily crosses the blood-brain barrier and naturally converts into serotonin. It extends the length of time the neurotransmitter serotonin stays active in your brain.

*Principal health related actions:* It is a calming neuro-nutrient and mood enhancer. Aids sleep. Appetite suppressant. Stimulates platelet aggregation and regulates smooth muscle function in the gastrointestinal and cardiovascular system. Beneficial for relief of chronic pain. Decreased serotonin levels can cause many disorders: anxiety, depression, insomnia, obsessive compulsive disorders (alcoholism, eating, gambling), seasonal affective disorder (SAD), and migraine headaches.

*Suggested uses:* To normalize serotonin levels in the body. Clinical studies indicate 5-HTP has comparable or superior ability to antidepressants in treating obsessive compulsive disorders and endogenous depression (a severe form of internally derived depression often characterized by insomnia, weight loss, and inability to experience pleasure). In people suffering from insomnia, it promotes sleep. Serotonin is the 'satiety' neurotransmitter, shown by psychological and biochemical studies to control eating behaviors.

*Suggested dosage ranges:* 5-HTP is more beneficial when taken with 50 mg of vitamin $B_6$, 100 mg of vitamin $B_3$, and 250 mg of magnesium citrate or glycinate. It is more effective when taken on an empty stomach. Some individuals may need to use 50 mg of pyridoxine-5-phosphate, the active form of vitamin $B_6$. To treat depression or control appetite, take 50 to 100 mg of 5-HTP a half hour before each meal, three times a day. For insomnia, take 50 to 200 mg thirty minutes before bedtime, on an empty stomach.

***Cautions:*** Do not used antidepressants and 5-HTP at the same time. Individuals consuming high levels have reported side effects such as constipation, headaches and nausea. It is not recommended for children or lactating or pregnant women. Those with a medical condition or taking medications that affect the central nervous system – especially MAOI (monoamine oxidase inhibitor) antidepressants, alcohol and weight loss drugs, should see their doctor before using 5-HTP. Too much 5-HTP can cause 'Serotonin Syndrome,' signaled by agitation, confusion, lethargy, muscle jerks, sweating and tremors. If these symptoms appear, immediately stop taking 5-HTP and consult with your naturopath or holistic doctor. If you are severely depressed or suicidal, see a health care professional immediately. Do not stop taking any antidepressants without first discussing this with your doctor or health care professional.

### *Agrispet*

Also known as ***Agrispet-L®***.

It is a 100 percent citrus extract of grapefruit, tangerine and lemon. It is a proprietary and exclusive product manufactured by Essentially Yours Industries. In vivo and in vitro lab tests have shown it to be effective.

*Principle health related actions:* Antibacterial, anti-fungus, antiseptic, anti-virus.

*Suggested uses:* Kills the following disease and illness causing agents: Candida albicans, streptococcus, staphylococcus, E. Coli, fungus, herpes, influenza, parasites, salmonella. Conditions it works on: Yeast infections, parasites, herpes simplex I and II, sore throats, gum disease (gingivitis), nail and skin fungus problems, athlete's foot, poison ivy, warts. Household uses include put it in drinking and rinse water for vegetables, fruits, fish, poultry, and meats. Use in bath water for pets to control fleas, ticks, and odor. Preventing algae in water bottles and fish tanks.

*Dosage:* Use the liquid internally or externally. Amount of drops dependents on use. Follow label directions. Available in health food stores.

***Caution:*** It is an non-toxic all-natural product, without harmful side-effects. Not recommended for pregnant or lactating women.

### *Acidophilus (Lactobacillus acidophilus)*

Also see ***Probiotics.***

Acidophilus or lactobacillus acidophilus are friendly bacteria that inhabit the intestines.

*What it does:* Aids and maintains intestinal tract. Supports normal intestinal flora levels as well as the immune system.

*Principle health related actions:* Helps get rid of bad breath caused by putrefied food in the gut, constipation, digestion or ear infection. The overgrowth of the fungus Candida albicans, can be eliminated after taking large doses of acidophilus for a few days. Beneficial for internally rebalancing the system to treat skin problems, such as acne. Alleviates PMS. Aid for menopausal women, to keep vaginal yeast infections, due to vaginal dryness from lower estrogen levels, in check.

*Dosage:* Take 2 capsules, three times a day, half an hour before or after meals. With liquid supplements, take 2 tablespoons (30 ml) three times a day, half an hour before or after meals. Acidophilus is also available in a granular form. This supplement is usually kept refrigerated, otherwise the bacteria will rapidly die off, rendering the product ineffective. Follow package directions for use and storage.

***Caution:*** If you have allergies to dairy products, make sure you only use dairy-free lactobacillus acidophilus

*Suggestion:* Ask your doctor about using acidophilus in conjunction with antibiotics. Antibiotics destroy the beneficial bacteria in your stomach, which can lead to diarrhea and/or an overgrowth of monila albicans fungus, which grows in the intestine, lungs, mouth (thrush), vagina (yeast infection), under the nails, and on the fingers.

*Food sources:* Kefir and yogurt with active bacterial cultures.

### *Alpha Carotene*

A member of the carotenoid family, it is the substances that give fruits and vegetable their natural colors. Alpha carotene, like its family member, beta-carotene, also becomes vitamin A.

*What it does:* Carotenoids protect plants and humans against environmental carcinogens, such as UV radiation from sunshine. It possess powerful anticancer and antioxidant properties. In vivo studies have shown its ability to significantly reduce the number of cancerous tumors in animals. It appears to be far more powerful than beta-carotene in protecting against free radical damage to eyes, liver, skin and lung tissue.

*Dosage:* Take 3 to 8 mg of a variety of carotenoids each day.

*Food sources:* Cooked pumpkin and carrots. Dark green leafy vegetables. Orange and red colored fruits.

### *Apple Cider Vinegar with 'mother'*

This vinegar is produced from apples, preferably certified organically grown apples. 'Mother' refers to the natural sediment, which hovers at the bottom of the bottle. This sediment contains trace minerals, such as potassium, as well as pectin, good bacteria and enzymes. Mother signals that you are getting unfiltered and unpasteurized apple cider vinegar containing beneficial nutrients.

*Principal health related actions:* Aids the digestive system by stimulating the flow of saliva and inhibiting the growth of bad bacteria in your digestive system. If you suffer from heartburn (indigestion), your stomach is probably not producing enough acid. Try apple cider vinegar and you may be pleasantly surprised. Other conditions and parts of the body it has been helpful for include: arthritis, asthma, maintaining bone mass, providing antioxidant and anticancer properties (beta-carotene and alpha carotene are in apple cider vinegar), its pectin (a water-soluble fiber) content can help lower high blood cholesterol levels, cold constipation, coughs, cramps, diabetes, diarrhea, detoxification of the body, depression (possibly due to its amino aid content or liver cleansing abilities), low energy, eye health, hiccups, may help body rid itself of gallstones and kidney stones, headaches, high blood pressure, muscle soreness, sinus and nasal congestion, sore or itchy throat, ulcers, Candida albicans yeast infections, bleeding, burns, abrasions and cuts, hair and scalp, herpes, insect stings and bites, poison ivy, poison oak, herpes zoster (shingles), sunburn, weight control, varicose veins, vaginal douche, corns and calluses.

In addition, it is an inexpensive beauty aid and cleaning agent. The list of uses is so extensive for this age-old remedy that we recommend you get one of these books *Apple Cider Vinegar* by P. Bragg or *Folk Medicine* by Dr. D. C. Jarvis.

*Dosage:* To aid digestion, take 1 or 2 capsules or 1 to 3 teaspoons (5 to 15 ml) in a glass of water before meals. Only use organically grown products with mother. Great in salad dressings, sauces and other condiments. Use for marinades and pickling. It is an acid-alkaline balancer.

### *Artichoke concentrate (Cynarin)*

A botanical cousin of the liver protecting herb milk thistle.

*Principal health related actions:* Helps reduce risk of heart disease and stroke by lowering high LDL (bad) cholesterol and triglyceride levels (blood lipid levels) and increasing HDL (good) cholesterol levels. Helps increase the liver's bile production, thereby aiding in the metabolism of fats.

*Dosage:* In capsule form, take 2000 mg a day on an empty stomach, for at least three months. Lower cholesterol and triglyceride levels should be detectable by this time.

### *Banaba leaf (Lagestroemia Speciosa L.)*

It is another wonder herb from Asia. In 1988, a clinical double-blind Japanese trial discovered a significant reduction in blood sugar levels between diabetics given banaba leaf and those given a placebo. Those taking the herb went from 153.9 to 133.1 mg/dl.

*Principal health related action:* Contains colosolic acid which helps transport glucose into cells, thereby reducing blood sugar levels.

*Dosage:* Take 15 mg daily, along with gymnema sylvestre, chromium, vanadium, alpha lipoic acid and 1500 mg of evening primrose or borage oil for their gamma linolenic acid (GLA).

**Caution:** Consult with your doctor or health care professional, before you stop taking any medication or insulin, or take natural remedies and supplements.

### *Baker's yeast* – See Beta-1,3 Glucan

### *Bee Pollen*

A source of life-enhancing nutrients – amino acids, enzymes, vitamins and minerals.

*Principal health related actions:* Combats fatigue. Helps build resistance to diseases. Soothes stomach problems. Facilitates better hormonal system function.

*Suggested uses:* Provides essential nutrients and energy. Take as a preventative measure to help your body resist disease. Raises blood pressure. Helpful in dealing with allergies, exhaustion, hay fever, hormonal imbalance, stomach ailments. Lessens negative impact of radiation treatments, such as chemotherapy.

*Dosage:* Depends on quality and source. Take as directed.

**Caution:** Some people have allergic reactions to bee pollen. To test for such a reaction, open a capsule and put, several of the granules under your tongue. If you have no reaction, take 1 or 2 capsules before each meal, gradually increasing your intake to a maximum of 6 a day. Not recommended for people with a tendency to or having high blood pressure.

### *Bee Propolis*

Also called ***bee glue***.

This is the sticky material bees gather from trees to seal their hives and protects against infection and intruders. It is a source of bioflavonoids, vitamins, minerals, resins and other substances.

*Principal health related actions:* Beneficial for gum disease, mouth ulcers, sore throats and initial stages of a cold. Effective against herpes virus when applied to lesions. It relieves pain, aids wound healing and heals urinary tract infections.

*Suggested dosage:* Externally use in a salve and massage into inflamed areas, such as sore gums and herpes lesions, to prevent infection, soothe and reduce inflammation. Use as a gargle for mouth ulcers and sore throats. Internally you can take 100 to 300 mg per day to stimulate the immune system.

### *Beta-1,3 Glucan*

Distilled from the cell walls of baker's yeast it fortifies and activates macrophages, very important cells in the immune system. Macrophages hungrily attack bacteria, cancer cells, fungi, viruses and other parties that invade the body. Beta-1,3 glucan protects against free radical damage from radiation, such as X-rays and the sun's UV rays. As such, it is a powerful antioxidant and immune system protector.

*Principal health related actions:* Protects and boosts immune system function. Reduces and prevents radiation damage. Lowers high blood cholesterol and triglyceride levels without the side effects of prescription drugs, thereby decreasing the potential for strokes and heart disease. Used in complementary medical treatments for chronic conditions such as herpes, Candida albicans, Epstein-Barr Virus, HIV and to counteract age-related decreases in immune system functioning. Since extreme or strenuous exercise by athletes causes a decrease in their immune systems' functioning, they use Beta-1,3 glucan to counteract this affect.

*Dosage:* Either half an hour before or two hours after a meal, take a 2.0 to 2.5 mg capsule with water. When treating serious conditions, consult your primary health care provider.

## *Betaine*

Also known as ***Trimethylglycine (TMG)***

Found in animals and plants it is part of the methyl group of substances which turns the potentially dangerous amino acid, homocysteine, into the beneficial compound methionine. Other substances that can help the process of methylation (turning homocysteine into methionine) are S-Adenosyl-L-Methione (SAMe), vitamin $B_{15}$, vitamin $B_3$, and folic acid. Methylation decreases as we age, which means homocysteine levels increase. Homocysteine is an indicator of increased chances of developing arthritis, cancer, depression, heart disease as well as other diseases. Fortunately, it is easy to reduce the homocysteine levels using one or a combination of these supplements: TMG, folic acid, vitamin $B_{12}$, vitamin $B_3$, fish oil omega-3 essential fatty acids, or S-Adenosyl-L-Methione (SAMe).

*Principal health related benefits:* Decreases chances of getting depression, Alzheimer's, heart disease and certain cancers. Lowers homocysteine levels, raises methane levels and brings all the beneficial consequences mentioned above.

*Dosage:* Take up to 300 mg a day.

*Food sources:* Spinach, beets and broccoli.

## *Bromelain*

An enzyme derived from pineapple juice.

*What it does:* Anti-inflammatory; digestive aid due to its protein-digestive and milk-clotting enzymatic properties; helps prevent blood clots.

*Principal health related actions:* Beneficial treatment for indigestion, some food sensitivities, asthma and urinary tract infections. Decreases swelling and pain resulting from inflammation. May help treat obesity, due to its digestive enhancing properties. Bromelain acts to prevent abnormally high levels of fibrinogen, a blood clotting agent in the body. Sudden blood clots can increase risk of heart disease and stroke.

*Dosage:* As a digestive aid, take up to 1000 mg after each meal. Combine with papaya to further enhance protein digestion. Inflammation reduction requires up to 1500 mg (1.5 grams) each day. For heart health, take one 500 mg tablet a day. If suffering from angina, nutritionally orientated health practitioners recommend 1000 to 1500 mg per day. Relief of angina or chest pain can take up to 90 days to occur. Consult with your primary heart care provider or doctor when you want to use alternative treatments.

***Caution:*** None for bromelain. Raw pineapple is not recommended for people with ulcers. Reports of increased heart rates have been made. For more information on enzymes refer to Chapter 4.

***Calcium pyruvaten*** – see Pyruvate

### *Cardiem*

A patented extract of rice bran, with the only single nutrient shown in published studies and clinical trials, to reduce three major risk factors for cardiovascular disease.

*Principal health related actions:* Reduces LDL (bad) cholesterol levels. Antioxidant properties that are significantly more effective than vitamin E for protecting against the oxidation of LDL. Effectively reduces thromboxane levels producing subsequent reductions in platelet aggregation (clumping) and clotting. May be effective against a broad range of cancers.

*Dosage:* Follow label directions.

### *Celery Seed extracts*

It contains over eighteen different anti-inflammatory factors, which may account for their effectiveness as a treatment for arthritic conditions, such as gout. See also Cherry Juice below. May use it in conjunction with cherry juice.

*Principal health related actions:* Diuretic. Regulates blood pressure. Lowers uric acid (hypouremic) levels in the blood, thereby relieving gout. No toxic effects from the long term use of celery seed extract have been reported. May prevent certain cancers.

***Caution:*** People with kidney disease and pregnant women should not use celery seed extract, since it has diuretic properties. Consult with your health care provider if in doubt about trying it.

### *Cherry Juice*

Nature's gout remedy.

Gout is an arthritic condition that suddenly attacks joints, causing intense pain, redness and swelling. Chronic inflammation can lead to chronic pain. Gout usually afflicts the big toe, but feet, ankles, knees and small hand joints can also suffer from gout. If not dealt with, gout can cause the kidneys to become diseased. Painkillers are used to reduce the high levels of uric acid in the blood.

*Principal health related actions:* Lowers uric acid levels in the blood, relieving gout.

*Dosage:* Cherry juice is a food that has been safely used for hundreds, if not thousands, of years. Concentrated black cherry juice is found to be more effective than red cherry juice. No toxic effects from the long term use of either black or red cherry juice have been reported.

### *Chitosan*

A fat-absorbing fiber derived from the outer skeletons of shellfish (mainly crabs and shrimp). Chitosan promotes weight loss, since it blocks the absorption of fat when it journeys through the digestive tract and itself absorbs four to six times its own weight in fats, before being expelled from the body. May result in lower levels of cholesterol. May help prevent cancer of the colon.

*Dosage:* Take 250 to 750 mg of tablets with each meal and a cup of water per tablet. Drink plenty of water when taking any fiber.

***Caution:*** Not to be used by children or pregnant or lactating women. Not for use by people with sensitivities or allergies to shellfish. Make sure to drink enough water when supplementing with chitosan. Do not use for more than 10 days at a time, since it can deplete the body of fat-soluble vitamins. Take additional fat-soluble vitamins (E, K, D and beta-carotene or vitamin A) and essential fatty acids, when using chitosan. Do not use it as a long-term solution for weight loss.

### *Chlorella (Chlorella pyrenoidosa)*

A single-celled fresh water micro-algae plant. One of the many 'green foods' with exceptional healing qualities. When properly processed as a supplement, it is easily digestible and rapidly absorbed by the body. It comes close to being a perfect food. Chlorella is loaded with powerful disease-fighting nutrients, such as chlorophyll, nucleic acids (RNA/DNA), plus 19 amino acids (including all of the essential ones), as well as 20 vitamins and minerals. It has been widely researched and used in Japan for numerous health related benefits, such as detoxifying the body by removing harmful pollutants and heavy metals from it. It gives the body a better chance to use its own wisdom to maintain and heal itself, a major ingredient in most whole green super food supplements.

*Principal health related actions:* Excellent detoxifier that helps rid the body of harmful chemicals. Anticancer food. Tonic for the cardiovascular system. Raises protein albumin levels in the blood. Albumin is a powerful antioxidant and principal transportation system for minerals, vitamins, hormones, fatty acids and vital nutrients in the body, as well as the garbage collector of toxins. It transports toxins to the liver, for removal from the body. Essential for proper liver, kidney, other organs and immune system functioning. Low serum albumin levels are a predictor of high death rates due to heart disease and other organ failures in the body.

*Dosage:* Take two 500 mg tablets three times a day.

## *Chondroitin*

One of three inexpensive natural remedies used individually or synergistically for curing some of the more than 100 arthritic conditions. The other two are glucosamine and pregnenolone. Chondroitin is produced from the specialized chondrocyte cells found in cartilage. In animals it is highly concentrated in the connective tissue and gristle surrounding the joints, which draws lubricating fluids that enhance the smooth movement of bone points. Other substances that also reduce inflammation and have painkilling properties which can be used in conjunction with these remedies.

*Principal health related actions:* Relieves arthritic pain and helps regenerate cartilage. One of chondroitin additional benefits is that it does not cause the unpleasant side effects, such as stomach distress that the painkilling NSAID drugs (non-steroidal anti-inflammatory drugs) can produce. Chondroitin has lipid (fat) clearing properties in the blood. Improves fatty acid metabolism. Helps connective tissue heal.

*Dosage:* In tablets or caplets of 300 mg, take 1 to 2 a day. With more severe arthritic conditions, take to 1000 mg twice a day. Usually a noticeable difference will be felt in a few weeks or months. However results can take up to a year to occur. The longer a condition has persisted, the longer it takes the body to rebalance and heal itself, once the appropriate remedy is used.

### *Coenzyme Q10 (Ubiquinone)*

Also known as ***CoQ10***.

The principle source is from Japanese producers, who extract it from ubiquinone, a vegetable source. Some experts believe it is a vitamin. It has powerful antioxidant properties.

*Principal health related actions:* Critical role in energy production at the basic cellular level. Delivers energy and oxygen to cells. Antioxidant. In Japan, it is used for heart problems. It is recommended for treating cardiovascular disease. Supports muscles. Revitalizes and boosts the immune system. Beneficial for heart disease, angina, aging, gum disease, high blood pressure, hypertension, hyperthyroidism, infections, irregular heartbeats (arrhythmia), athletic performance, mitral valve prolapse, periodontal disease. Due to its powerful antioxidant properties it is being tested to slow the effects of degenerative neurological diseases such as ALS (amyotrophic lateral sclerosis), Huntington's disease, Parkinson's disease. In addition, coenzyme Q10 is being researched and used to aid breast cancer therapies such as chemotherapy, radiotherapy, and with tamoxifen. The dosages are in the 90 mg to 390 mg range and usually include supplementation with other powerful antioxidants and fatty acids.

*Dosage:* A fat-soluble supplement, coenzyme Q10 is absorbed when taken with fat. The body absorbs soft gel capsules better than dry forms of tablets or caplets. Take one or two 60 mg capsules a day. For heart disease, 50 to 300 mg a day may be needed, depending on the severity of the problem. Some experts suggest that for every 2.2 pounds (1 kg) of body weight, you take 2 mg of coenzyme Q10. The key is to raise the level of coenzyme Q10 in the blood. In those who have survived heart failure, it normally takes two to 10 weeks before supplementation with coenzyme Q10 produces results. Supplementation must continue, if you want to maintain the heart strengthening effects.

***Caution:*** Not toxic. In matters of the heart and cancer, always consult with your doctor or naturally orientated health care provider. To date, no drug contraindications have been reported.

*Food Sources:* Present in very small amounts in all foods, especially seafoods. Japanese producers of coenzyme Q10, extract it from a vegetable source.

### *Conjugated Linoleic Acid (CLA)*

A fat that can help you lose weight and help your body work better. Modern diets no longer include enough of this good fat.

*Principal health related actions:* Promotes weight loss by regulating the body's protein and fat metabolism. The result is a reduction in body fat and increase in muscle mass and tone, which burns more calories than fat to maintain itself in the body. May help prevent and reduce incidence of heart disease, as well as offer protection against some types of cancer.

*Dosage:* Take up to 1200 mg before each meal.

*Food sources:* Lamb, red meats and dairy products. Modern farming and processing methods have lead to a significant reduction of the CLA fat content in these sources, estimated to be 1/5 of what it was.

### *Coriolus versicolor extract*

For over 20 years, it has been used by the Japanese medical establishment as part of a non-toxic cancer treatment, known as 'PSK' or 'Crestin'. It is used in conjunction with surgical and radiation therapies.

*Principal health related actions:* Normalizes and boosts immune system functioning and in vitro (in test tubes) has been found to reduce tumor growth. May be useful in treating AIDS and other diseases that result from a weak immune system. Useful as part of a cancer treatment program. Beneficial for auto immune system (the immune response of an organism against any of its own cells or tissues) functioning, helping to prevent some arthritic conditions, lupus and similar diseases. Increases T-cells, the immune system's disease fighters.

*Dosage:* Currently 3000 mg (3 grams) capsules are available for medical treatments. Until smaller dosages become available, we suggest you use other herbs to boost your immune system.

### *Creatine (Creatine monohydrate)*

It combines with phosphorus to become phosphocreatine, an energy source for muscular contractions. It increases the reserves of energy that adenosine triphosphate (ATP) stores in the muscles.

*Principal health related actions:* Improves performance and recovery time of muscles. Increases muscle stamina and energy supply to the muscle. Helps prevent muscle fatigue. By increasing muscle mass and strength, it enhances athletic performance. Helps those who exercise develop better muscle tone and lose fat. Lowers high blood lipid levels, cholesterol and triglycerides in the blood, which may reduce the risk of stroke and heart disease. Being studied as a treatment for muscle atrophy (sarcopenia) which begins around age 30.

*Dosage:* Use creatine monohydrate since it is the most absorbable form of this supplement. Initially, take 1 teaspoon (5 grams) of the powder, three times a day for three days, then reduce to one teaspoon, twice a day. Take with water or juice, on an empty stomach or with meals.

*Food sources:* Found in many meats.

***Caution:*** Excessively high doses may lead to liver or kidney conditions.

### *Cryptoxanthin*

A Carotenoid that the liver and intestines can convert into vitamin A. Very important for women and those who smoke or use other tobacco products. Smokers and those who chew tobacco have lower levels of cryptoxanthin.

*Principal health related actions:* May protect against cervical cancer.

*Dosage:* Consume 4 to 6 mg of many carotenoids each day. Eat three to five fruits each day.

*Food sources:* Papaya, peaches, oranges, tangerines.

### *Curcumin*

Spice up your life with this powerful antioxidant that is found in turmeric. Curry powder derives its unique yellow color from turmeric. Indian Ayurvedic medicine consider turmeric an important healing spice.

*Principal health related actions:* anti-inflammatory especially effective against rheumatoid arthritis, without the potential side effects of prescription non-steroidal anti-inflammatories (NSAIDs) or over-the-counter drugs. Appears to reduce cancer cell activity and benefit treatment programs for breast, colon and skin cancers. Protects against the free radical damage caused by smoking. Offers heart and stroke protection by it ability to reduce high blood cholesterol levels and chances of blood clots. Beneficial for strengthening and reducing inflammation in the liver. May promote weight loss in the obese. Used by naturopaths in the treatment of liver problems, such as hepatitis C and to treat gallbladder diseases.

*Dosage:* Take up to 1500 mg of capsules a day, with food. Only purchase 15:1 or higher concentrations.

*Food sources:* Eat curried foods. Add turmeric to your foods.

***Caution:*** Do not use if taking anticoagulants or have a blood clotting problem. Women of childbearing age or having fertility problem, should only use therapeutic doses of curcumin, unless under the direction of a doctor, naturopath, or naturally oriented healer.

***Cynarin*** – see Artichoke concentrate.

## *DHEA (Dehydroepiandrosterone)*

A steroid hormone produced in the adrenal gland, brain and skin. By our mid-forties we produce about half the DHEA our bodies made when we were twenty. Considered a master hormone, it is responsible for starting and promoting numerous bodily functions that make our bodies youthful and vibrant.

*Principal health related actions:* Boost energy levels. In males promotes and maintains youthful testosterone levels, helping to prevent the loss of libido. Low levels of DHEA in men, have been found to correlate with a decreased sexual function and other sexually related problems. Strengthens and supports the immune system. Supplementation may reverse age-related diseases since it stimulates natural killer cell activity, critical for optimal immune system function. Beneficial for diabetes, obesity and those with multiple sclerosis. Fosters positive emotional, psychological and physical states. Improves ability to cope with stress, and reduces the negative affects of the 'fight or flight' response hormone, cortisol. Studies indicate that high levels of cortisol present in the body for more than two weeks, cause food to be stored as fat around the waist. Lupus patients treated with DHEA, under medical supervision, have experienced positive results. This offers promise with other autoimmune diseases, such as rheumatoid arthritis.

*Dosage:* Have your doctor test your DHEA and testosterone levels before supplementation. Your health care provider should monitor your DHEA levels. To ensure purity, only DHEA products that are labeled 'pharmaceutical grade' should be used. In the morning, men over 40 can take up to 50 mg each day, women over 40 can take up to 25 mg a day.

Dr. Michael Colgan, author of *Hormonal Health,* recommends taking DHEA in the morning, since this corresponds with the mid-morning peak production of testosterone; as well, DHEA's reported stimulating properties may affect sleep patterns. He suggests taking it only for five days a week. When supplementing with DHEA, have your physician or health care provider measure your DHEA levels every three to six months. The optimal levels a middle-aged or older person should supplement to, are those of a 25-year old's mid- to normal range. For women that is 1600 to 3000 ng/ml; for men it is 2800 to 4000 ng/ml.

***Cautions:*** Do not take DHEA if you have had breast or prostrate cancer, unless under medical supervision. At daily dosages of 25 mg or more, DHEA can trigger heart palpitations, irregular heart beat and heart attack. If in doubt, the prudent course of action is to take DHEA under the supervision of a doctor, naturopath or naturally oriented medical practitioner.

### *Emu oil*

Emu oil is another treasure from Australia. It is processed from the fat of a close relative to the ostrich, the emu bird. Aboriginal's use it to for wounds, joint pain and as a sunscreen. Emu oil is an excellent source of linolenic acid. Dr. Peter Ghosh, of Sydney's Royal North Shore Hospital, researched and verified the relief it offers arthritic patients.

*Principal health related actions:* The linolenic acid helps reduce arthritic inflammation, swelling and stiffness. Reduces the effects of muscle aches and pains as well as sprains. Excellent skin moisturizer. Beneficial for burn treatments and faster wound healing. It offers superior protection for the skin against the sun's harsh rays and provides a treatment for sunburn. It may protect against radiation burns.

*Dosage:* Available in natural health food stores and some pharmacies, as a cream and lotion. Massage it into painful muscles and joints, up to three times a day. Use as per label directions for burns, sunburns and wounds.

### *Fertilized chicken egg*

Also known as ***Ardor, Libido*** or ***Virilite*** in a powder form.

*Possible health related benefits:* Anticancer properties. In the 1940s, the

Canadian doctor John Ralston Davidson, used a powder derived from fertilized chicken eggs along with dietary supplementation to successfully treat many cancer patients, who lived five, 10 and more years beyond the treatment periods.

In men and women, it has been found to counteract the loss of sex drive experienced with antidepressant drugs such as Prozac. This ancient Chinese aphrodisiac was rediscovered by Dr. Bjodne Eskeland of Norway while researching far eastern sexual stimulants. In a double blind study he conducted in Norway, 83 percent of the men reported results ranging up to "a very pronounced increase" in sex drive. Similar results were found with women. No negative side effects were reported.

*Principal health related actions:* Improves low or nonexistent sex drive in men and women. Successfully used to treat some types of cancer, in conjunction with nutrient supplementation.

*Dosage:* Follow physicians or pharmacists directions.

*Sources:* In the United States and Canada, it may be available through physicians on a prescription basis, and is known as Ardor, Libido or Virilite.

### *Flaxseed oil*

A source of lignans (a soluble fiber), alpha-linolenic acid (ALA), oleic acid, linoleic acid plus other essential omega-3 fatty acids, which are missing in our highly processed foods. The essential fatty acids found in flaxseed are also known as vitamin F. It offers the following benefits: antioxidant, anti-inflammatory, demulcent, emollient, and purgative. For a fuller explanation on the role of fats in your health, see Chapter 5.

*Principal health related actions:* Beneficial for digestive and urinary disorders. Lowers cholesterol, blood triglycerides and helps prevent blood clot. Decreases homocysteine levels in the blood; high levels of this protein are thought to be a critical risk factor and therefore a good predictor of heart disease. Soothes and reduces muscle soreness and helps reduce their recovery time. Keeps skin youthful and vibrant. Bacteria in the stomach change the lignan fiber into cancer fighting substances. May help in weight reduction, since the brain is getting nutrients essential to your well-being, and lets it know you are satiated, giving you the feeling of fullness. Maintains hormone balance. Eases premenstrual syndrome (PMS). Alleviates menopausal symptoms such as vaginal dryness, which can lead to recurrent yeast infections, and lessens hot flashes.

***Note:*** Ground flax seeds are a superior source of lignans.

*Dosage:* Only use certified organically grown and cold-pressed flax seed oil or flax seed powder, preferably with a high lignan content. High temperatures destroy the beneficial properties of the oil, so using a food blender or processor on the seeds may destroy much of the oil's therapeutic properties. Use 1 to 3 teaspoons (5 to 15 ml) of oil on your foods (salads, potatoes, vegetables, pasta, rice, tofu, et cetera) or in a drink each day. In 1000 mg capsules, take 1 to 3 with each meal, up to three times a day.

***Caution:*** Flaxseed oil, if not properly processed, can easily become rancid. It is important to refrigerate it. Make sure to follow the storage directions on your bottle. If unsure, refrigerate it.

*Source:* Seeds.

## *Fructo-oligosaccharide (FOS)*

Also known as ***neosugar*** or ***inulin***

It is a complex sugar derived from plants, that is good for you! Jerusalem artichokes are the most abundant source of FOS.

Regular refined sugars are broken down by digestive juices. FOS bypasses this mechanism, where it is digested by the good bacteria in the gut. In turn, this promotes the growth of these health enhancing good bacteria. Some of the bodily functions the good bacteria are vital for include the efficient functioning of your immune system, cancer prevention, utilization of B vitamins, preventing an overgrowth of bad bacteria and fungi, regulating blood sugar levels, decreasing high cholesterol levels, and digestion. (For more information on these good bacteria, refer to Probiotics, Acidophilus, and Lactobacillus G.G.

It is believed that as we age, the reduction of good bacteria in our systems leaves us more susceptible to the illnesses and diseases of old age. FOS may be the answer.

*Principal health related actions:* Improves the immune system. Increase good bacteria levels. Reduces chance of gastrointestinal cancers. Can help the body deal with gastrointestinal problems such as chronic yeast infections like Candida albicans, bloating, and flatulence. Beneficial in the treatment of diarrhea and constipation. Normalizes blood sugar and cholesterol levels. Aids the utilization of the stress-alleviating B vitamins, which in turn help the body deal with stress.

*Dosage:* Take 1 gram a day to support your body. With acute or chronic conditions, increase the up to 5 grams a day. It can be taken with probiotics.

## *GE 132*

Also known as ***Germanium,*** it is a naturally occurring trace element found in foods and herbs. Also see page 129 – Germanium.

## *Glucosamine*
### *(Glucosamine sulfate or glucosamine hydrochloride)*

It is a naturally occurring sulfur nutrient in the body. It is a basic building block of key connective tissue components needed to replenish and maintain cartilage and joint function. Chock full of beneficial nutrients such as the amino group, glucose, glycoproteins, mucopolysaccharides and the sulfate group. It is an effective way to deal with some of the 100 arthritic conditions – particularly rheumatoid arthritis.

It usually takes from one to 12 months of supplementation to maximize the benefits. The longer arthritic condition has existed, the longer it usually takes to alleviate it.

Those on a tight budget may want to try finely ground dried chicken bones. The active ingredient in glucosamine is found in the bone marrow. A Harvard Medical School study reported that within two weeks of starting supplementation with finely ground dried chicken bones, all patients originally scheduled for hip-replacement surgery, no longer suffered significant amounts of pain.

*Principal health related actions:* Helps the regeneration of cartilage, ligaments and intervertebral discs. It is a mild anti-inflammatory. Promotes synthesis of cartilage in the joints. Beneficial in osteoarthritis for relief of pain and inflammation. Helpful for mild inflammation due to sports injuries, such as cartilage trauma, as well as degenerative joint disease, osteoarthritis and inflammation in joints.

*Dosage:* According to Dr. George Grant, glucosamine hydrochloride is almost 50 percent more potent than glucosamine sulfate. In addition it has none of sulfate's side effects (see cautions below.) As the main stomach acid, hydrochloride eases the work of the digestive system in getting more active components into your body. Reducing your consumption of refined sugar, red meat, caffeine and alcohol, in addition to lowering your cholesterol and exercising moderately, will greatly increase your chances of improving and, more importantly, decrease the time to see positive results. Take one 500 mg caplet three times a day. Formulations are now available with Devil's Claw, an anti-inflammatory herb, chondroitin, pregnenolone, and methylsulfonylmethane also called MSM.

**Caution:** High doses have been known to cause gastric irritation, and occasionally nausea or heartburn. Avoid these problems by taking it with meals. Regular and salt-free supplements are not recommended for people on potassium-reduced diets, with severe renal diseases, on heart medications or suffering from high blood pressure due to salt intake. Not for those who react adversely to sulfate.

*Source:* Crab shell

### Glutathione

A powerful antioxidant the body produces from within. It is a powerful detoxifier that also aids and improves pancreatic function.

*Principal health related actions:* Beneficial in treating diabetes. Helps reduce liver toxicity and/or congestion. Effective for prevention of oral cancers, particularly when combined with vitamins C, E and beta-carotene.

**Caution:** Not for use during chemotherapy. Do not use glutathione supplements in children under 12 years of age. Not for use by pregnant or nursing women.

**Note:** Researchers of attention deficit disorder (ADD) and attention deficit hyperactivity disorder (ADHD) believe that the nutritional deficiencies stemming from our modern processed food diets may be one of the many causes for these memory-related problems, since the lack of proper and sufficient nutrients may interfere with the body's ability to produce glutathione. Restoring the body's internal chemical balance naturally, may resolve the problems, but counseling and behavioral modification may be needed to deal with any inappropriate behavioral problems that have arisen.

*Food sources:* Asparagus, avocado, broccoli, watermelon.

### Glycerol

The key ingredient in sports fluid replacement drinks, occurs naturally in all cells of your body. Its main function is to retain the water in the cells. It carries water to and from cells, maintains the body's fluid balance.

Strenuous physical activity depletes our bodies of fluids. The hotter and more humid the weather is, the faster you lose fluids. This can cause dehydration, resulting in lower blood plasma, which means there is less blood to carry critical nutrients and oxygen to your muscle cells. Your stamina decreases and you tire more quickly. In addition, you now risk heat stroke and heat exhaustion, since your body's ability to cool down is severely hampered. Drinking water may help, but may not meet your body's complete fluid needs.

*Principal health related actions:* During exercise, glycerol prevents dehydration. After exercise, it dehydrates the body. Glycerol is better than just water during strenuous physical activity, since it helps keep body temperature lower, and less strain on muscles means a lower heart rate.

*Dosage:* Have a sports drink containing glycerol about 30 to 45 minutes before strenuous physical activity, and upon completion of the activity. Always drink lots of water during the activity. If exercising for a prolonged period of time, drink a glycerol sports drink during the activity.

### *Grapefruit pectin*

It is a unique form of a water soluble fiber derived from the membranes, rinds and juice sacs of grapefruit. The University of Florida and Dr. J. Cerda developed and own the patents on the product ProFibe™. The formula also contains guar gum, another soluble fiber. Double-blind studies have proven its effectiveness in reducing arterial plaque and lowering cholesterol.

*Principal health related actions:* Powerful artery unclogging powers. Excellent cholesterol lowering abilities with none of the side effects of pharmaceutical drugs, such as Mevacor and Zocor. Helps overweight people lose weight, without any changes to their diet and exercise habits.

*Dosage:* The supplement is in a powder form that can be sprinkled onto food. In double-blind studies, to achieve plaque-removing results, at least 15 grams a day of grapefruit pectin fiber were taken in three doses of 5 grams, at each meal. For cholesterol lowering effects, take 5 to 10 grams a day. Available in American health food stores, drugstores and supermarkets. To order by mail in the U.S., call 1 (800) 756-3999. In Canada, it is only available by mail order; call (877) 396-9690.

***Caution:*** Gas is the usual problem experienced by people who suddenly increase their fiber intake. Occasionally loose stools or diarrhea can result. This will pass with time, as the body adjusts to an increase in fiber consumption. Grapefruit pectin is not toxic and considered a safe food product.

### *Grapefruit Seed Extract*

A powerful antibacterial, antifungal, anthelmintic (fights worms) and antiviral substance. It contains health promoting nutrients, such as bioflavonoids and the natural immune system booster, hesperidin. Primarily used for yeast infections due to Candida albicans.

*Principal health related actions:* Fights bacterial, fungal (especially Candida albicans) and viral infections, as well as worm infestations and other fungal infections. Can be applied externally for toenail fungal infections, or try tea tree oil which is also very effective.

*Dosage:* For tinctures or extracts, use 10 to 15 drops in water or juice, taken two to five times a day, or as per directions. For toenail fungal infections, apply once in the morning and just before bed, until the infection disappears.

### *Grape Seed OPC*

In combination with pine tree bark extract, produces a powerful group of antioxidants that Europeans have been using for decades. These antioxidants are known as Pycnogenol™, generic pycnogenols, proanthocyanidolic oligomers, procyanidins, oligomeric procyanidins and simply grape seed extract. They help build better capillaries and veins, which can have profound effects upon your body's vascular system.

*Principal health related actions:* Since it strengthens and helps blood vessels such as veins, which become more resilient, it is used by Europeans to treat varicose veins among others things. Reduces swelling due to edema, a build up of fluids. In turn this may be beneficial for congestive heart disease, high blood pressure and injuries involving swelling. Used to treat eye problems, such as macular degeneration, cataracts, night blindness and glare. While it does not cure macular degeneration, it appears to significantly slow and sometimes stop its progress. This supplement's anti-inflammatory properties combined with its antihistamine abilities, prevent histamine-induced inflammation. Reduces and may cure allergies, hay fever, and some types of arthritis. People with attention deficit disorder (ADD) and attention deficit hyperactivity disorder (ADHD) have found it helpful in alleviating or completely eliminating their problem. It may work as well as Ritalin (methylphenidate). Additional benefits that have been reported include lower heart rates, remission of tennis elbow, disappearance of acne, enhanced moods, better sleep quality.

*Dosage:* Try the less expensive but just as, if not more, effective grape seed extract rather than Pycnogenol™. The Europeans mainly use grape seed extract in their research studies. To maintain the integrity and health of your vascular system, take 50 to 100 mg a day. For diseases take 150 to 400 mg a day. For ADD and ADHD children should take 1 milligram per pound of body weight. Adults should take 2 mg per pound of body weight.

***Caution:*** No adverse or toxic affects have been reported or found in studies. While it may be effective with young children, only use it in consultation with a medical or naturally orientated health care practitioner.

*Source:* Derived from grape seeds.

***Green Concentrates*** – see Whole Green Super Food Supplements.

***Green Drinks*** – see Whole Green Super Food Supplements.

### *Green Tea Extract*

Green tea is a pleasant beverage with potentially powerful cancer fighters called polyphenols, which may have more effective anticancer and antioxidant properties than vitamin C or E. Adding milk or cream to green tea drinks, negates its beneficial properties.

*Principal health related actions:* Stimulates repair of sun damaged skin. Inhibits cancerous tumor formation. Reduces the odds of getting esophageal, lung, stomach, pancreatic and colon cancer. Smokers should definitely drink green tea frequently, to lessen some of the potential deadly affects of smoking. May prevent heart disease, high blood pressure, high cholesterol, improve HDL (good) cholesterol levels and stop abnormal blood clotting.

*Dosage:* Combine green tree extract with grape seed extract for a powerful, yet gently acting, healing combination. Take 1 tablet twice a day. Drink 3 cups of green tea a day, to equal the active ingredients in 2 green tree extract tablets. For sunburns, use a cup of green tea that has cooled to room temperature, then dip a cotton ball in it and gently apply to the area affected. Available in skin creams.

***Green food supplements*** – see Whole Green Super Food Supplements.

### *Gugulipid*

It comes from the mukul myrrh tree and has been used by India's Ayurvedic medical healers for hundreds of years. The active ingredient in it is the steroid-like compounds called gugulsterones.

*Principal health related actions:* Lowers bad cholesterol (LDL) and triglyceride levels while raising good cholesterol (HDL) levels. Beneficial for cardiovascular health and decrease risk of strokes.

*Dosage:* When using 250 mg capsules, standardized to contain 2.5 percent guggulsterone, take two capsules, twice a day, with meals.

**Caution:** Not recommended for pregnant or lactating women.

### *Gymnema sylvestre*

Used in the Indian Ayurvedic healing system it lowers type I and type II diabetic blood sugar levels, and appears to regenerate the pancreas' insulin-producing beta cells. For other diabetic natural options refer to the index.

*Principal health related actions:* Normalizes blood sugar levels and reduces the urge to eat sweets. May help heal the pancreas.

*Dosage:* Take a 200 mg capsules, twice a day. For liquid gymnema extracts mix five to ten drops in water, tea or juice, drink one cup a day. Take along with banaba leaf, chromium, vanadium, alpha lipoic acid and 1500 mg of evening primrose or borage oil for their gamma linolenic acid (GLA).

**Caution:** Consult with your doctor or health care professional, before you stop taking any medication or insulin, or take natural remedies and supplements.

***HCA*** – see Hydroxy citric acid.

### *Hemp oil*

An excellent source of essential fatty acids, which are needed for optimal health. Among it potential benefits are pain relief, reduction of arthritic inflammations, antidepressant possibilities (since the brain is mainly made up of fats), protection from heart disease, anticancer benefits.

Though banned for decades due to its hallucinogenic properties, it is making a comeback, since it is fast growing, environmentally beneficial and can be used in foods, clothing, shoes, paper plus a host of other products. Over 100 million dollars worth of legal products are made from hemp and hemp oil. The Canadian government allows farmers to grow Cannabis sativa, the hemp plant, with very low amounts of the hallucinogenic chemicals. Just thought we would whet your appetite for those good, bad and ugly fats. For additional information on fats and oils, refer to Chapter 5.

### *Hesperidin (Hesperidin methyl chalcone-HMC)*

A bioflavonoid immune system builder and powerful antihistamine.

*Principal health related actions:* Beneficial in treating environmental allergies, bruising and circulatory problems, such as weakness, night leg cramps, and varicose veins. Reduces edema.

*Dosage:* More effective when taken with other bioflavonoids, such as quercetin and rutin. Take with an equal amount of vitamin C as it helps boost this vitamin's effectiveness. Take between 25 and 1000 mg a day to maintain health. To deal with health-related problems, take between 1000 to 6000 mg (1 to 6 grams) a day. Consult with your health care provider if unsure. No known cautions.

*Food sources:* Fruits, vegetables, grains, legumes (especially soybean products), nuts, seeds. Found in some teas and wines.

### *HMB (Beta-hydroxy beta-methylbutyrate)*

A by-product of the amino acid leucine. It is found in animal and plant food. A four-week study of weight lifters taking HMB showed increased strength due to more muscle mass, combined with a loss of body fat. To benefit from HMB you must exercise when taking it; the more vigorous the workout, within reason, the greater the results will be. HMB is a less expensive and safer choice than the illegal and potentially dangerous anabolic steroids that some athletes take.

*Principal health related actions:* Improves your body's ability to lose fat and build muscle, while vigorously exercising. Efficient treatment for uremia patients.

*Dosage:* In powder or capsule form, take 2 to 3 grams a day with food.

**Caution:** Consult with you doctor or primary health care provider, before taking supplements if you are pregnant or lactating. Some athletes take many substances together, hoping it will improve the results. Multiple food or naturally occurring substances in the body, that have not had any reported negative effects, may peacefully coexist. Take a cautious approach of watchful waiting for matters such as this.

### *HMP-33*

For additional information, refer to Ginger.

HMP-33 is a standardized extract from ginger. Europeans use it to treat the pain and stiffness of osteoarthritis and rheumatoid arthritis. Recently, Americans have discovered this powerful healing substance, which has been used for hundreds of years in the Ayurvedic Indian system. Gingeroles are an anti-inflammatory substance of ginger present in HMP-33, without the substance shogaoles that may cause stomach upset.

*Principal health related actions:* HMP-33 interferes with the production of prostaglandins, a chemical responsible for causing arthritic pain. In addition, it prevents leukotrines from causing a chronic inflammatory response. Consequently, it alleviates the pain and inflammation often accompanying osteoarthritis and rheumatoid arthritis. It takes about three to four weeks for these benefits to occur. Possibly beneficial for pain relief of muscle injuries and strains. Used to treat bursitis and fibromyalgia.

The relief offered by HMP-33 comes without any of the potentially hazardous side effects of the NSAIDs used as arthritic pain killers. For example, ginger and even more so its extract HMP-33 soothes and protects the stomach's mucous membrane, whereas NSAIDs may cause gastric irritation leading to internal bleeding in the digestive tract. In addition, long-term use of NSAIDs can eventually render them ineffective, as the body adjusts to them.

*Dosage:* Take 1 capsule twice a day.

***Caution:*** People with gallstones should consult with their doctor prior to use. Not recommended for pregnant or lactating women.

### ***Human Growth Hormone***

For more information refer to the amino acids ***Arginine, Glutamine*** and the ***Human Growth Hormone*** sections in Chapter 13.

***Hydrocitric acid*** – see Hydroxy citric acid.

### *Hydroxy citric acid (HCA)*

Also known as 'hydrocitric acid' is extracted from the rare tropical fruit, garcina cambogia, found in Asian jungles. Used in curries and by Ayurvedic Indian healers for centuries, for its appetite-suppressing qualities and aid to digestion. It is a lipogenesis inhibitor, which means it reduces the rate that proteins and carbohydrates are turned into fat. This happens when the muscles' and liver's stores of excess energy are turned into glycogen, leaving no room for more glycogen. Excess calories from proteins and carbohydrates, then get turned into fat. HCA tells the muscles and liver to store more glycogen and stops the brain from asking the stomach for more food. The result is you burn more calories and eat less, because you do not feel hungry.

*Principal health related actions:* Used as a weight loss aid, because of its appetite-suppressing and digestive aid properties. By reducing high triglycerides levels, it may have heart healthy benefits.

*Dosage:* Take between 1500 to 2250 mg a day. Best results obtained by taking 500 to 750 mg half an hour before your main meals. When taking HCA, it is important to drink at least eight or more glasses of water each day. Sold in capsules and as an ingredient in weight loss bars, drinks and formulas.

***Caution:*** Not for use by pregnant or lactating women. It is not addictive nor habit forming. As with all weight loss programs, it is important to make lifestyle changes if you want permanent health enhancing benefits. HCA is most effective if you eat right and exercise.

***Note:*** This demonstrates the potentially powerful and healing opportunities that await us in our jungles. It is critical that we rapidly seek and find a balance between immediate economic gain and what is in the long-term best interests of humanity and the planet. If not for ourselves, then for our children, all children.

***Hydroxyapatite*** – see Calcium

### *Infopeptides*

They are polypeptides, short chains of amino acids that are too small to be called proteins. They are found in the colostrum (yellowish liquid) of mother's milk. The *Journal of Orthomolecular Medicine* (Vol 13, No. 2, pp 110-118, 1998) reported on this recently discovered powerful pain-reliever. It has natural antiviral properties and powerful abilities to regulate the immune system by activating low functioning areas and suppressing overactive ones. A case of a woman with the rare progressive muscle weakening condition, spinal-muscular atrophy (SMA), showed significant improvement in muscle tone, strength and coordination using infopeptides under her physician's guidance, at higher dosage levels than below.

*Principal health related actions:* Beneficial in treating inflammatory conditions such as fibromyalgia, arthritis and sciatica. Helpful for immune system deficiencies, for example cancers and AIDS. Indications are that it improves autoimmune problems, such as lupus and multiple sclerosis. As an antiviral, it may help short (acute) and long (chronic) term viral problems, such as shingles, viral pneumonia, influenza and chicken pox. Physicians have topically applied it to speed wound healing in infants and for childhood eczema cases.

*Dosage:* Available in spray form – 4 to 6 sprays equals 1 teaspoon (5 ml). In liquid form, take 1 to 2 teaspoons. One teaspoon (5 ml) for maintenance, two teaspoons (10 ml) for therapeutic purposes. Swish in mouth for two to three minutes, then swallow. The mouth's mucous membranes absorb liquids.

***Caution:*** In rare cases, people who are extremely milk sensitive or very lactose intolerant may be allergic to infopeptides.

## *Kudzu*

Is an herb used by ancient Chinese healers to treat alcoholism and prevent hangovers. A tenacious legume, this traveling vine grows in the wilds, all over the southeastern United States and is native to Japan. It does not have any of the negative side effects of alcohol treatment drugs such as Naltrexone, which work by causing nausea and vomiting and unfortunately can damage the liver.

*Principal health related actions:* Kudzu suppresses the desire for alcohol, thereby breaking alcohol addictions. When taken before drinking alcohol, it may prevent hangovers. It also may relieve hangovers. Enhances vital organ functions that are affected by alcohol. May have cardiovascular benefits since it dilates cerebral and coronary vessels, improving blood flow and oxygen levels in the blood. May have antioxidant properties to prevent clogged arteries. The Chinese use it for chest pains (angina), high blood pressure, allergies, diarrhea, headaches, upset stomach and mild fevers.

*Dosage:* Drink kudzu tea as part of a treatment program for chronic alcoholism. Take up to 1500 mg in pill form or rectangular cubes before or after drinking alcohol. You can break it down into 500 mg doses taken three times a day. If using a tincture, follow directions on the label. Chinese herbal shops sell it as an extract or root.

**Caution:** The major appeal of kudzu is the fact it has no toxic side effects, reported to date and no liver toxicity. Do not use kudzu in combination with prescription drugs, unless your health care provider or doctor okays such use. Not recommended for pregnant or lactating women.

### *Lactoferrin*

A protein found in breast milk it promotes the growth and maintenance of the good bacteria in a baby's digestive system and attacks the bad bacteria.

*Principle health uses:* Used as a natural antibiotic by Japanese pediatricians to treat ear infections, rather than pharmaceutical antibiotics which indiscriminately kill both good and bad bacteria. Pharmaceutical antibiotics suppress the human immune system. According to Japanese and European professionals, lactoferrin boosts the weakened immune system of cancer patients undergoing chemotherapy, with fewer side effects.

*Dosage:* Available in chewable wafers and capsules. Take up to 500 mg in wafers or capsules each day, for up to 14 days.

### *Lecithin (Phosphatidyl choline)*

This is a good fat, vital to your well-being. The brain, for example is mainly composed of fat, of which choline is a principal component. For more information about good and bad fats, refer to Chapter 5.

*Principal health related actions:* treats brittle hair and nails. Improves the balance of LDL (bad) to HDL (good) cholesterol. Reduces high cholesterol. Beneficial fat in long-term weight loss or weight management programs. It also improves brain and nerve function. Increases HDL, the good cholesterols' levels.

**Caution:** Not for use by those with liver diseases, e.g. fatty liver disease.

*Food source:* High quality soya lecithin granules.

### *Lipoic Acid (Alpha-Lipoic Acid or Lipoec acid)*

Is a naturally occurring essential non-vitamin produced in the body. It is both water and fat soluble. Powerful and unique antioxidant, free radical destroyer. Vital for an efficient kreb cycle – the reactions that occur in the body to produce up to 95 percent of the energy required for optimal functioning and vitality. Aging reduces lipoic acid production by the body. Supplementation becomes necessary, since it is a vital protector of your health. It can replace other antioxidants, such as vitamin E and C, when they are in short supply. In addition, lipoic acid increases the effectiveness of vitamins E and C.

*Principal health benefits:* Heavy metal detoxifier, such as mercury toxicity from dental amalgams. Excellent antioxidant. Europeans use it to treat diabetic complications and normalize blood sugar levels. It is particularly effective in preventing complications from diabetes, particularly insulin-resistant Type 2 diabetes. It helps prevent nervous system conditions such as nerve damage, atherosclerosis (hardening of the arteries) and blindness. Athletes indicate it prevents muscle soreness the morning after a vigorous workout. Lipoic acid has been used to cure liver disease due to eating the highly poisonous amanita mushroom; without treatment there is a 90 percent chance of death. Since it can pass through the blood-brain barrier, lipoic acid is a promising treatment for reversing the damage caused by a stroke. It may prevent or reverse open-angle glaucoma, diabetes, AIDS, liver diseases and heart disease.

***Note:*** Lipoic acid was effectively used to treat children exposed to radiation from the Chernobyl accident in the former Soviet Union.

*Dosage:* Take one or two 50 mg tablets a day, or as per your health care provider's directions. It is used in many antioxidant formulas.

***Caution:*** No toxicities are known. Diabetics should be closely monitored when taking lipoic acid. Not recommended for pregnant or nursing women.

### *Lutein*

A powerful antioxidant, one of the more than 600 members of the carotenoid family that can save your sight. Aging can result in macular degeneration, where the central part of the eye's retina, the macula, is destroyed. Until recently, there were no known treatments for this problem, which is a leading cause of blindness.

*Principal health benefits:* Preserves vision and prevents blindness due to macular degeneration. Zeaxanthin is another carotenoid that may also prevent macular degeneration. A Harvard study revealed that people getting a minimum of 6 grams of lutein in their daily diet, had significantly lower rates of macular degeneration. Lutein inhibits mammary tumor growth.

*Dosage:* Take 6 to 20 mg of lutein per day. Combination products with zinc and/or zeaxanthin, and possibly other sight savers, such as bilberry or ginkgo biloba, may be more beneficial, but is is important that they contain at least 6 mg of lutein.

*Food sources:* Collard greens, corn, kale, mustard greens, spinach. Starting around our mid-40s, our bodies are less able to derive the maximum nutritional benefits from the foods we eat as our digestive systems become less efficient. These types of foods can be difficult to fully digest and derive the benefits they offer. Consider adding digestive enzymes to your diet, so you can get greater nutritional value from your foods. For more information on digestive enzymes refer to Chapter 4 and the index.

### *Lycopene*

Another powerful member of the carotenoid family is found in that most versatile of fruits, the tomato. It gives tomatoes their red color. Lycopene is believed to be a more powerful antioxidant than beta-carotene and has powerful anticancer properties. Researchers at Ben Gurion University, in Israel, found that lycopene restrained cancerous growths in endometrial, breast and lung cancers. The greater the dose, the more effective lycopene was. Lycopene also appears to protect skin from UV sun damage and offer some protection from tobacco smoke's carcinogens. Researchers at John Hopkins found patients with pancreatic, bladder and rectal cancer, have significantly lower levels of lycopene in their blood. Women with cervical intraepithelial neoplasia, a precancerous indicator, have also been discovered by American researchers to have low lycopene levels.

*Principal health benefits:* Preservation of and protection for the prostrate gland. Cancer protection for the breasts, lungs, pancreas, endometrium plus other parts.

*Dosage:* Take one 5 to 10 mg capsule a day, with food. When using a combination formula for prostate protection, make sure it contains at least 5 mg of lycopene along with saw palmetto and pumpkin seed extract.

*Food sources:* By weight, watermelon is the best source at 4.1 grams per 100 grams. Next are tomatoes at 3.1 grams per 100 grams. Small amounts are also found in apricots. The best source is cooked or steamed tomatoes, with a dash of extra virgin olive oil or other fat to make it more easily digestible. Fresh or juiced tomatoes are not as good a source of lycopene as tomatoes that are cooked, steamed or processed into a lycopene supplement. Since the body doesn't absorb lycopene very well, from raw tomatoes the USDA has indicated that steaming and cooking does not hurt lycopene levels. By the mid-40s, our bodies are less able to derive the maximum nutritional benefits from foods like tomatoes. Consider adding digestive enzymes to your diet, so you can get greater nutritional value from your meals. For more information on digestive enzymes refer to Chapter 4 and the index.

### *Maitake mushroom extract*

Maitake mushroom extract is another powerful healer from the Orient. Japanese researchers examined the folklore behind this ancient remedy and found it activated the body's natural defenders against cancer and viral cells, the T-cells. Mitake's beta-glucan content make it a superior medicinal mushroom. When taken in time, tumors shrunk more than they did with just chemotherapy. When combined with chemotherapy, the shrinkage was 99 percent within 14 days. It increases the benefits from chemotherapy while decreasing the extreme fatigue and nausea that chemotherapy can cause.

*Principal health benefits:* Has cancer fighting properties; alleviates extreme fatigue and nausea caused by chemotherapy. Take with vitamin C to increase its immune system boosting properties, which means increased resistance to disease. Beneficial for HIV-infected AIDS patients. It is being used by some doctors and naturally orientated healers since it significantly reduces the destruction that the AIDS virus can cause to body's T-cells.

*Dosage:* Take one or two standardized extract 100 milligram tablets each day. Take with vitamin C to boost its immunity building properties. People with tumors take four to ten caplets a day; cancer or AIDS patients take eight to ten caplets a day; diabetics take ten caplets per day until blood sugar levels are reduced, then take a maintenance dose of three to six caplets a day; hypertensive people take six caplets a day, once blood pressure levels are lowered take a maintenance dose of two to four caplets a day.

*Suggestion:* Inform your doctor or health care provider when using it. The information may help save or improve another patient's life.

## Malic acid

This is an alpha hydroxy acid (AHA), which is vital for the body's normal production of energy. It is believed to accomplish this by aiding the delivery system of oxygen to muscle cells, thereby preventing hypoxia (below normal oxygen levels). Researchers found malic acid combined with magnesium was beneficial for fibromyalgia sufferers. May help improve endurance and stamina of athletes by increasing the muscles' ability to receive and use oxygen.

*Principal health benefits:* Alleviates symptoms of fibromyalgia. Potentially offers increased athletic stamina and endurance.

*Dosage:* For fibromyalgia, take 6 capsules a day with water. The dose is 1200 mg of malic acid, in combination with 300 mg of magnesium hydroxide. Take 3 capsules, twice a day, one hour before breakfast and at bedtime, or as directed by your doctor or naturopath.

*Food sources:* Apples, cranberries, grapes, plus other fruits and vegetables.

## Melatonin

A hormone produced in your brain, by the pineal gland. During sleep the amount of melatonin increases, during the day the amount falls. It appears to be a master hormone, controlling the circadian rhythm, our body's 24 hour sleep/wake cycle, plus a host of vital activities in our bodies. Around our mid-forties the reduction in the pineal gland's production of melatonin becomes noticeable, as our sleep patterns change. It is a powerful antioxidant that protects cells from the damage free radicals cause.

*Potential health benefits:* Treatment for jet lag. May be an anti-aging supplement that reverses signs of aging, in turn increasing the quality and length of life. Melatonin offers relief to some sufferers of cluster headaches. It prevents the formation of the amyloid plaque which kills brain cells, and can lead to Alzheimer's disease. Increases immune system functioning. In tests with melanoma skin cancer patients, after the surgical removal of metastasized tumors, the placebo group had a significantly lower survival rate than those given 20 milligrams of melatonin each night. Major benefits of melatonin are that you wake up without feeling groggy and that it is not addictive, like most of the over-the-counter drugs for sleeping.

*Dosage:* For a better night's sleep or insomnia, try 1 mg of melatonin a half hour before going to bed. If that is not enough, then increase the dosage by 1 mg each day, up to a maximum of 4 mgs. The sublingual (under the tongue) type is faster acting, since the melatonin gets into the blood stream, through the mouth's mucous membrane.

To prevent the side effects of jet lag, once you arrive at your destination, take 1 to 3 mg of the sublingual form of melatonin, about thirty minutes before you want to sleep.

For melatonin's cancer fighting properties, under your doctor or natural health care provider's supervision, try 10 to 20 mg a day of melatonin, taken sublingually.

For cluster headaches, under your doctor or health provider's supervision, try 10 mg of melatonin.

If over 40 years of age, take 0.5 to 1 mg before going to sleep, for its powerful antioxidant and anti-aging properties.

***Caution:*** Do not drive or operate heavy machinery if you have just taken melatonin. Do not take melatonin if you are suffering from an autoimmune disease. If you are taking medications, speak with your doctor and tell your pharmacist before taking it, since it can interact with tranquilizers, antidepressants and other drugs. Do not take melatonin if pregnant, nursing, trying to become pregnant, suffer severe mental illness, have immune system cancers, have an autoimmune disease, or severe allergies. Not recommended for children.

## *Methionine (S-adenosyl methionine-SAM)*

Methionine is an anti-inflammatory, anti-depressant and liver detoxifier. For additional information and the most bio-available form, refer to 'S-Adenosyl-L-Methione (SAMe)'. It may have anti-aging properties as well as be helpful for rheumatoid arthritis, mild depression, liver congestion and many other health problems. It is not toxic.

## *Methylsulfonylmethane (MSM)*

Organic sulfur, an essential nonmetallic mineral, found in every cell and critical for almost all bodily functions. It is nonallergenic, whereas synthetic manufactured sulfa drugs may cause allergic reactions. The body uses it to produce antibodies, enzymes, amino acids, the powerful antioxidant glutathione, hair, skin, nails, and connective tissue such as collagen and cartilage. MSM is critical to protein synthesis and stability.

*Potential health benefits:* Very effective in treating sever allergic reactions and asthma. Promotes wound healing, since it helps form connective tissue and thereby helps skin renew itself. As a health and beauty aid, it improves the condition of your nails and hair. MSM, especially when used with glucosamine, is a powerful treatment for arthritis. Other helpful substances you may want to combine with MSM for arthritis are: Devil's Claw (an anti-inflammatory herb), chondroitin, and pregnenolone.

*Dosage:* Take one 1000 mg tablet with breakfast and supper. For allergies, take MSM with bioflavonoids and vitamin C. Within four weeks, the watery eyes and runny nose will disappear. MSM is also available in skin lotions, apply it as directed.

*Food sources:* Dairy and dairy products, eggs, garlic, meat, onions, poultry. MSM is very difficult to obtain through foods, since processing frequently destroys it.

***Mushrooms*** – see entries under Maitake, Reishi, Shiitake mushrooms.

### *N-Acetylcysteine*

Also known as ***N-Acetyl Cysteine, NAC, HMG-CoA reductase*** or ***HMGR***

This amino acid helps athletes and the chronically ill. You may use N-acetylcysteine or cystine instead of cysteine for supplementation. N-acetylcysteine and cysteine are beneficial in reducing or preventing side effects from radiation (X-rays, nuclear radiation) and chemotherapy. N-acetylcysteine more effectively boosts glutathione levels than cystine or even glutathione supplementation. Its potential benefits include better recovery after strenuous exercise, protection from cigarette smoke's carcinogens, increased production of the powerful antioxidant glutathione, less lung and ear infections. NAC reduces sinus inflammations that can cause sinus headaches and prevent damage due to radiation. For more information about amino acids and cysteine refer to Chapter 13.

*Dosage:* Take one 500 mg capsule, three times a day, with each meal. If lung and ear infections plague you, speak to your doctor or naturally orientated healer about using NAC.

***Caution:*** Not for use if you have peptic ulcers or are taking drugs that cause gastric sores.

### *Pectins*

Fractionated or separated fruit pectins

This nutraceutical food substance inhibits tumor growth and metastasis in 'sticky cell' type carcinomas. It may aid other types of cancer therapies. It is not toxic and has no known negative side effects.

### *Phosphatidylserine (PS-30 Complex, PS)*

Is a phospholipid, an important fat needed by the brain to relay messages and help retrieve and store information in brain cells.

Aging reduces this and other powerful memory chemicals in the brain, so we tend to forget or lose our train of thought, in essence have sluggish brains that are no longer as efficient as they used to be. PS can improve memory and restore brain function. It is not available in common foods and is usually made from soy phospholipids.

*Possible health related actions:* Improves poor concentration. Enhances short term memory and prevents memory loss. Alleviates attention deficit disorder (ADD).

*Dosage:* Use a 30 percent standardized PS extract. Take 200 to 600 mg a day.

**Caution:** None known. Consult with your doctor or natural healer before using it for children with ADD and for memory problems.

### *Pregnenolone*

A hormone produced by the adrenal glands and the brain. Aging reduces production of this and other hormones that affect our memory, ability to concentrate, perform tasks and learn. It helps deal with some of the more than 100 arthritic conditions, particularly rheumatoid arthritis. Significant alleviation of pain, swelling and stiffness have been reported by patients taking it for two to four weeks. Additionally, it can make you feel happier and smarter and may benefit those suffering from depression.

*Possible health related actions:* Better memory and improved ability to concentrate. Alleviates rheumatoid arthritis symptoms.

*Dosage:* Take 5 to 10 mg a day.

**Caution:** Consult with your doctor or naturally orientated healer before taking it, since pregnenolone may increase your sex hormone levels.

### *Proanthocyanidins (PCOs)*

PCOs are powerful antioxidants found in stems, leaves, skins and bark of plants. They were first discovered in the mid-1940s in the red skin of peanuts. It has since been noted they occur naturally in vegetables and fruits. To discover more about their heart healing and antioxidant properties, refer to Grape Seed extract, Grape Seed OPC, Pine tree bark extract and Pycnogenol.

### *Probiotics*

The word 'probiotic' means 'for life'. Probiotics provide a full spectrum of good bacteria needed to maintain optimal health and internal balance in the body, primarily the digestive system's florae. Overuse of antibiotics, birth control pills and corticosteroids (steroids) can cause a loss or imbalance of these intestinal florae. This leaves you susceptible to bacterial, viral and fungal diseases. Aging also reduces our levels of these health-promoting bacteria, rendering us easier prey for disease. Probiotics help keep hormone levels normal and offer protection against pollutants. They produce some B vitamins and may reduce or rebalance cholesterol levels. They also inhibit the growth of harmful bacteria such as Salmonella, Candida albicans and Staphylococcus aureus.

*Possible health related actions:* Boosts the immune system. Aid for controlling yeast infections. Possibly offers protection against cancer. Being used for prevention of salmonella in chickens and their eggs.

*Dosage:* Look for probiotics containing at least these bacteria: bifidobacterium, Lactobacillus acidophilus and lactobacillus bulgaricus. Look for them in the freezer section of your health food stores or ask your pharmacist to recommend one they are carrying. Some of the better brands are kept refrigerated. Available in capsules, powders and liquids. Follow label directions. Take half an hour before meals. For more information about the benefits of friendly bacteria, see Acidophilus, Lactobacillus G.G., and the digestive system section in Chapter 3.

*Food sources:* Eat food rich in fiber because dietary fiber is consumed by intestinal bacteria, transformed into organic acids, which reduce and inhibit the growth of bad bacteria.

***Caution:*** When you start taking probiotics, you may develop bloating or gas. This means the good bacteria are fermenting. Your body will adjust to this within 10 to 14 days.

## *Prune juice*

Mother nature's laxative. Aaaahhhh! *News flash:* The FDA does not recognize the laxative properties of prune juice.

## *Puncturevine (Tribulus terrestris)*

Also spelled Puncture Vine

It has been a part of Indian and Chinese healing systems for over 5000 years. Studies indicate it increase production of the luteinizing hormone, which stimulates testosterone production in men and estrogen in women. This is very beneficial to the female and male reproductive systems. In turn, these benefits help burn fat and build muscle.

*Principal health related actions:* In men puncturevine boosts the benefits of workouts and the ability to perform sexually. May increase sperm production and fertility levels. Its ability to increase estrogen levels may help reduce the symptoms of fatigue and hot flashes that can accompany menopause.

*Suggested uses:* Nature's answer to Viagara, puncturevine can improve male sex life and muscle mass. It offers a long-term, comparatively inexpensive natural option to prescription drugs.

*Dosage:* Available in tablets and capsules. Get products with a standardized potency of 40 percent furostanols. Use as directed.

**Caution:** Some puncturevine supplements contain DHEA and a metabolite of DHEA, androstenedione, which may increase testosterone levels. For this reason, it should not be used by men with a history of prostate cancer.

## *Pycnogenol generic and Pycnogenol™ (Pine bark extract)*

Pycnogenol is derived from the bark of pine trees. This powerful antioxidant contains bioflavonoids, glucose, natural soluble organic acids and proanthocyanidins. It is an excellent free radical scavenger and protects cells from free radical damage, which is believed responsible for many diseases. For additional information refer to Grape Seed Extract and Grape Seed OPC.

*Principal health related actions:* Useful for allergies, chronic degenerative diseases, ADD, ADHD, weakening eyesight. It is an anti-inflammatory and anti-aging substance. Neutralizes free radicals in the blood. Strengthens blood vessels, which is beneficial for heart health and sexual function.

*Dosage:* Try the less expensive but just as, if not more, effective grape seed extract rather than Pycnogenol™. The Europeans mainly use grape seed extract in their research studies. To maintain the integrity and health of your vascular system, take 50 to 100 mg a day. For diseases, take 150 to 400 mg a day. For ADD and ADHD, children should take 1 mg per pound of body weight. Adults should take 2 mg per pound of body weight.

***Cautions:*** None known. Ensure that children use it in consultation with a medical or naturally orientated health care practitioner.

### *Pyruvate*

Also known as ***Calcium pyruvaten***

This could be the weight loss supplement for the 21st century. It burns fat and increases muscle tone without exercising. Pyruvate is a normal by-product of your body's metabolism. It is vital to energy production since it releases the fuel ATP, which your cells produce, and provides energy to your whole body.

*Principal body system it benefits:* Cardiovascular.

*Principal health related actions:* Aids in weight loss and burns fat. Increases stamina and energy levels. Beneficial for the cardiovascular system's health and helps reduce the chance of heart disease by lowering blood pressure and cholesterol levels.

*Dosage:* For athletes, take between 3000 to 4000 mg in capsules or powder each day, before a meal or exercise, on an empty stomach. For weight loss, take 4000 to 5000 mg in capsules or powder, on an empty stomach.

***Caution:*** For long-term weight loss, lifestyle changes may be needed. Check with your health care provider to see if an ongoing or sudden weight gain indicates an underlying problem.

### *Quercetin (Quercitin)*

A bioflavonoid and cousin of rutin it is used in cromolyn sodium, a prescription anti-allergy drug. As well as being anti-allergic (a natural antihistamine), it is a powerful antioxidant and natural anti-inflammatory. Studies indicate it has powerful anticancer properties. Improves circulation and strengthens the tiny blood vessels called capillaries.

*Principal health related actions:* Helps treat food allergies and allergies transmitted by air. Use with bromelain to boost the bio-availability (amount of active ingredient the body absorbs) of quercetin for the body.

*Dosage:* Take a 400 mg standardized extract capsule, three times a day before meals.

***Caution:*** Not recommended for use in children seven years of age or younger.

*Food sources:* Apples, onions.

### *Red wine polyphenols*

Powerful antioxidants found in red wine protect your cardiovascular system against the ravages of bad LDL cholesterol. They prevent the buildup of plaque, help blood oxygenation and slow blood clot formation, which are major causes of stroke and heart attack. Recently, they have been discovered to reduce the rate of cancer tumor growth.

*Dosage:* In capsules, take up to 60 mg a day. This avoids the potential problems of headaches that red wine can cause, alcohol-induced liver damage and lots of calories.

### *Reishi mushroom (Ganoderma lucidum)*

In studies using mice, reishi extracts have stopped the growth of cancerous tumors. It is a heart tonic, thought to oxygenate systems and body parts. A potent natural mood elevator.

*Health conditions it may be useful in treating:* Stop growth of cancerous tumors. Its antihistamine action is beneficial for allergy control. Aids in lowering cholesterol and preventing blood clots. Used to greatly lessen the symptoms of altitude sickness. Valuable heart tonic, which is used as a preventative measure and treatment for arrhythmia. It eases chest pains from angina. Elevates one's mood.

*Sources:* Reishi mushrooms, capsules, tinctures and extracts. In tea, use 3 to 6 teaspoons per 8 ounces of boiling water; drink daily.

### *Resveratrol*

Found in grapes and peanuts it offers antifungal properties, reduces the rate and formation of blood clots, prevents plaque formation in arteries and may be anticarcinogenic. It may help restore malignant cells to their normal state.

*Principal health related actions:* Lessens chances of heart disease. Beneficial for the treatment of cancer tumors.

*Dosage:* If undergoing treatment for cancer, consult with your health care provider to decide on the best dosage levels for you. A 1000 mcg capsule a day is suitable for preventative purposes. A glass of wine equals 640 mcg.

## *Royal Jelly*

It is the milky white secretion of a specialized group of nurse bees during the first 12 days of their life. It contains all the B vitamins, vitamin A, C, D, E, minerals, hormones, essential amino acids, fatty acids, simple carbohydrates, pantothenic acid, iron, calcium, silicon, sulfur, potassium, antibacterial and antibiotic elements. It may have anti-aging and beauty enhancing properties. It stimulates the adrenal glands, which are critical for mood, appetite, metabolism and sex drive. All bee larvae eat royal jelly during the first three days of life. After that, only the future queen bee continues eating it. Comparatively, queens are much larger than other female bees, living up to 45 times longer, and are very fertile.

*Principle health related actions:* May slow aging process. Can improve texture and quality of skin, reducing fine lines and wrinkle formation. Sexual tonic for restoring sexual energy and drive. Useful for treating menopausal symptoms. Helpful for asthma, pancreatitis, insomnia, liver disease, kidney disease, stomach ulcers, bone fractures, and immune system functioning.

*Dosage:* Take between one to three 300 mg capsules a day.

***Caution:*** If you are allergic to bee pollen, check with your allergist or health care provider, before taking royal jelly. The jelly may have bee pollen contaminants.

## *Rutin*

A bioflavonoid usually derived from eucalyptus. It is a member of C-complex, working synergistically with vitamin C and other bioflavonoids, such as hesperidin and quercetin. It has anti-inflammatory, antiviral, anticancer and antimicrobial properties.

*Principle health related actions:* Offers allergy relief by slowing histamine production, the chemical responsible for triggering allergic symptoms. Vital for vitamin C absorption. Aids and maintains the collagen layer, which is critical for supporting the outer layer of skin, the epidermis. Facilitates wound healing. Strengthens the tiniest blood vessels, the capillaries; because of this it may help treat varicose veins, bruises and hemorrhoids. Prevention of cancer. May enhance body's ability to fight viral infections.

*Dosage:* Take between 100 to 1500 mg a day, at least 30 minutes before a meal. The amount depends on the severity of the condition. For maintenance purposes, 100 mg a day is sufficient.

## S-Adenosyl-L-Methione (SAMe)

A combination of two amino acids it is part of the methyl group of substances which turns the potentially dangerous amino acid, homocysteine, into the beneficial compound, methionine. Other substances that can help the process of methylation (turning homocysteine into methionine) occur are trimethylglycine, vitamin $B_{12}$ and folic acid. Homocysteine indicates increased chance of developing arthritis, cancer, depression, heart as well as other diseases. Methylation increases metabolite levels of SAMe, from methionine, which decrease as we age. SAMe is vital for melatonin production, the powerful hormone that regulates our 24-hour circadian rhythm (waking and sleeping patterns), and is an anti-aging hormone with numerous benefits.

*Principle health related actions:* Anti-aging properties. Beneficial as an anti-inflammatory treatment for osteoarthritis, providing as much relief as NSAIDs, such as Ibuprofen, without damage to the stomach lining. Heals and restores cartilage, which help the joints work better, without wearing away the bones. Possibly beneficial for treating elderly sufferers of dementia. Improves cognitive abilities. May be helpful in treatment of fibromyalgia, by reducing the joint pain and lifting patients' moods. Possibly helpful for other types of chronic pain, as well. Its antidepressant qualities are effective in about 75 percent of patients, without any harmful side effects. Soothes the pain of migraines. Stabilizes DNA and prevents harmful mutations that could become cancers. Helps the liver detoxify and keep the body clean. May neutralize the potentially harmful amino acid, homocysteine.

*Dosage:* Take up to 1500 mg of capsules a day. Entric-coated SAMe has the longest shelf-life and is the most absorbable product. For osteoarthritis, test subjects were successfully treated with 600 mg in a capsule, each day. For fibromyalgia, speak to your health care provider or doctor about trying SAMe. For mild to moderate depression take 200 mg two times daily, on an empty stomach, half an hour before breakfast and lunch or two hours after these meals. Some have to increase their dosage to 400 mg twice a day. Doctors Bottiglieri and Brown, authors of *Stop Depression Now*, suggest you try SAMe from four to nine months. Most note an improved mood within days.

***Note:*** For depression if SAMe is too expensive, or does not help, refer to St. John's Wort or 5-HTP, excellent herbal antidepressants.

***Caution:*** At the above dosage levels SAMe may cause an upset stomach or mild headache. If you are severely depressed or suicidal, see a health care professional immediately. Do not stop taking any antidepressants without first discussing this with your doctor or health care professional.

### *Shark Cartilage*

It contains calcium, collagen, protein, and an important family of microproteins called glycosaminoglycans. These nutrients become part of the synovial membranes of our joints. Years of use wear away the cartilage cushion used by the joints. By reinforcing the chemical composition of the synovial membranes, we reduce the effects of wear and tear.

In addition, shark cartilage contains an anti-angiogenesis component, which enhances immunity, slows and may stop the growth of blood vessels into tumors. It may be beneficial for many diseases, such as psoriasis, arthritis, cancer, rheumatism, melanoma, shingles, hemorrhoids.

*Dosage:* Before each meal, take two to three 750 mg capsules.

***Caution:*** Not recommended for small children, pregnant or lactating women or anyone who has recently had surgery or a heart attack.

### *Shark Liver Oil*

It has the highest naturally occurring level of alkylglycerols. These substances are found in our liver, spleen, bone marrow and human breast milk. They are part of the white blood cell production process. The oil stimulates production of leukocytes and thrombocytes, antibodies in the immune system. It also has antifungal and antibiotic properties that speed wound and sore healing. Fishermen have used it for centuries to sooth irritated respiratory tracts and reduce the size of swollen lymph nodes.

Dosage: Take one to two 500 mg soft gel capsules with every meal. It is not toxic.

### *Shiitake mushroom (Lentinus edodes)*

It is used in Japan to fight cancerous growths due to its beneficial effects upon the immune system.

*Principle health related actions:* Fights infections. Lowers cholesterol. Prevents heart disease. Boosts the immune system. Has cancer fighting properties. Beneficial for the heart.

*Dosage:* Can be eaten raw or lightly cooked, so as not to destroy its beneficial components. In capsules, take 1 to 3 a day, or as per label directions. The active cancer-fighting ingredient is thought to be lentinan.

***Caution:*** Speak to your doctor or naturally orientated healer about incorporating shiitake mushroom capsules into your cancer fighting program.

## *Silymarin*

It is a combination of three bioflavonoids extracted from the milk thistle plant. They are silydianin, silybin and silychristin and offer powerful antioxidant properties. They increase superoxide dismutase and glutathione antioxidant levels in the body. This extract helps boost liver function, protects the liver from free radical damage, cirrhosis of the liver and viral hepatitus. See Milk thistle, for more information on liver protection.

*Dosage:* Take up to 1.5 grams a day, in tablets or capsules.

## *Soy Concentrates (Isolates)*

Derived from the soybean they exhibit unique and powerful health and healing properties. They contain the powerful substances diadzein, genistein, phytic acid and isoflavones. Sprouted soy is an excellent source of plant estrogens (phytoestrogens).

*Principal health related actions:* Plant estrogens in soy alleviate menopausal symptoms. The protease inhibitor and antioxidant in soy, phytic acid, slows and stops enzymes that promote tumors. Daidzein, an isoflavone in soy, may be beneficial in breaking the growth cycle that promotes breast, prostate and other cancer cells. A daily intake of soy protein reduces triglyceride levels and lowers total cholesterol.

*Dosage:* Make sure the soy supplement you take contains diadzein and genistein. To lower cholesterol levels, drink between 45 to 50 grams daily of soy protein or as per package directions. Take 2 capsules a day.

### *Spirulina*

A protein-rich microalgea it has a higher concentration of nutrients than any other plant and is easily digestible. Here are some of its components: essential amino acids, iron, vitamin $B_{12}$, chlorophyll, gamma-linolenic acid (GLA), linoleic acid, arachidonic acid, nucleic acids RNA and DNA. It is a nutrient-dense powerhouse of food substances.

*Principal health related actions:* Detoxifies and cleanses the body. Take it when fasting. Improves absorption of minerals. Protects and supports the immune system. Aids in stabilizing blood sugar levels. Helps reduce cholesterol levels. An excellent aid to weight loss since it curbs one's appetite. Reduces insulin need. Beneficial in treatment of obesity.

*Dosage:* Take up to 5 grams a day or more, as per package directions. For hypoglycemic's, take it between meals to keep your blood sugar levels balanced.

***Caution:*** Once the container is opened, spirulina requires refrigeration to maintain its high nutrient levels, even though some labels do not say so.

### *Tiger Balm®*

Medicinal ingredients in the regular strength white balm ointment are camphor, menthol, cajeput oil, mint oil, and clove oil. The extra-strength red balm ointment also contains cinnamon oil and may stain clothing.

*Principal health related actions:* It is a powerful pain relieving ointment, used by athletes worldwide. It is found in health food stores and some pharmacies. If you suffer from minor muscular aches and pains due to arthritis, overexertion, joint pains or backaches, it offers excellent temporary relief. Use sparingly.

***Trimethylglycine*** – see Betaine.

***Vanadyl sulfate*** – see Vanadium.

### *Whey*

A protein-rich concentrate derived from milk protein. It does not contain undesirable ingredients, such as lactose, the difficult-to-digest milk sugar. It raises levels of the powerful antioxidant glutathione.

*Principal health related actions:* Protects against degenerative and age-related diseases. It is an immune system booster that has been shown to be very effective against Streptococcus pneumonia, Salmonella and other common infections. Helps build and maintain muscle mass. May have anti-aging properties. Aids weight loss and weight management programs.

*Dosage:* Take 1 ounce (2 tablespoons, 30 ml) in 8 ounces of juice or water each day.

## *Whole Green Super Food Supplements*

Also known as 'green drinks' or 'super vitamin' drinks, usually contain 16 to 80 nutritional substances and include combinations of a few or all of the following: nutrient rich foods, juice blends, fiber blends, vegetable powder blends, sprouted multi-grains, multi-algae blends, multistrain probiotic blends, standardized herbal and fruit extracts, organic fruit polyphenol blends, digestive enzymes.

They generally offer antioxidant protection, immune system support, increased energy, gastrointestinal reinforcement and a diverse and extensive nutrient supplementation option. From detoxifying your body to cardiovascular and blood sugar system support, these are the wave of the future. If you are like most people, you do not eat enough fruits and vegetables on a daily basis and probably do not receive enough of the nutrients needed for optimal health. Try one of the many brands of these powerful multiple nutrient drinks.

You may take a multi-vitamin and mineral complex with this, or target a specific ailment with herbs, homeopathic or aromatherapy remedies. For about a dollar a day, you are inexpensively protecting your body from the ravages of our highly stressful society. These make a solid foundation upon which to build a healthy diet and a sound natural remedy and supplement support program. Enjoy a renewed sense of vitality and youthfulness today.

*Dosage:* Usually 1 tablespoon (15 ml) per day, on an empty stomach or 15 to 30 minutes before you eat. Follow package directions.

***Caution:*** Not recommended for pregnant or lactating women.

## *Zeaxanthin*

A powerful antioxidant carotenoid that may prevent macular degeneration, the leading cause of of age-related blindness. It is a condition caused by the destruction of part of the retina, called the macula. Eventually you no longer can do the daily activities of life, such as reading, watching television, driving, using a computer, cooking and walking unassisted.

*Principle health related actions:* May prevent blindness due to macular degeneration. May provide cancer prevention properties and decrease growth rates for tumors.

*Food sources:* Beet greens, chicory leaf, okra, Swiss chard, watercress.

*Dosage:* Take it as part of an antioxidant or mixed carotenoid formula, from 25 to 150 mg per day. Combination formulas for vision may contain lutein, ginkgo biloba, bilberry and taurine.

# chapter 19

# A Model of Health and Healing for the New Millennium

## Complementary Alternatives That Enhance Natural Remedies and Supplements

As a specialist in Physical Medicine and Rehabilitation, Dr. Ko treats conditions characterized by chronic pain, numbness, stiffness and/or fatigue. The following are descriptions of some evidence-based-"physical remedies" that he has found effective in clinical practice.

### *Acupuncture*

The World Health Organization defines acupuncture as "The procedure of inserting needles through the skin or mucous membranes at one or more specific points, without the injection of any substance, to effect a therapeutic and/or analgesic response in a patient, with the intent to stimulate the neuroendocrine system."

### *Types of Acupuncture*

**Traditional Chinese medicine** (TCM) was originally developed over 2000 years ago as part of a whole system of medicine for diagnosing and treating disease and pain disorders. In recent years, scientific medical research has begun to demonstrate and explain its effectiveness.

**Anatomical Acupuncture** (AA) involves the modern approach which integrates current knowledge of anatomy, physiology and neuroendocrine mechanisms with acupuncture techniques. For more information, contact the Traditional Acupuncture Institute, American City Building, 10227 Wincopin Circle, Suite 100, Columbia, MD 21044-3422 at (301) 596-3675 or Acupuncture Foundation of Canada at (416) 752-3988.

**Intramuscular stimulation**, (IMS) or Chan Gunn "dry-needling" based on Dr. Chan Gunn's work uses dry needling of muscle trigger points for pain relief. May be combined with electrical stimulation.

**Electroacupuncture** according to Voll (EAV) is now often used to stimulate the inserted needles with gentle electrical impulses. TENS (Transcutaneous electrical nerve stimulation) involves a no-needle approach where rubber electrodes convey the impulses over acupuncture points. Laser can also be used over these points.

### *Acupuncture works by*

- Direct nerve stimulation with resultant "gating" of pain impulses at the spinal cord level.
- Stimulating the production of endorphins, the body's own hormones that mimic morphine in attaching to opiate receptors resulting in pain relief, general relaxation and homeostasis (internal stability).
- Stimulating descending neural pathways that work to inhibit pain transmission (neurotransmitters include serotonin, norepinephrine, substance P).

### *What conditions respond to acupuncture treatments?*

The World Health Organization reports acupuncture is beneficial for:

- Pain disorders including headaches, neck and back pain, neuralgia, tennis elbow, tendinitis, frozen shoulder, sciatica, and arthritis.
- Digestive problems including: gastritis, hyperacidity, constipation, diarrhea, irritable bowel syndrome.
- Respiratory conditions including: sinusitis, bronchitis, asthma.
- Urinary, menstrual and reproductive problems.
- Addictions, insomnia.

### *Considerations when undergoing acupuncture*

- Patients with pacemakers should avoid electrical stimulation.
- Certain points are contraindicated during pregnancy.

- Caution must be used in bleeding disorders (e.g. hemophilia) and when taking anticoagulants.
- Special care must be taken over the chest wall to avoid lung or heart puncture, and over the base of the skull.
- Only sterile disposable needles should be used to avoid transmitting HIV and hepatitis.
- Needle phobia is a contraindication. Use Acupressure/TENS instead.
- Local discomfort from the needles is usually minimal.

## *Biofeedback*

### *What is biofeedback?*

*"The technique of using equipment (usually electronic) to reveal to human beings some of their internal physiological events, normal and abnormal, in the form of visual and auditory signals, in order to teach them to manipulate these otherwise involuntary or unfelt events by manipulating the displayed signals."*

– John V. Basmajian M.D., F.R.C.P.C.

### *Types of Biofeedback include*

Reading of the autonomic nervous system such as skin temperature, galvanic skin response, blood pressure, heart rate, respiration rate.

Surface EMG (electromyography) to:

(1) relax tense, tight muscles.

(2) restrengthen weak, atrophied muscles.

(3) retrain proper muscle recruitment patterns.

Check out the "back-in-action Physiotherapy" web site at: http://members.home.net/backinaction

EEG (electroencephalography) for Optimizing appropriate brain wave patterns. This may be enhanced by using photic (light) and audio (sound) stimulation to facilitate proper entrainment (neurotherapy).

### *How does biofeedback work?*

It teaches self-awareness of internal physical cues which then allows the individual to modify/control involuntary functions.

## *What conditions respond to biofeedback?*

The Association for Applied Psychophysiology and Biofeedback [(303) 422-8439] has compiled literature supporting the use of biofeedback for:

- Neuropsychological disorders including Attention deficit disorder (ADD), minor brain injury, anxiety, insomnia and stress-related conditions. Check out "Advanced Wellness Programs" at web site: www.totalmastery.com
- Musculoskeletal pain, such as carpal tunnel syndrome, myofascial pain disorder, repetitive strain injury, patellofemoral syndrome, shoulder instability, migraine and tension headaches.
- Neuromuscular diseases including urinary incontinence, digestive system problems (irritable bowel), partial nerve injuries and paralysis, facial nerve palsy (Bell's palsy), movement disorders.
- Cardiovascular conditions including Raynaud's disease (cold hands), high and low blood pressure.

## *What are the risks or potential adverse effects of biofeedback?*

The use of phototherapy may precipitate or aggravate seizures in predisposed individuals (e.g. those with epilepsy or who have had a recent stroke).

### *Orthopaedic Medicine with Manipulation & Prolotherapy*

## *What is Orthopaedic Medicine?*

Orthopaedic Medicine was founded by the British physician, Dr. James Cyriax, (1904-1985). This field of medicine focuses on nonsurgical therapies for musculoskeletal conditions. The key concepts are:

#1. Referred pain:

pain may be felt distal to (away from) its source.

pain radiates segmentally and does not cross midline.

pain is usually felt deeply.

pain does not necessarily include the source (area of lesion).

pain is referred distally within the dermatome.

pain is felt anywhere in the dermatome; not necessarily in all of it.

#2. Selective tension: an injured structure hurts when tension is placed on its fibers.

#3. Manipulation therapy: Manipulation is defined by the Ontario Medical Association (June 1983 Policy statement) as follows: "A forced movement applied directly or indirectly to an articulation, or a collection of articulations, which suddenly carries the articular elements beyond their usual physiological range of movement without passing the limit imposed on their anatomical range of movement."

Professionals who can legally manipulate include:

- Chiropractors – a health specialty started in 1885 by Dr. D. Palmer
- Osteopaths – started by Dr. T. Still (1828-1917)
- Physiotherapists – many use the Maitland protocol
- Physicians – trained as osteopaths D O. or through the American Association of Orthopaedic Medicine

Craniosacral therapists offer a gentler form of manipulation originated by an American osteopath William Sutherland in the 1930s and developed by osteopathic physician and surgeon John E. Upledger in the 1970s. Craniosacral therapy emphasizes the bones of the skull, face, mouth, sacrum and coccyx.

#4. Prolotherapy: From the Latin "Proles", which means to "stimulate growth", this therapy involves the injection of proliferants (e.g. dextrose, phenol, sodium morrhuate) at bone ligament junctions. This results in a localized inflammatory response leading to fibroblast proliferation and collagen formation. The latter is the building block of ligaments. In proper hands, this is an excellent means for treating musculoskeletal pain from ligamentous laxity (loose ligaments). Injections are usually done about once a month for three to six sessions.

#5. Neuraltherapy: Neuraltherapy is a treatment approach that originated with German physicians (including Dr. Ferdinand Huneke in the 1920s) for chronic pain and illness. It involves the injection of local anesthetics (Dr. Ko prefers preservative-free Hydroxide-buffered procaine) into "interference fields" (such as scars, autonomic ganglia, nerves, glands, muscle trigger points) which have lower electrical potentials than surrounding tissues.

### *What conditions respond to these treatments?*

Prolotherapy is helpful in chronic pain arising from ligaments (associated laxity, instability, popping/cracking sensation).

Manipulation for acute and chronic musculoskeletal pain conditions (low back pain, neck pain, TMJ (temporomandibular joint) dysfunction, tennis elbow, plantar fasciitis, rotator cuff instability, et cetera).

Neuraltherapy for post-surgical pain conditions and post traumatic pain syndromes.

Nonresponders include: severe diabetics, smokers, those with poor immune function, extreme obesity, fibromyalgia, psychogenic pain or chronic disability.

### *What are the risks and/or potential adverse effects?*

Increased pain (normally expected for the two to three days after injection).

Neuritis and sensory dysethesias (impairment of sensation but short of anesthesia) with injection into nerve/muscle.

Manipulations/injections of the cervical spine: dizziness, fainting, convulsions, stroke.

Organ puncture (over chest wall, abdomen).

Infection abscess, cellulitis, sepsis minimized by sterile technique.

Fish allergy contraindicates for sodium morrhuate use.

### *How many of the above treatments are needed?*

### *Dr. Ko's Six-to-Eight Rule*

Generally, six to eight sessions to determine whether acupuncture, biofeedback or orthopaedic medicine will be effective in significantly improving your condition. Treatment sessions usually last between 15 and 30 minutes. Relief may be immediate or occur within a few hours to days. Better results will occur if you:

1. Optimize nutrition.
2. Detoxify (e.g. stop smoking).
3. Exercise (daily stretching, regular aerobic conditioning).
4. Control stress.
5. Get restorative sleep.

For traditional medications (such as NSAIDs), Dr. Ko usually recommends six to eight days before making any changes.

For longer acting drugs (e.g. antidepressants), herbal therapies and nutraceuticals, six to eight weeks may be required before medication can be reevaluated.

The Biological Terrain Assessment is a technology that may objectively monitor progress with naturopathic and dietary approaches.

### *The best clinical results are achieved by*

A. Using the "Four Component Balance Approach" from the Neural therapy paradigm created by Dr. Dietrich Klinghardt. This approach emphasizes that optimum results are obtained by concurrently using the best working modalities in each of the four areas:

  i) Structure

  ii) Biochemistry

  iii) Psychoemotional

  iv) Electromagnetic (autonomic nerve function).

  *Examples of modalities in each area are:*

  Structure – Exercise, manipulation, prolotherapy, surgery.

  Biochemistry – Medication, hormone replacement, nutrition, naturopathy.

  Psychoemotional – Biofeedback, psychotherapy, spiritual counseling.

  Electromagnetic – Acupuncture, bioflex magnets, neural therapy.

B. Applying the six to eight rule.

C. Transition to a home-based program:

  1. Acupuncture: Acuhealth TENS unit [Telephone 1 (800) 567-PAIN].

  2. Biofeedback: Thought Technology devices [Telephone 1 (800) 361-3651].

  3. Orthopaedic Medicine: exercise especially spray and stretch, aquajogger, movement therapies such as feldenkrais, pilates, tai-chi, and yoga.

  4. Nutrition and lifestyle changes. Excellent quality brands include PhytoPharmica, Thorne and Seroyal.

In treating any condition, a proper medical diagnosis must first be made. More serious conditions such as cancer, ALS, HIV should first be excluded. Following this, a qualified, knowledgeable practitioner, who ideally is also conflict-of-interest free, can advise whether such treatment is appropriate.

> *"Doing everything for everyone is neither tenable nor desirable; what is done should ideally be inspired by compassion and guided by science, and not merely reflect what the market will bear."*
>
> – David Grimes, *Journal of the American Medical Association*, 1993

# Appendix A

## Key Information Resources for health care professionals and consumers

Use these resources to get scientific and other studies related to natural remedies mentioned in this book. For additional information or references, check the listing of books and studies in the bibliography. It is up to you and your health care provider to arrange a mutually beneficial relationship, in your quest for optimal health.

The National Center for Complimentary and Alternative Medicine, located in Silver Springs, Maryland, is underwritten by the American federal government. Initially they were given a 25 million dollar budget to handle grants for researchers into the safety and effectiveness of alternative medicine. They offer professionals and consumers health related information through their

Toll free telephone: 1 (800) 644-6226.
Internet home page: www.altmed.od.nih.gov

Medical and alternative health information services that charge fees.

They tell you what you want to know about a treatment and/or product based on the studies and information available. They take the time to explain to you what the information means. This empowers you, so you can present it to your health care provider or your health care provider can access it for your benefit. Two excellent ones are:

Health Resources in Conway, Arkansas.
Toll free telephone 1 (800) 949-0090.

Institute for Health and Healing Library offers an information service through the Plaintree Health Resources Center, 2040 Western Street, San Francisco, California
Telephone (415) 923-3681.
Fax (415) 673-2629.

Consumer Health Information Service, Toronto Reference Library, 789 Yonge Street, Toronto, Canada. Open to the public.
Telephone (416) 393-7056.

York University complementary medicine and resource site:
E-mail: wellness@yorku.ca

An internet wellness database for alternative and complementary medicine information and products:
Internet site: www.wellcard.com

Other health Internet communities and sites;

Health AtoZ (includes MEDLINE): www.healthatoz.com

Yahoo Health: www.yahoo.com/health

American Medical Association: www.ama-assn.org

Centers for Disease Control and Prevention Home Page: www.cdc.gov

Free MEDLINE: PubMed and Internet Grateful Med: www.nlm.nih.gov/databases/freemedl.html

Health Canada Online: www.hc-sc.gc.ca/english

HealthWorld Online: www.healthy.net

Mayo Clinic Health O@sis: www.mayohealth.org

News and opinions: www.rath.nl/GB/olhealth.htm

Self-health care wellness site: www.wellcard.com

Some of the key reference books used, that provide information with references to medical reports and scientific studies:

*The Physicians Desk Reference*: Can be found in resource and medical libraries, at pharmacies, and doctors' offices. It is updated annually and is the principle American and Canadian pharmacological reference book. Older editions reported on herbal remedies, but as the infatuation with synthetic drugs grew, the recording and reporting on natural remedies has effectively disappeared from current issues.

*Martindale: The Extra Pharmacopeia*. It is the United Kingdom's pharmacological and herb reference book. The pharmaceuticals and herbs are well referenced and very conservatively dealt with. In terms of herbs it gives superior supporting documentation compared to its North American equivalent, which is clearly slanted to pharmacological drugs only. In the U.S.A. and Canada you can access it at most university medical libraries.

*Alternative Medicine: The Definitive Guide.* 380 leading edge physicians explain their treatments. A user friendly reference book, that clearly explains and gives treatment protocols for a wide assortment of complementary medicines. Extensive documentation. Available in health food stores, bookstores and libraries. Available for $59.95 through Future Medicine Publishing.

Toll free telephone 1 (800) 720-6363.

*German Commission E Monographs* translated into English, it is the German medical professions herb reference book. The detailed information gives the recognized uses for health care providers of herbs and other substances, supported by scientific studies. Available for $189 through The Herb Research Foundation.

Toll free telephone: 1 (800) 307-6267 or (303) 449-2265.

For herbal medicine information you can write to these two organizations and/or subscribe to *Herbalgram,* a top notch magazine they jointly publish, that reviews the most recent botanical medicine developments.

The American Botanical Council, P.O. 201660, Austin, Texas 78720

The Herb Research Foundation, 1007 Pearl Street, Suite 200, Boulder, Colorado 80302

*Herbalgram* subscription toll free telephone number: 1 (800) 748-2617 or (303) 449-2265.

# Appendix B

# Glossary of Terms

## – A –

**Abscess** - is due to an infection of a sebaceous gland. This results in an inflammation of the skin and localized painful swelling.

**Absorption** - the process by which a substance passes into the bloodstream.

**Acid** - a sour substance that is usually water-soluble. Has a pH reading of less then 7.

**Acute** - a sudden onset, sharp rise and of short -duration.

**Adrenals** - glands above the kidneys, that manufacture adrenaline , DHEA and other vital substances that affect the quality of life.

**Alkali** - a substance having marked basic properties, which can neutralize acid.

**Alcohols** - are pungent colorless liquids, forming esters in reaction with organic acids, sometimes used as a solvent when extracting essential oils or as a carrier base for essential oils.

**Alterative** - agents that gradually and favorably alter the body' s condition. Blood purifiers.

**Alzheimer's disease** - a degenerative disease of the central nervous system, usually exhibiting premature mental deterioration.

**Amenorrhea** - the condition after the onset of menstruation where there is the abnormal absence of the menstrual cycle.

**Amino acids** - the organic components from which proteins are made.

**Amoebic dysentery** - ulcerative inflammation of the colon causing severe diarrhea, often with blood and mucous.

**Analgesic** - pain relieving without affecting consciousness.

**Anthelmintic** - stimulating herbs or substances that work against parasitic worms, which may be in the digestive system.

**Antibacterial** - see Antibiotic.

**Antibiotic** - substances which can inhibit the growth of microorganisms and are capable of destroying or weakening bacteria, et cetera.

**Anti-catarrhal** - herbs and substances which eliminate or counteract mucous formation.

**Anticoagulant** - a substance that prevents or delays blood clotting.

**Anti-depressant** - an agent or substance used to treat depression.

**Anti-fungal** - battles or is antagonistic to fungi.

**Antigen** - any substance normally not present in the body, which stimulates an immune response.

**Antihistamine** - a drug or substance that counteracts or blocks the physiological action of histamine.

**Anti-inflammatory** - helps the body to combat the inflammation manifested by redness, pain, heat and swelling in the body, usually due to disease or injury.

**Anthelmintic** - works against worm infestations.

**Antilithic** - herbs and substances that help remove or prevent the formation of gravel or stones in the urinary tract.

**Anti-microbial** - substances used to rid the body of micro-organisms that have intruded into it or act on the skin.

**Anti-neoplastic** - those herbs or substances that have the precise action of inhibiting and fighting the development of tumors.

**Anti-oxidant** - an agent or material that inhibits oxidation and thereby prevents rancidity of fats or oils or the deterioration of other substances caused by the oxidative process.

**Antipyretic** - reducing, removing, or preventing fever.

**Anti-rheumatic** - herbs and substances that have a reputation for prevention, relief and/or curing rheumatic problems.

**Antiseptic** - substances that counteract or prevent the growth of disease causing germs and infections.

**Anti-spasmodic** - herbal remedies and substances which rapidly relax nervous tension, which may be resulting in colic or sudden involuntary digestive contractions.

**Antiviral** - that which checks the growth of a virus, by weakening or abolishing its action.

**Aphrodisiac** - arouses and/or increases sexual appetite and/or drive.

**Aromatherapy** - the practice and art of using the essential oils derived from plants, for healing purposes.

**Aromatic** - the oils of aromatic herbs can penetrate into muscles and increase circulation.

**Aromatic baths** - baths in which oils are used for cosmetic or healing purposes.

**Arthritis** - an inflammation and/or pain in a joint or joints. Symptoms include swelling, redness of the skin and impaired motion. Two types of arthritis are: Osteoarthritis due to wear and tear of cartilage of the joints, especially those that are weight-bearing. Rheumatoid arthritis is chronic and manifested by inflammatory changes in joints which can be crippling. It is a degenerative joint disease.

**Astringent** - that which contracts blood vessels and body tissues, reducing blood flow or having a biting or harsh quality.

**Auto immune** - the immune response of an organism against any of its own cells or tissues.

**Ayurvedic medicine** - "Ayurvedic" is the Sanskrit term for "science of life and longevity". The system is based on the idea that health is a balance between emotional, physical and spiritual states.

## – B –

**Bactericide** - an agent that kills germs or bacteria.

**Base oil** - the main, essential or principal ingredient, acting as the vehicle for an essential oil. For therapeutic uses, such as aromatherapy, usually odorless high quality cold-pressed light vegetable oils are used.

**Bio-availability** - the rate and degree to which a substance is absorbed by the body or is available at the site of the physiological activity.

**Bioflavonoids** - biologically active flavonoids, usually sourced from lemon and orange rinds. It maintains blood-vessel walls plus other health benefits. Also known as vitamin P complex.

**Bitter** - an herb that aids digestion and promotes appetite.

**Boil** - a boil is technically called a 'furuncle'. It is due to an infection of a sebaceous gland. This results in an inflammation of the skin and localized painful swelling.

## – C –

**Calmative** - any agents or substance which reduces ones level of excitement or agitation. Promotes a state of sedation.

**Candida albicans** - is also know as moniliasis or candidiasis, which can show itself in many forms. Candida albicans is a fungi which an excess of causes a yeast-like fungal infection. It thrives in the warm moist parts of the body such as the mouth (candidiasis), penis (balanitis), vagina (thrush), beneath the breasts and between folds of the buttock (diaper rash). Each condition manifests itself in a slightly different way, yet all are caused by the Candida albicans fungi.

**Carbuncles** - a collective mass of boils caused by the staphylococcus aureaus. Characterized by a painful node, covered with tight red skin that later thins and discharges pus. Commonly found on buttocks, upper back and nape of the neck. Extensive sloughing of the skin occurs when it is healing.

**Carcinogen** - a cancer-causing substance or event (e.g, X-ray treatments).

**Carrier oil** - see Base oil.

**Carminative** - substances, usually herbs and spices, taken to relieve gas and griping.

**Carotene** - the yellow-orange pigment from plants, that can become vitamin A in the body.

**Catalyst** - a substance that causes change, usually increasing the rate of a chemical reaction, and at the end of the reaction it is unchanged.

**Catarrh** - is an inflammation of a mucous membrane. especially one chronically affecting the nose and air passages.

**Cathartic** - substances that have a laxative effect.

**Chelation** - the use of an agent to bind with a mineral so that it is more easily absorbed by the body.

**Chicken pox** - is an acute, highly contagious viral disease, especially during childhood. It is caused by the *herpes zoster* virus, the same one responsible for shingles.It is characterized by skin eruptions of itchy spots, that blister, then turn to crusts. Also called Shingles or Zona.

**Cholagogue** - promotes the flow and evacuation of the bile into the small intestine.

**Cholestatic** - a failure or checking of bile flow.

**Chronic** - a long-term, or slow definite course of indefinite duration..

**Coenzyme** - the nonprotein component that produces the active part of an enzyme system.

**Collagen** - the principle organic component of bone, cartilage, and connective tissue. When collagen is exposed to prolonged heated with water it becomes gelatin and glue.

**Cold-pressed** - mechanical method of extracting oil, by crushing the whole plant or part of the plant, without using heat. The oil is then filtered. This produces "virgin" oil.

**Cold sore** - is a viral infection, brought on by the herpes simplex type 1 virus, causing inflammation to the skin, usually the lips, mouth and face. It is characterized by small blisters. Herpes simplex type 1 is highly infectious and can spread to other parts of the body.

**Colitis** - inflammation of the colon.

**Colloidal** - is a description used for a substance made up of small particles, insoluble, nondiffusible particles that remain suspended in a different type of medium, such as water, alcohol, et cetera.

**Compress** - a pad folded cloth pad, often moist or medicated that is applied to part of the body for healing, pressure , or to change the temperature, either up or down, of the area.

**Conjunctivitis** - an inflammation of the mucous membrane that covers the front of the eye and lines the inside of the eyelid.

**Corn** - is an area of thickened hard skin between or on the toes. Sometimes it forms an inverted pyramid, which causes pressure in deeper layers of skin, resulting in pain.

**Cuticles** - are the hardened layer of outside skin, at the base and sides of a fingernail.

**Cystitis** - is a bladder infection caused by bacteria, that results in an inflammation of the bladder.

## – D –

**Dandruff** - is a condition affecting the scalp. Overactive sebaceous gland secretions in the scalp cause scales to form, which may itch and burn. It may be caused by poor diet, inadequate stimulation of the scalp, poor blood circulation,

**Decongestant** - a medication or treatment the relieves congestion, especially in the nose.

**Demulcent** - substances that sooth and protect damaged tissue.

**Dermatitis** - is an inflammation of the skin. Characteristics may include flaky skin, redness, itchiness and rashes resulting in blisters, sores and scabs.

**Diaphoretic** - substances used to induce sweating.

**Diffuser** - an apparatus that spreads out an essential oil, in the air, throughout a room.

**Digestive** - assists and aids in the process of digestion.

**Distillation** - a process of heating a mixture, using steam and high pressure to separate the components of the mixture, and condensing the resulting vapors, to produce a concentrated purer essential oil.

**Diuretic** - a substance that increases the flow of urine.

**DNA** - deoxyribonucleic acid. The nucleic acids that are usually the chemical molecular basis of hereditary.

**Dysmenorrhea** - a menstrual condition, with cramping pains, whose intensity may be incapacitating.

### – E –

**Eczema** - is a skin disorder characterized by inflammation, itching and scaliness.

**Emmenagogue** - herbs that promote menstruation.

**Emollient** - something that when applied to skin, soothes or softens it. Acts as lubricants to the intestinal wall and softens feces.

**Emphysema** - is a condition of the lungs, in which the air sacs become distended and lose elasticity.

**Endogenous** - produced internally from the body.

**Endogenous depression** - a severe form of internally derived depression often characterized by insomnia, weight loss, and inability to experience pleasure.

**Enteric coated** - a pill treated so it passes through the stomach unaltered and disintegrates in the intestines.

**Enzyme** - a complex protein substance that initiates chemical changes. Vital for digestion and other processes in the body.

**Expectorant** - a medicine or agent that helps to bring up phlegm or mucous, so it is expelled from the respiratory tract.

**Exogenous** - produced outside of the system or body.

**Extra-virgin** - used to describe the highest quality grade of olive oil from the first pressing of the olives.

### – F –

**FDA** - Food and Drug Administration.

**Febrifuge** - reducing, removing, or preventing fever.

**Fever** - is an abnormally increased body temperature, which is a vital part of your bodies defense mechanism.

**Flatulence** - passing gas through the anus. Usually due to improper or incomplete digestion of sugars.

**Flu** - is an acute, contagious viral disease, characterized by inflammation of the respiratory tract, fever and muscular pain. It is also known as 'influenza'.

**Flower remedies** - a healing system founded by Dr. Edward Bach, based on the principle that a negative state of mind had to be replaced with the opposite virtue, to regain the inner harmony needed to heal. Using plants and trees, he created a revolutionary therapeutic system that is safe, natural and gentle. Through observation, he classified 38 negative states of mind common to most people. He discovered the corresponding flower from plants or trees, for each state of mind, which helped to alleviate the specific negative mood. There are hundreds of other homeopathic flower remedies.

**Free radical** - is one or more atoms, that have at least one electron missing. Electrons are negatively charged components of an atom. The missing electron(s) create an unstable atom, which seeks a component to complete it. This causes a chemical reaction to occur with other molecules or atoms attracted to the free radical atom and easily able to bond with it. The process can cause a lot of damage to the body.

**Fungal infections of the skin** - fungal organisms are found on all healthy skin of humans, cats and dogs. Fungal infections occur when the natural balance is disturbed. In humans, by taking advantage of a persons weakened immune system, infections by opportunistic fungi become present. Examples of common one's include Tinea pedis (see Athlete's Foot), Tinea cruris (see Dhobi Itch and Jock Itch), Tinea ungium (see Ringworm), Tinea capitis (see Ringworm), Tinea corporis (see Ringworm).

**Fungicidal** - that which checks the growth of fungi, molds or spores.

## – G –

**Gastritis** - inflammation especially of the mucous membrane of the stomach.

**Gingivitis** - is a build up of bacterial plaque, that causes the gums to swell, redden and bleed easily.

**GLA** - gamma-linolenic acid; produced from linoleic acid in the body, it is an Omega-6 fatty acid.

**Glucose** - the form in which carbohydrates are usually assimilated by animals; the blood sugar.

## – H –

**Halitosis** - is bad smelling breath.

**HDL** - high-density lipoprotein, that transports cholesterol and fats through the blood system. HDL is the 'good' cholesterol.

**Hemolytic anemia** - red blood cells dying at a faster rate than that of replacement by the body.

**Hemorrhoid** - is a painful swelling of a vein, in the region of the anus or rectum, often with bleeding. It is a varicose vein. Also known as Piles.

**Hemostatic** - an agent that shortens the clotting time of blood.

**Hepatic** - tones, strengthens and stimulates the secretive functions and nature of the liver.

**Herbs** - a plant or plant parts prized for their savory or medicinal qualities.

**Hives** - are an allergic skin condition or hypersensitive reaction characterized by itching, burning and the formation of smooth patches.

**Homeopathy** - a therapeutic system founded by Samuel Hahnemann, in which diseases are treated with remedies having a minute amount of the disease, to illicit the symptoms similar to the diseases and thereby the healing response from the body. Hahnemann's' idea is "like heals like".

**Hormone** - a product of living cells, in the endocrine organs, transported by body fluids and producing a specific effect by activating receptive cells remote from the point of origin.

**HPB** - Health Protection Branch (Canada's FDA).

**Hypercalcemia** - excessive amounts of calcium accumulation in the blood.

**Hypervitaminosis** - a state resulting from ingesting an excessive amount of a vitamin(s).

**Hypoglycemic** - a state brought about by abnormally low blood sugar levels.

**Hypouremic** - lowers uric acid levels in the blood.

**Hypovitaminosis** - a deficiency disease due to a lack of vitamins in the diet.

**Hypoxia** - below normal oxygen levels.

## – I –

**Immune** - protected and not susceptible to disease.

**Influenza** - commonly known as flu, is an acute, contagious viral disease, characterized by inflammation of the respiratory tract, fever and muscular pain.

**Inhalation** - to breath in a vapor, using the lungs and respiratory system as the delivery system for the essential oil into the blood stream.

**Insulin** - the hormone involved in the metabolism of sugar in the body. It is secreted by the pancreas.

**IU** - International units, standard of measurement for supplements. Refer to Appendix C.

## – K –

**Keratolytic** - causing or relating to keratolysis.

**Ketosis** - an acidic environment in the blood occurs, which renders your own body fat as the main energy source.

**Kreb cycle** - the reactions that occur in the body to produce up to 95 percent of the energy the body requires for optimal functioning and vitality.

## – L –

**Lactating** - milk producing.

**Laxative** - a substance that makes the bowels loose and relieves constipation. Results in a moderate evacuative effect.

**LDL** - low-density lipoprotein: the component that when oxidized, causes cholesterol deposits along arterial walls.

**Leg ulcer** - is an open sore on the leg, discharging pus.

**Legumes** - are plants having seeds that grow in pods, such as beans or seeds.

**Leucorrhoea** - is an inflammation of the vagina that is caused by an excessive amount of bacteria or fungi. Often

there is a thick yellow or white discharge accompanied by severe itching to the vagina.

**Lignans** - a fiber that friendly bacteria in the gut changes to a cancer-fighting substance.

**Linoleic acid** - a polyunsaturated fat, that is a component of lecithin. It is a key member of the Omega-6 family. Vital for life. Linoleic acid can only be obtained from foods. Also known as vitamin F.

**Lipid** - organic compounds consisting of fats or fatty substances.

**Lipophilic** - means fat loving.

**Lipoprotein** - a transporter of fatty substances, characterized by weight (e.g., low-density, high-density, et cetera)

**Lipotropic** - inhibits excessive or abnormal accumulation of fat in the liver.

**– M –**

**Macular degeneration** - a condition caused by the destruction of a part of the retina, called the macula. A leading cause of age related blindness.

**Megavitamin therapy** - the use of large doses of vitamins to treat illness.

**Meningitis** - an inflammation of the three membranes that envelop the brain and spinal column.

**Menorrhagia** - Gastritis - acid indigestion, colitis, duodenal ulcers.

**Metabolize** - the physical and chemical reactions in living cells that undergo changes, by which energy is provided for critical processes and activities, and a result is new material is assimilated.

**Miscible** - to mix, or can be mixed.

**Mucilage** - a thick sticky substance, gelatinous constituent, in certain plants.

**Myelin sheathing** - the outer protective layer of the nerves.

**– N –**

**Nasal ulcer** - is an open sore in the nose, discharging pus.

**Naturopathy** - a system of treatment of disease that uses natural agents (e.g., water, vitamins, minerals, air, herbs, homeopathy, nutrition, et cetera) and physical methods (e.g. acupressure, acupuncture, manipulation, et cetera) with underlying principles such as doing the patient no harm, using the bodies natural wisdom to heal itself, disease prevention and maintaining optimal health.

**Nutraceuticals** - are substances from natural sources that can positively affect one's health. These unusual healing products are not herbs, minerals or vitamins. In the proper dosage and concentration, they may stimulate and support the body's healing process. It is their wide range of effectiveness and safety which offers benefits for a variety of health conditions. Properly used, they can eliminate the need for prescribed drugs and, most importantly, the potential side effects prescription drugs can cause.

**Nervine** - substances used to ease anxiety and stress, as well as nourish the nerves.

**– O –**

**Omega-3** - a part of an essential fatty acid group, usually deficient in modern diets. External food sources supply the body's needs. Alpha-linolenic acid is the main Omega-3 fatty acid.

**Omega-6** - a part of an essential fatty acid group, usually abundant in modern diets. External food sources supply the body's needs. Linolenic acid is the main Omega-6 fatty acid.

**– P –**

**Paronychia** - is a fungal infection that affects toenails and fingernails. Cuticles become painful and red, with a small discharge. Skin below nails becomes discolored.

**Phenylketonuria** - an inherited inability to oxidize a metabolic product of phenylalanine and severe mental retardation.

**Phlebitis** - inflammation of the walls of a vein.

**Phytochemicals** - refer to the medicinal qualities of plant life, such as the vitamins, minerals, and thousands of healing substances in the herbs and foods we eat. Some of these remedies have been passed down through the ages, others are recent discoveries.

**Piles** - see Hemorrhoids

**Plantar Wart** - are small, usually less than 1/4 inch, sometimes larger. They are caused by a virus invasion through an abrasion or microscopic cut on the sole of the foot. The warts grow inward and under the skin. The pressure exerted by walking causes the area to become flattened until it becomes callused. The location has a tiny black on on the surface. They can be very painful. They are difficult to get rid of and may reappear.

**Poison Ivy** - is a plant having leaves of three leaflets and ivory -colored berries. When the sap from the plant comes in contact with the skin, it causes a severe rash, redness, swelling, blistering, and intense itching in sensitive people.

**Poison Oak** - is a climbing vine, related to poison ivy.

**Polyunsaturated fats** - vegetable sourced highly non-saturated fats, which may lower blood cholesterol levels.

**Prickly heat** - is a skin eruption caused by inflammation of the sweat glands.

**Pruritis** - or itching is a most irritating condition, generally accompanying a mild vaginal infection, such as cervicitis or trichomonal vaginitis.

**Psoriasis** - is a chronic skin disease, characterized by scaly, reddish patches and itching. The inflammation sometimes shows up as silvery scales that appear on elbows, knees, scalp and torso. It is not contagious. The cause is generally unknown.

**Pulmonary embolism** - obstruction of pulmonary arteries carrying blood from the heart to the lungs.

**Purgative** - substances which promote increased contractions and dilations of the alimentary canal, moving things onward as well as promoting bowel movement.

## – R –

**Rash** - an eruption of spots on the skin.

**RDA** - Recommended Dietary Allowance. Established by the National Academy of Sciences, National research Council and the Food and Nutrition Board.

**RDI** - Recommended Daily Intake. It is the recommended nutrient intake levels, regardless of age, sex, weight, lifestyle, et cetera and is based on the Recommended Dietary Allowance. On food labels it appears as the Percent of Daily Value (%/DV).

**Rhinitis** - is an inflammation of the nose or its mucous membrane.

**RNA**- abbreviation used for ribonucleic acid.

## – S –

**Salpingitis** - is caused by the streptococci and staphylococci bacteria. It is an inflammation of the Fallopian tubs. Symptoms can include fever, vaginal discharge and vomiting.

**Saturated fatty acids** - Typically solid at room temperature. Predominately found in animal food sources. Saturated fatty acids tend to raise blood cholesterol levels.

**Scabies** - is a highly contagious, itching skin disease caused by the itch mite, sarcoptes scabiei. The female mite burrows under the skin to lay its eggs. The newly hatched mites burrow out of the skin and this causes severe itching and irritation. Possible signs include small red pimples and scratching, which may result in sores, that can become infected. Secondary infections are of great concern with scabies. Easily transmitted from person to person. Area's commonly affected by this condition include the groin, penis, nipples and skin between the fingers. Disinfect bed linens, mattress and clothing to prevent reinfection.

**Sedative** - calms and/or quiets nervous excitement.

**Shingles** - is the nontechnical term used for the *herpes zoster virus*, the same one responsible for chicken pox.

**Sinusitis** - is an inflammation of the sinuses. The mucous membranes that line the cavities above, behind and to each side of the nose become swelled.

**Sitz bath** - is a therapeutic bath in which only the hips and buttocks are immersed.

**Stimulant** - enliven and/or quicken the physiological functioning of the body.

**Stye** - a small inflamed swelling on the rim of an eyelid.

**Sublingual** - under the tongue.

**Synergistic** - when the combination of two or more substances is greater in the total effect than their individual effects.

**Synthetic** - artificially produced or manufactured.

**Systemic** - affecting the body generally. Able to spread through the whole body.

## – T –

**Tachycardia** - relatively rapid heart rate due to physiological or pathological conditions.

**T Cells** - are the white blood cells produced in the thymus. T cells protect the body against viruses, bacteria, cancer-causing substances. At the same time they control the manufacture of B cells, the antibody producers. T cells also control the unwanted manufacturing of potentially harmful T cells.

**Tinea** - is a fungal infection, caused by a microscopic fungal mold.

**Tocopherols** - the group of substances that make vitamin E. Known as alpha, beta, delta, episilon, eta, gamma, and zeta. They are derived from vacuum distillation of edible vegetable oils.

**Tonic** - herbs that enliven or strengthen either specific organs or the whole body.

**Toxic** - a deadly, lethal, or poisonous affect caused by a toxin.

**Toxicity** - the state or nature of being noxious, poisonous, or destructive.

**Toxin** - any poison produced by living or dead animals, plants or organisms.

**Trans-fatty acids** - artificially created fatty acids, produced by the process of hydrogenation. They are unsaturated, yet act like saturated fats. They extend the shelf-life of processed foods, and are very unhealthy.

**Triglycerides** - are an ester formed by the reaction between an alcohol and an acid. They are derived from glycerol, the principle element in fats and oils.

## – U –

**Ulcers** - are open sores on the skin or mucous membrane, that discharges pus.

**Unsaturated fatty acids** - usually liquid at room temperature. Found mainly in vegetable, nut and seed fats.

**Urethritis** - a bacterial infection of the urethra which usually precedes an attack of cystitis.

## – V –

**Vaginitis** - an inflammation of the canal from vulva to the uterus.

**Vagotonic** - tones and strengthens veins.

**Vaporization** - to change something into a steam suspension (vapor) or mist for dispersion through the air. The air is used a delivery system for an essential oil. It can be done by heating, spraying or evaporating an essential oil.

**Varicose ulcers** - are enlarged veins abnormally and irregularly swollen, that form on the lower legs, often as a result of varicose veins. The slightest break in the skin, can cause a sore or ulcer to develop that takes a long time to heal. The aged, usually suffering from poor circulation, are very prone to this condition.

**Vasopressin** - a pituitary hormone, that helps the pancreas release insulin.

**Virgin oil** - highest quality vegetable oil extracted from the first pressing of the plant. Extra-virgin used to describe the highest grade of the first pressing of olive oil.

## – W - Z –

**Warts** - a small, usually hard, tumorous growth on the skin, caused by a virus.

**Xerophthalmia** - excessive dryness of parts of the eye.

**Zona** - is also called shingles, it is caused by the herpes zoster virus, the same one responsible for chicken pox.

# Appendix C

## Conventional American Fluid Measurements and Their Standard International Equivalents

### Fluid Measurements

| | | | | | | |
|---|---|---|---|---|---|---|
| 1 tsp | = | 1/3 tbsp | = | 1/6 oz | = | 4.9 ml |
| 3 tsp | = | 1 tbsp | = | 1/2 oz | = | 14.8 ml |
| 2 tbsp | = | 1 oz | = | 29.6 ml | = | .0296 l |
| 1 c | = | 16 tbsp | = | 8 oz | = | 236.6 ml |
| 1 l | = | 1.0567 qt | = | 33.814 oz | = | 4.2268 c |
| 1 l | = | 1000 ml | = | 2.113 pt | | |

Essential oils are measured in drops,
due to their high concentration.

20 drops = 1/30 oz = 1 ml

| | | | |
|---|---|---|---|
| tsp – teaspoon | tbsp – tablespoon | c – cup | pt – pint |
| oz – fluid ounce | qt – liquid quart | ml – milliliter | l – liter |

### International System of Units for Liquid and Dry Weights of Mass

IU = International Unit
an agreed to standard of measurement for supplements

| | | | | |
|---|---|---|---|---|
| 1 g | = | 1,000 mg | = | 0.03527 oz |
| 1 mg | = | 1,000 mcg | = | .00003527 oz |

g - gram mg - milligram mcg - micrograms oz - ounce

# Appendix D

# Bibliography

## and Recommended Reading

These four medical reference books were vital to the preparation of this book: *The Physicians Desk Reference, Martindale: The Extra Pharmacopeia, Alternative Medicine:The Definitive Guide* and *German Commission E Monographs*. The following journals supplied vital information: Journal of the American Medical Association (JAMA), Lancet and the New England Journal of Medicine. In addition to these and the following materials, the scientists, doctors, health care providers, researchers, and many others were instrumental in the preparation of this book. For specific information regarding specific supplements, treatment modalities, protocols or research information, refer to the key information resources in Appendix A. The bibliographical information on Chapter 19 for Dr. Ko's treatment protocols are grouped at the end of the bibliography. Self-health care is about taking back control of your health, the suggested readings should help you succeed.

Alberts, Bruce, Dennis Bray, Julian Lewis, Martin Raff, Keith Roberts, James Watson, *Molecular Biology of the Cell,* 3rd Edition, New York, New York, Garland Publishing, 1994

Ali, Elvis and George Grant, Selim Nakla, Don Patel, Ken Vegotsky, *The Tea Tree Oil Bible,* 2nd edition, Niagara Falls, New York, AGES Publications, 1999

Ambau, G.T., *The Importance of Good Nutrition, Herbs & Phytochemicals*, Mountain View, California, Falcon Press International, 1997

*American Medical Association Family Medical Guide*, revised and updated 3rd edition, 1994

Anderson, Jean and Barbara Deskins, *The Nutrition Bible*, New York, New York, William Morrow and Company, Inc., 1995.

Asimov, Isaac, *The Intelligent Man's Guide to the Biological Sciences*, New York, New York, Washington Square Press, 1968

Balch, James F. and Phyllis A., *Prescription for Dietary Wellness,* Garden City Park, New York, Avery Publishing Group, 1998

, *Prescription for Nutritional Healing,* Garden City Park, New York, Avery Publishing Group, 1990

Bettschard, R,, Edzard Ernst, et al, *The Complete Book of Sympyoms and Treatments*, Boston, Massachusetts, Element Books, Inc. 1998

Blackburn, G. "Safe Amounts of Vitamins," article in *HealthNews* National Research Council, 10th Edition, August 26, 1997

Bourre, Jean-Marie, *Brainfood: A Provocative Exploration of the Connection Between What You Eat and How You Think*, Boston, MA, Little, Brown and Company, 1993

Bowes, Anna De Planter, *Bowes and Churches Food Values of Portions Commonly Used*, 17th edition, Philadelphia, Pennsylvania, Lippincott, 1998

Burton Goldberg Group, *Alternative Medicine: The Definitive Guide*, Fife, Washington, Future Medicine Publishing, 1994

Carper, Jean, *Food Your Miracle Medicine*, New York, New York,, HarperCollins Publishers, 1998

, *Miracle Cures*, New York, New York, HaperCollins Publishers, 1997

Chopra, Deepak, *Ageless Body, Timeless Mind: The Quantum Alternative to Growing Old*, New York, New York, Harmony Books , 1993

Cichoke, Anthony, *The Complete Book of Enzyme Therapy*, Garden City Park, New York, Avery Publishing Group, 1999

Colgan, Michael, *Hormonal Health*, Vancouver, British Columbia, Apple Publishing, 1996

, *Optimum Sports Nutrition*, Ronkonkoma, New York, Advanced Research Press, 1993

Collinge, William, *American Holistic Health Association Complete Guide to Alternative Medicine*, New York, New York, Warner Books, 1996

*Compendium of Pharmaceuticals and Specialties*, Canadian Pharmaceuticals Association, Ottawa, Ontario, 1999

Consumer Reports, Editors of, *The Medicine Show*, Mount Vernon, New York, Consmuers Union, 1981

Copper, Kenneth, *Overcoming Hypertension*, New York, New York, Bantam Books, 1990

Cummings, Stephen & Dana Ulman, *Everybody's Guide to Homeopathic Medicines*, New York, New York, Jeremy P. Tarcher,/Perigee Books, 1991

Cunningham, Donna, *Flower Remedies Handbook*, New York, New York, Sterling Publishing Company, 1992

Diamond, John, W. Lee Cowden, Burton Goldberg, *An Alternative Medicine Definitive Guide to Cancer*, Tiburon, California, Future Medicine Publishing, Inc., 1997

Diamond, Harvey and Marilyn, *Fit for Life II: Living Health, The complete Health Program*, New York, New York, Warner Books, 1988

Duke, James, *The Green Pharmacy*, New York, New York, St. Martin's Press, 1998

Dunne, Lavon, *Nutrition Almanac*, Toronto, Ontario, McGraw-Hill, 1990

*Encyclopedia of Alternative Medicine*, Don Mills, Ontario, Stoddart, 1996

*Encyclopedia of Vitamins, Minerals, and Supplements*, New York, New York, Facts on File, 1996

Erasmus, Udo, *Fats the Heal Fats the Kill*, Burnaby, B.C., Alive Books, 1993

Feltman, John, *The Prevention How-To Dictionary of Healing Remedies and Techniques,* Emmaus, Pennsylvania, Rodale Press, 1992

Fratkin, Jake, *Chinese Herbal Patent Formulas,* Portland, Oregon, Institute for Traditional Medicine, 1989

French, R and P. Jones, *Nutritional aspects of vanadium*. Nutr Rep 1993;11:41,48.

, Role of vanadium in nutrition: Metabolism, essentiality and dietary considerations. *Life Science* 1993; 52: 339-346.

Fulder, Stephen, *The Garlic Book*, Garden City Park, New York, Avery Publishing Group, 1997

Garrison, Robert and Elizabeth Somer, *The Nutrition Desk Reference,* New Canaan, Connecticut, Keats Publishing, 1995

, *The Nutrition Desk Reference*, 3rd edition, New Canaan, Connecticut, Keats Publishing, Inc., 1995

*German Commission E Monographs*, English edition, Austin, Texas, American Botanical Council, 1998

Gottlieb, Bill, and Susan Berg, Patricia Fisher and Doug Dollmore, et al., *New Choices in Natural Healing*, Emmaus, Pennsylvania, Rodale Press, Inc., 1995

Graci, Sam, *The Power of Superfoods*, Scarborough, Ontario, Prentice-Hall Canada Inc, 1999

*Great Saint Ormand Street Hospital Study: Hyperactivity and the Role of Food in Children,* London: Great Saint Ormand Street Hospital – Refer to *Little Monsters,* Television video.

Holt, J.D. *Journal of Investigative Medicine*, volume 46, 1998 edition.

Kipple, Edward and the Editors of Consumer Reports, *How to Clean Practically Anything*, 4th edition, Mount Vernon, New York, Consmuers Union, 1996

Kloss, Jethro, *Back to Eden*, New York, New York, Benedict Lust Publications, 1990

Kordich, Jay, *The Juiceman's Power of Juicing*, New York, New York, Warner Books, 1993

Lambert-Lagace, Louise & Michelle Laflamme, *Good Fat Bad Fat*, Toronto, Ontario, Stoddart Publishing Co., 1995

Lee, John and Virginia Hopkins, *What Your Doctor May Not Tell You About Menopause*, New York, New York, Warner Books, 1996

Lee, Lita, and Lisa Turner and Burton Goldberg, *The Enzyme Cure,* Tiburon, California, Future Medicine Publishing, 1998

Lee, William H. and Lynn Lee, *The Book of Practical Aromatherapy*, New Canaan, Connecticut, Keats Publishing, Inc., 1992

Levinson, Harold N., *Smart But Feeling Dumb*, New York, New York, Warner Books, 1994.

Lieberman, Shari and Nancy Bruning, *The Real Vitamin & Mineral Book*, Garden City Park, New York, Avery Publishing Group, 1997

*Little Monsters,* Television video show, London: British Broadcasting Corporation (1992)

Lust, John, *The Herb Book,* New York, New York, Bantam Books, 1974

Mabey, Richard, *The New Age Herbalist,* New York, New York, Macmillan Publishing Company, 1988

Mart, James, *The Ultimate Consumer's Guide to Diets and Nutrition*, Boston, Massachusetts, Houghton Mifflin, 1997

Marti, James and Andrea Hine, *The Alternative Health and Medicine Encyclopedia,* Detroit, Michigan, Gale Research Inc., 1995

*Martindale: The Extra Pharmacopeia,* 31st ed., James Reynolds, Editor, London, England, Royal Pharmaceutical Society, 1992

*Merck Manual, The,* 17th Edition, West Point, Pennsylvania, The Merck Publishing Group, 1999

Mindell, Earl, *Earl Mindell's HerbBible*, New York, New York, Simon & Shuster Inc., 1992

, *Earl Mindell's Supplement Bible*, New York, New York, Simon & Shuster Inc., 1998

, *Vitamin Bible,* New York, New York, Warner Books, 1991

, *Vitamin Bible for the 21st Century*, New York, New York, Warner Books, 1999

Mindell, Earl and Larry Johns, *Amazing Apple Cider Vinegar*, New Canaan, Connecticut, Keats Publishing Inc., 1996

Moyer, Bill, *Healing and the Mind*, New York: Bantam Doubleday Dell Audio Publishing, 1993

Murray, Michael, Joseph Pizzorno, *Encyclopedia of Natural Medicine,* Second Edition, Rocklin, CA, Prime Publishing, 1998

National Research Council, *Recommended Dietary Allowances*, 10th edition, Washington D.C., National Academy Press, 1989

Ornish, Dr. Dean, *Dr. Dean Ornish's Program for Reversing Heart Disease*, New York, New York, Random House, 1990

Papadogianis, Peter, *Treat the Cause*, Scarborough, Ontario, Prentice Hall Canada, 1998

Passwater, Richard, *The New Supernutrition*, New York, New York, Simon & Schuster 1991

*Physician's Desk Reference*, 49th Edition, Medical Economics Company, Montvale, New Jersey, 1995

*Physician's Desk Reference*, 53rd Edition, Medical Economics Company, Montvale, New Jersey, 1999

*Prevention Pain-Relief System, The: A Total Program for Relieving Any Pain in Your Body*, Edited by Alice Feinstein, Emmaus, Pennsylvania, Rodale Press, 1992

Reid, Daniel P., *Chinese Herbal Medicine*, Boston, MA, Shambhala Publications, 1996

Reiter, Russel and Jo Robinson, *Melatonin*, New York, New York, Bantam Books, 1995

Robbins, John, *Diet for a New America,* Walpole: Stillpoint Publishing, 1987

, *May All Be Fed: Diet for a New World,* New York, New York, Avon Books, 1993

Rosenfeld, Isadore, *Doctor, What Should I Eat,* New York, New York, Warner Books, 1995

Royal, Penny, *Herbally Yours,* Third Edition, Hurricane, Utah, Sound Nutrition, 1982

Sahelian, Ray, *DHEA: A Practical Guide*, Avery Publishing Group, Garden City Park, New York, 1996

Salaman, Maureen and James Scheer, *Foods that Heal,* Menlo Park, California, Statford Publishing, 1989

San Francisco Bay Area Regional Poison Control Center, *Community Newswire*, Poison Prevention and Hazardous Materials Information , Vol. 9, No. 1, Winter 1993

Sears, Barry, *Mastering the Zone*, New York, New York, HarperCollins, 1997

Somer, Elizabeth, *The Essential Guide to Vitamins and Minerals*, 2nd Edition, New York, New York, Harper Perennial, 1995

Stoffman, Phyllis, *The Family Guide to Preventing and Treating 100 Infectious Diseases*, New York, New York, Wiley, 1995

Teeguarden, Ron, *Radiant Health*, New York, New York, Warner Books, 1998

Tierra, Michael, *The Way of Herbs*, New York, New York, Simon & Shuster, 1990

*Trace Elements in Human Nutrition and Health*, World Health Organization, Geneva, 1996

Tracy, Lisa, *The Gradual Vegetarian,* New York, New York, Dell Publishing, 1993

Tyler, Varro E., *The Honest Herbal*, 3rd edition, New York, New York, Pharmaceutical Products Press, 1993

Van der Zee, Barbara, and Barbara Griggs, *Green Pharmacy: The History and Evolution of Western Herbal Medicine*, Rochester, Vermont, Healing Arts Press, 1991

Vegotsky, Ken, *The Ultimate Power*, Los Angels, CA, AGES Publications, 1995

Vitamin-Mineral Safety, Toxicity and Misuse," *Journal of the American Dietetic Association*, 1978

Wades, Carlson, *Amino Acids Book,* New Canaan, Connecticut, Keats Publishing, 1985

Walker, Morton, *Sexual Nutrition,* Garden City, New York, Avery Publishing Group, 1994

Whitaker, Julian, *Dr. Whitaker's Guide to Natural Healing,* Prima Publishing, Rocklin, California, 1996

Whitney, Eleanor Noss & Sharon Rady Rolfes, *Understanding Nutrition,* 7th ed., St. Paul, MN, West Publishing Company, 1996

Williams, Sue Rodwell, *Nutrition and Diet Therapy,* 8th edition, Mosby, St. Louis, 1997

Williams, Tom, *The Complete Illustrated Guide to Chinese Medicine,* Element Books, Rockport, MA, 1996

Women's Network on Health & The Environment Newsletter, *Bioech Corn Kills Butterflies,* 1999

Worwood, Valerie Ann, *The Complete Book of Essential Oils & Aromatherapy,* San Rafael, California, New World Library, 1991

Worwood, Valerie Ann, *The Fragrant pharmacy,* Ealing, London, Transworld Publishers/Bantam Books, 1994

Wright, Jonathon and John Morgenthaler, *Natural Hormonal Replacement,* Petaluma, California, Smart Publications, 1997

Lavalle, James, Allan Spreen and Janet Zand, *Smart Medicine for Healthier Living,* Garden City park, New York, Avery Publishing Group, 1999

## Bibliography for Chapter 19 for Dr. Ko's treatment protocols

The following evidence-based research of randomized controlled trials and reviews guiding the use of these therapies, is supplied to assist your physician or health care provider, in your mutually beneficial quest for optimal health and healing.

### Acupuncture:

Ernst, E and AR White. Acupuncture for back pain: A meta-analysis of randomized controlled trials. Arch Intern Med. 1998; 158: 2235-41.

Vickers, AJ. Can Acupuncture have specific effects on health? A systematic review of acupuncture antiemesis trials. J R Soc Med. 1996; 89: 303-11.

### Biofeedback:

Donaldson, CCS, et. al. Randomized study of the application of single motor unit biofeedback training to chronic low back pain. J Occup Rehab. 1994; 4: 31-44.

Linden, M et al. A controlled study of the effects of EEG biofeedback on cognition and behavior of children with attention deficit disorder and learning disabilities. Biofeedback and Self-Regulation. 1996; 21: 35-49.

Zwart, JA, Sand T. Exteroceptive suppression of temporalis muscle activity: a blind study of tension-type headache, migraine and cervicogenic headache. Headache 1995;35:338-43.

**Orthopaedic Medicine/Prolotherapy:**

Chang-Zern, et al. Difference in pain relief after trigger point injections in myofascial pain patients with and without fibromyalgia. Arch Phys Med Rehab 1996; 77: 1161-66.

Klein, RG, et al. A randomized double-blind trial of dextrose-glycerine-phenol injections for chronic low back pain. J Spinal Disord. 1993; 6: 23-33.

Ko, GD. Prolotherapy: a new "old" treatment for chronic back pain. Nat Med J. 1998; 1(6): 12-15.

Koes, BW, et al. Spinal manipulation for low back pain: An updated systematic review of randomized clinical trials. SPINE. 1996; 21: 2860-73.

# Index

— H —

## To Write to the Authors

If you wish to write the authors, please send your correspondence to AGES Publications™ and we will forward your request. Both the authors and publisher appreciate hearing from you and learning of the benefits and enjoyment you received from this book. AGES Publications™ cannot guarantee that every letter written can be answered by the authors, but all will be forwarded.

If you want to get a more extensive reference list and copies of Dr. Ko's articles and protocols send your request along with a $10.00 check to cover materials, shipping and handling to.

**In the U.S. write to:**
AGES Publications™
Attn: Ken Vegotsky
1623 Military Road, Suite 203-NR
Niagara Falls NY 14304-1745

**In Canada write to:**
AGES Publications™
Attn: Ken Vegotsky
1054-2 Center St., #153-NR
Thornhill ON L4J 8E5 Canada

Please enclose a self-addressed, stamped envelop for reply, and $3.00 (for Canada, $4.00) to cover costs. If outside the U.S.A. or Canada, enclose an international postal reply coupon with a self-addressed envelope and $3.00 U.S. to cover costs.

On the Internet – http://www.800line.com/ages/
E-Mail – ages@800line.com

## About the Authors

**Dr. Elvis Ali**, B.Sc., N.D., Dipl. Ac., M.R.N.

...is a licensed Naturopathic Doctor and a Registered Nutritional Consultant, R.N.C.. He graduated with a B.Sc. in Biology in 1979, and became one of Canada's first full time registered undergraduates in the field of Naturopathic Medicine. He received a Doctorate in Naturopathic Medicine in 1987 from the Canadian College of Naturopathic Medicine, one of only five accredited schools offering a four year, full time program in Naturopathic Medicine in the U.S.A. and Canada. Elvis has been in private practice for over 12 years specializing in Chinese Medicine, Nutrition and Sports Medicine.

"My mission is to educate the public, to be a spokesperson for complementary health and wellness options and continued research in the field of herbal remedies, and to bring safe and non-intrusive options into the public domain," says Dr. Ali. He has written numerous articles on nutrition, stress and alternative healing options. Dr. Ali makes numerous radio and TV appearances as he strives in his commitment to increase the health and wellness of every man, woman and child in the U.S.A. and Canada.

One of Canada's premier natural remedy and supplement companies, Swiss Herbal Remedies, retains Dr. Ali as their resident Naturopath with ongoing responsibility for product research and development. He is currently involved in conducting seminars throughout the U.S.A. and Canada.

He is married and the father of Hassan, Kareem and Azeeda.

To arrange a keynote, seminar and/or workshop presentation by Dr. Ali, send e-mail to ages@800line.com or write to AGES Publications™ Attention Dr. Ali at the address on page 382.

## **S. David Garshowitz**, BSc. Phm., F.A.C.A.

...graduated from the University of Toronto Faculty of Pharmacy in 1955, majoring in drug manufacturing and hospital pharmacy administration. He is the President of San Pharmacy Limited, operating York Downs Pharmacy, 3910 Bathurst Street, Toronto, Ontario, 1 (800) 564-5020, and San Total Health Pharmacy, 5954 Highway 7 East, Markham, Ontario, 1 (888) 993-3666.

Garshowitz's pharmacies specialize in the compounding of sterile injectable medications, natural hormone replacement therapy, preparation of allopathic medications – integrating mainstream and complementary medicine (supplementation, enzymes, homeopathic remedies, et cetera). These pharmacies act as information centers to the community and to health practitioners concerning drug/drug, drug/herb, and herb/herb interactions.

Garshowitz is a member of the following professional pharmaceutical organizations: Professional Compounding Centers of America, Fellow American College of Apothecaries, American Nutraceutical Association, American Academy of Anti-aging Medicine, Ontario College of Pharmacists, Ontario Pharmaceutical Association, Canadian Pharmaceutical Association, Drug Information and Research Center, Metro Toronto Pharmacists Association, an the Rho Pu Phi International Pharmaceutical Fraternity.

He can be contacted from the U.S.A. or Canada by calling 1 (800) 564-5020 or 1 (888) 993-3666, sending e-mail to ages@800line.com or writing to AGES Publications™ Attention David Garshowitz at the address on page 382

## **Dr. George Grant**, M.Sc., M.Ed., Ed.D., C. Chem., R.M.

...is a multi-talented scientist (Biochemist) who pioneered the research on: Beta Endorphins, anticancer drugs; Lactobacillus viridescens model system to investigate microbial greening; HPLC analysis of B vitamins; GC-MS drug identification of potential drugs for prostate cancer; and, indoor air quality problems as related to Tight Building Syndrome. He is well known for his research on Stress Management and Wellness and is listed in the *International Who's Who of Professional's*. Dr. Grant holds two patents on Modified Atmosphere Packaging (MAP) and Liposomal Weight Management spray.

Dr. Grant is the author of over fifty published research articles, and he is noted across North America for his conference presentations and hundreds of public speaking engagements. Dr. Grant is an active member of professional organizations in the U.S.A. and Canada. He is a licensed Analytical Chemist, Food/Nutrition Scientist, and Consultant for several international firms.

He is married and a father of two boys.

Dr. Grant is known nationally and internationally as a wellness coach. He makes presentations in the U.S.A. and Canada. To contact Dr. Grant, send e-mail to ages@800line.com or write to AGES Publications™ Attention Dr. Grant at the address on page 382.

**Dr. Gordon D. Ko**, MD, CCFP(EM), FRCPC, FAAPMR, CIME, N.MD.

...is a medical graduate from the University of Toronto, Canada. He completed additional residency training in Family Practice, Emergency Medicine and his current specialty of Physical Medicine & Rehabilitation (Physiatry). He is an active member of the American Association of Electrodiagnostic Medicine and the Association for Applied Psychophysiology and Biofeedback. He serves on the executive committee for the Canadian Association of Orthopaedic Medicine and as advisor/past president for the Chinese Canadian Medical Society. Dr. Ko is also on the editorial review board for the Natural Medicine Journal (Fairfax Publications). In addition, he is board certified in the American Board of Physical Medicine and Rehabilitation, the American Board of Independent Medical Examiners and the American Naturopathic Medical Association.

Dr. Ko is currently the medical director for the Canadian Center for Integrative Medicine, 5954 Highway #7 East, Markham, Ontario L3P 1A2. The facility's specialists practice neurology, physiatry, rheumatology and anaesthesiology working alongside allied health professionals in physiotherapy, psychotherapy, naturopathy, acupuncture and pastoral counseling. This center focuses on integrating conventional and complementary approaches in optimizing health and wellness. Dr. Ko's clinical focus is on electrodiagnosis and multidisciplinary treatment of pain, numbness and/or fatigue disorders.

Website: http://www.integrativemedicine.on.ca/

At Sunnybrook and Women's College Health Sciences Center, Dr. Ko conducts research on complementary medicine for chronic pain, fibromyalgia and neuromuscular disorders with emphasis on acupuncture, biofeedback, naturopathy, and orthopaedic medicine. His peer-reviewed articles have been well received by the medical community. As a respected lecturer and teacher, Dr. Ko is helping the next generation of medical students and residents have a better understanding of their role in the healing process. He is an Associate Professor and Lecturer in the Division of Physiatry, Department of Medicine, University of Toronto.

Media activities include articles in the Globe and Mail, live radio and TV interviews such as the popular phone-in show, *"Doctor-on-Call"* on The Women's Network. Dr. Ko lectures extensively to professional and lay public groups on topics ranging from *"Overcoming Pain, Fatigue and Stress at Your Workplace"* to *"Alternative Medicine Overview: What the public wants and what physicians think."*

Dr. Ko enjoys a busy family life as the married father of three children along with community church involvement. He uses a practical, down-to-earth approach when treating patients, lecturing and teaching.

To contact Dr. Gordon Ko, send e-mail to gordon.ko@swchsc.on.ca, fax (416) 480-6885, send e-mail to ages@800line.com or write to AGES Publications™ Attention Dr. Ko at the address on page 382.

**Dr. Joseph Levy**, BA., B.PhE., MSW., PhD.

...is an internationally respected scientist and researcher. He has lectured at universities, hospitals, clinics, spas and health-related venues in the United States, Europe, South America, Asia, Middle East and Canada.

Professor Levy has three books, over 50 scientific articles and hundreds of professional and trade articles to his credit. Since 1995, Dr. Levy has been developing one of the most innovative interactive multimedia wellness web sites in the world, www.yorku.ca/admin/wellness/. INFOHEALTH is the name of this web site resource, which brings together a sophisticated computer, Internet, telephone video and CD-ROM interactive milieu, for the retrieval, storage and dissemination of health related information and programs.

As a researcher and program consultant, Dr. Levy has participated in over $2.5 million of externally funded health research. The sponsorships have come from government and private organizations in the United States, Canada, Europe, Israel and Japan.

His academic activities blend well with his consulting in the Integrated Health and Health Promotion field. He has worked with such international corporations as IBM, General Motors, General Foods, Global TV, CTV, CBC, CN Railroads, Ontario Day Hospital Association, The Mutual Group plus dozens of American, Canadian, European and Asian organizations.

Contact Dr. Joseph Levy via http://www.yorku.ca/admin/wellness/, send e-mail to ages@800line.com or write to AGES Publications™ Attention Dr. Levy at the address on page 382.

**Ehab Mekhail**, B.Sc. Pharm., B.ph., ph.ch.

...is a pharmacist, a member of the Ontario College of Pharmacists, Canadian Pharmacists Association, Drug Information and Research Center, and owner of a Medicine Shoppe Pharmacy. He pursues his life long interest in natural remedies and homeopathic remedies, and gives public presentations on medications and herbal products in his pharmacy and at health clinics.

Ehab is married and an active member of his community.

To contact Ehab, send e-mail to M1W2T1@aol.com, send e-mail to ages@800line.com or write to AGES Publications™ Attention Ehab Mekhail at the address on page 382.

## **Dr. Selim Nakla**, M.D.

...is a medical graduate from the oldest university in the world, Alexandria University, Egypt. He has been published in the American Journal of Obstetrics, Gynecology and Neunatology. For the past twelve years he has been practicing a blend of traditional and holistic medicine for health management in his practice. His primary focus includes physiotherapy, rehabilitation medicine, acupuncture and complementary medicine modalities.

Dr. Nakla's presentations in the U.S., Canada, Italy and Egypt, focus on nutrition and complementary/alternative medicine. He helps people help themselves, using as non-intrusive a style as possible for their health and wellbeing.

To contact Selim, send e-mail to ages@800line.com or write to AGES Publications™ Attention Selim Nakla at the address on page 382.

## **Dr. Alvin Pettle**, M.D., F.R.C.S. (C) (OBS GYN)

...is a pioneer Canadian gynecologist who practices integrative medicine. He graduated from the University of Toronto medical school in 1969 and received his fellowship in obstetrics and gynecology in 1974.

He practiced obstetrics and gynecology for twenty-five years at The Etobicoke General Hospital in Toronto, where from 1990 to 1994, he was Chief of Obstetrics and Gynecology.

During his active years in obstetrics, he was the Canadian pioneer in the Leboyer Gentle Birth Technique, which incorporates a soothing and joyous atmosphere, using dim lights and warm baths, for a gentle birthing process.

Over the last seven years he has opened two wellness centers in Toronto. The Ruth Pettle Wellness Center is named in memory of his mother. He is joined in his work by his wife, Carol, a registered nurse and formally Head Nurse of the Labor and Delivery Department at The Etobicoke General Hospital.

His medical and community affiliations include the American College of Infertility, Canadian Medical Association, Physicians for Peace, Society of Obstetrics and Gynecology (Canada), Ontario Medical Association, and the Royal College of Physicians and Surgeons (Canada).

Dr. Pettle has published numerous articles on natural hormones and his adaptations to the birth process. They include: *Gentle Birth,* a feature article in the Canadian Family Physician Journal, November 1978; *Gentle Questions of Birth,* in Issues of Health, MacLeans Magazine, April 1982; *Endometriosis: Doctor Travels 4000 Miles for Patients Surgery,* a feature article in the Medical Post. He is also a contributor to the Women's Wellness Network, www.wwn.on.ca on the Internet.

His television presentations include the nationally syndicated morning show, Canada AM, a TV show segment *Dr. Alvin Pettle on Gentle Birth* as well as The Women's Network's *Body, Mind and Soul* in 1998 and *Beyond Medicine* in 1999. Dr. Pettle is in demand for radio, TV and print media interviews as an authority on natural hormone and integrative medical therapies for women. He lectures to doctors, nurses, and the public on *The Integrative Management of Premenstrual Syndrome (PMS) and Menopause*. He is the preeminent specialist in natural hormone replacement therapies for women.

Dr. Pettle is a father of five children and grandfather to Jory, Mathew, Andrew, Meagan, Rachael and Mitchell. *"All that I have or need in this world is within their eyes."*

To contact Dr. Pettle, send e-mail to ages@800line.com or write to AGES Publications™ Attention Dr. Pettle at the address on page 382.

**Ken Vegotsky**, B.Sc.

...is the team leader on this project. Ken is a professional speaker, author and entrepreneur who has given keynote addresses and seminars in the U.S.A. and Canada. He has been featured in print, radio and TV in the U.S.A., Canada, Australia, New Zealand, United Kingdom and a host of other countries.

***"Ken is the Victor Frankl of our day,"*** noted Dottie Walters, President Walters Speakers Bureau International and author of *Speak & Grow Rich.*

Mark Victor Hansen, New York Times #1 bestselling co-author of the *Chicken Soup for the Soul Series*, says Ken's work is, ***"Brilliant and illuminating."***

*"In recognition of being seen as a model of courage and hope for others, who demonstrates to all of us the nobility of the human spirit,"* begins the Clarke Foundation nomination of Ken for a *Courage to Come Back Award*. These awards were originated by the St. Francis Health Foundation of Pittsburgh, Pennsylvania.

Ken has served on the boards of NACPAC (affiliate of the American Chronic Pain Association), a community information service and a half-way home for mentally challenged people in transition.

After numerous inspirational speeches, he was encouraged by listeners to tell his story. In his National Bestseller, *The Ultimate Power,* Ken shares his captivating first-person account of his near-death experience, garnished with proven keys for unlocking your personal power. Discover *How You Can Unlock Your Mind-Body-Soul Potential.* You'll feel embraced by caring and compassion as you share his moving experience.

To contact Ken Vegotsky, send e-mail to ages@800line.com or write to AGES Publications™ Attention Ken Vegotsky at the address on page 382.

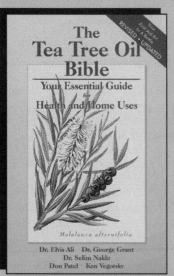

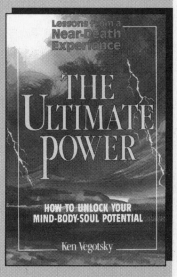

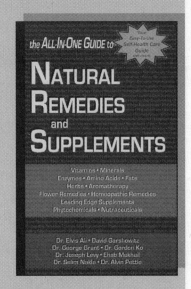

# Order Form

| | Qty | Price | Total |
|---|---|---|---|
| The Tea Tree Oil Bible<br>Your Essential Guide for<br>Health and Home Uses | | $7.95 | |
| *the All-In-One Guide to™*<br>Natural Remedies and Supplements<br>Vitamins, minerals, enzymes, amino acids,<br>fats, herbs, aromatherapy, homeopathy,<br>flower remedies, leading edge remedies,<br>phytochemicals, nutraceuticals, and<br>oldies but goodies | | $7.95 | |
| The Ultimate Power<br>How to Unlock Your<br>Mind–Body–Soul Potential | | $9.95 | |
| ••• Round-Up ••• *By E-Mail*<br>A Summary of the Best in<br>Health Newsletters from<br>Around the World.™ | | $18.97 | |
| ••• Round-Up ••• *By Postal Service* | | $36.97 | |
| ($3.00 for 1st + $0.50 for each additional book) | | Shipping | |
| | | Total | |

E-Mail ______________________________

Name ______________________________

Address ______________________________

______________________________

City ____________________ ZIP __________

Phone ______________________________

Please make certified check/money order payable to and send to
Adi, Gaia, Esalen Publications Inc.
1623 Military Rd. #203-NR, Niagara Falls, NY 14304-1745

VISA ❑ MasterCard ❑ American Express ❑

Card #: ____________________ Exp. Date: ________.

Signature: ______________________________

North America – Order Toll Free 1 888 545-0053
Trade and Bulk order enquiries welcomed